N⟨ ⟩l

Withdrawn

Reason:

Date:

By:

Question Everything

D1582549

Wounds and Lacerations

Wounds and Lacerations
Emergency Care and Closure

FOURTH EDITION

Alexander T. Trott, MD
Professor of Emergency Medicine
University of Cincinnati College of Medicine
Cincinnati, Ohio

1600 John F. Kennedy Blvd.
Ste 1800
Philadelphia, PA 19103-2899

WOUNDS AND LACERATIONS: EMERGENCY CARE AND CLOSURE,
FOURTH EDITION   ISBN: 978-0-323-07418-6

Notices

Knowledge and best practice in this field are constantly changing. As new research and experience broaden our understanding, changes in research methods, professional practices, or medical treatment may become necessary. Practitioners and researchers must always rely on their own experience and knowledge in evaluating and using any information, methods, compounds, or experiments described herein. In using such information or methods they should be mindful of their own safety and the safety of others, including parties for whom they have a professional responsibility.

With respect to any drug or pharmaceutical products identified, readers are advised to check the most current information provided (i) on procedures featured or (ii) by the manufacturer of each product to be administered, to verify the recommended dose or formula, the method and duration of administration, and contraindications. It is the responsibility of practitioners, relying on their own experience and knowledge of their patients, to make diagnoses, to determine dosages and the best treatment for each individual patient, and to take all appropriate safety precautions.

To the fullest extent of the law, neither the Publisher nor the authors, contributors, or editors assume any liability for any injury and/or damage to persons or property as a matter of products liability, negligence or otherwise, or from any use or operation of any methods, products, instructions, or ideas contained in the material herein.

Library of Congress Cataloging-in-Publication Data

Trott, Alexander.
  Wounds and lacerations : emergency care and closure / Alexander T. Trott.—4th ed.
    p. ; cm.
  Includes bibliographical references and index.
  ISBN 978-0-323-07418-6 (hardcover : alk. paper)
  I. Title.
  [DNLM: 1. Wounds and Injuries—therapy. 2. Emergencies. 3. Suture Techniques. 4. Wound Healing. WO 700]
  617.1—dc23   2011039845

Senior Content Strategist: Stefanie Jewell-Thomas
Content Development Specialist: Roxanne Halpine Ward
Publishing Services Manager: Patricia Tannian
Senior Project Manager: Kristine Feeherty
Design Direction: Steven Stave

Printed in the United States of America

Last digit is the print number: 9 8 7 6 5 4 3 2 1

Working together to grow
libraries in developing countries
www.elsevier.com | www.bookaid.org | www.sabre.org

ELSEVIER   BOOK AID International   Sabre Foundation

To Jennifer, who was the original inspiration for the text,
and for her endless patience and support

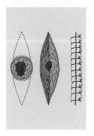

Editorial Coordinator

Shawn Ryan, MD, MBA
Assistant Professor
Emergency Medicine
University of Cincinnati
Cincinnati, Ohio

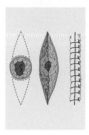

Contributors

Gregg A. DiGiulio, MD
Associate Professor
Department of Pediatrics
Northeast Ohio Medical University
Rootstown, Ohio;
Attending Physician
Division of Emergency Medicine, Department of Pediatrics
Akron Children's Hospital
Akron, Ohio

Javier A. Gonzalez del Rey, MD, MEd
Professor of Clinical Pediatrics
Department of Pediatrics
University of Cincinnati College of Medicine;
Director, Pediatric Residency Training Programs
Associate Director, Division of Emergency Medicine
Cincinnati Children's Hospital Medical Center
Cincinnati, Ohio

Carolyn K. Holland, MD, MEd
Assistant Professor of Clinical Pediatrics and Emergency Medicine
Pediatrics and Emergency Medicine
University of Cincinnati College of Medicine;
Attending Physician
Department of Pediatrics, Division of Emergency Medicine
Cincinnati Children's Hospital Medical Center;
Attending Physician
Department of Emergency Medicine
University Hospital
Cincinnati, Ohio

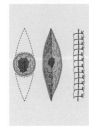

Preface

There are certain clinical skills basic to most practitioners: physicians, mid-level providers, nurses, wound care technicians, and medics. The care of surface injury and lacerations is one of them. Until the 1980s, suturing and other wound care procedures were taught at the bedside from one generation to the next. "Watch one, do one, teach one," was a common refrain heard by young students trying to glean knowledge that would give them the skills to clean, suture, and dress wounds.

With the growth of emergency medicine and its acceptance as a specialty came a rapid growth of textbooks and educational materials that organized and presented didactic material necessary for the students and residents training in emergency care. *Wounds and Lacerations,* now in its fourth edition, represents an effort to provide students and practitioners with a ready source of information and recommendations to care for a patient with surface injuries. All care recommendations are the product of the available evidence, science and literature, to back them up. In cases where no science exists, consensus of experienced practitioners and the authors is offered as support. The success of previous editions lends credence to this approach, as well as the straightforward and uncomplicated manner in which the content is presented.

The reader of this new edition will find a change in format and content. Each chapter will be introduced with the Key Practice Points covered in that chapter. The text has been edited for greater clarity, and more lists and tables are used for quick and easy reference. Each chapter has been updated with the most recent available science and literature. Many illustrations have been updated, and new ones have been added. There have been significant changes in several content areas. The use of absorbable sutures on the face and hand is now a common practice. The cosmetic outcome is the same as for nonabsorbable sutures, and visits for suture removal can be eliminated. The emergence of community-associated methicillin-resistant *Staphylococcus aureus* is a new challenge. The use of emergency department ultrasound to find and remove foreign bodies is becoming more common. Recommendations for tetanus and rabies prophylaxis have undergone significant changes.

Although this text originated from practices in the emergency department, it is clear that wound care crosses many specialties and disciplines. Wound care can take place in emergency departments, clinics, practitioners' offices, aid stations, and even in the field. Where this text is used and who uses it have no limits. If it can benefit one patient, under whatever circumstance, then it is a success.

Alexander T. Trott, MD

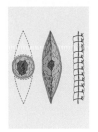

Contents

Wounds and Lacerations

CHAPTER 1
Emergency Wound Care: An Overview

Key Practice Points

- The average laceration cared for by emergency caregivers is 1 to 3 cm in length, with 13% of lacerations considered significantly contaminated.
- The most common complication of wound care is infection, occurring in 3.5% to 6.3% of lacerations.
- The most important step for reducing infection in wound care is wound irrigation.
- All wounds form scars and take months to reach their final appearance.
- 95% of glass in wounds is radio-opaque, and radiographs are recommended.
- The understanding of local practice when caring for wounds, such as the use of prophylactic antibiotics for wound care, is important.

Superficial wounds, including lacerations, bites, small burns, and punctures, are among the most common problems faced by emergency physicians and other providers of urgent and primary care. Each year in emergency departments (EDs) in the United States, 12.2 million patients with wounds are managed.[1] The most frequently performed procedure in the ED, other than intravenous-line (IV-line) insertion, is wound care.[2]

Of 1000 patients whose clinical findings were entered into a wound registry, 74% of the patients were male, with an average age of 23.[3] The average laceration was 1 to 3 cm in length, and 13% of lacerations were considered significantly contaminated. Most wounds (51%) occurred on the face and scalp, followed by wounds on the upper (34%) and lower (13%) extremities. The remaining wounds occurred on various sites of the truncal areas and proximal extremities.

The most common complication of wound care is infection. Approximately 3.5% to 6.3% of laceration wounds become infected in adults treated in the ED.[4-6] Infection is more likely to occur with bite wounds, in lower extremity locations, and when foreign material is retained in the wound. The rate of infection in children is only 1.2% for lacerations of all types.[7]

GOALS OF WOUND CLOSURE

Because wounding is an uncontrolled event and there are biologic limitations to healing, the wounded skin and related structures cannot be perfectly restored. Each step of wound care serves to achieve the best possible outcome with the fewest problems.

- *Hemostasis:* All bleeding from the wound except minor oozing should be controlled, usually with gentle, continuous pressure, before wound closure.
- *Anesthesia:* Effective local anesthesia before wound cleansing allows the caregiver to clean the wound thoroughly and to close it without fear of causing unnecessary pain.

- *Wound irrigation:* Irrigation is the most important step in reducing bacterial contamination and the potential for wound infection.
- *Wound exploration:* Wounds caused by glass or at risk for deep structure damage should be explored. Radiographs and functional testing do not always identify foreign bodies or injured tendons.
- *Removal of devitalized and contaminated tissue:* Visibly devitalized and contaminated tissue that could not be removed through wound cleansing and irrigation needs to be completely but judiciously débrided.
- *Tissue preservation:* At the time of ED or primary closure, tissue excision should be resisted. It is best to tack down what remains of viable tissue, especially in complicated wounds. Because of the natural contraction of wounds, cosmetic revisions done later can be accomplished successfully if sufficient tissue remains. Unnecessary tissue excision can lead to a permanent, uncorrectable, and unsightly scar.
- *Closure tension:* When laceration edges are being brought together, they should just barely "touch." Excessive wound constriction when tying knots strangulates the tissue, leading to a poor outcome. If necessary, tension-reducing techniques, such as the placement of deep sutures and undermining, can be applied.
- *Deep sutures:* Because all sutures act as foreign bodies, as few deep sutures as possible are to be placed in any wound.
- *Tissue handling:* Rough handling of tissues, particularly when using forceps, can cause tissue necrosis and increase the chance of wound infection and scarring.
- *Wound infection:* Antibiotics are no substitute for wound preparation and irrigation. If the decision is made to treat the patient with antibiotics, the initial dose is most effective when administered intravenously as soon as possible after wounding.
- *Dressings:* Wounds heal best in a moist environment provided by a properly applied wound dressing.
- *Follow-up:* Well-understood verbal and written wound care instructions and timely return for a short follow-up inspection or suture removal at the proper interval are essential to complete care.

PATIENT EXPECTATIONS

One of the most important aspects of wound care is understanding and managing the patient's reaction to a wound. Patients often have many preconceptions about wound care and expectations about the outcome, which are often unrealistic. Patients sometimes believe that wounds can be repaired without scar formation. All wounds leave a scar, which is a fact that has to be conveyed to all patients. Scar formation and wound healing will be more thoroughly discussed in Chapters 4 and 22.

Another patient misconception is the time it takes for wounds to heal. Ironically, when the sutures are removed, that is the weakest point in healing (see Chapter 4, Fig. 4-2). Sutures are removed when there is enough holding strength to keep the wound edges together and to prevent increased scarring that can be caused by leaving sutures in the wound too long. If there is concern that the wound might open after suture removal, Steri-Strips can be applied to give the wound time to become stronger. Final scar appearance may not be evident for several months because of the biologic complexity of wound healing.

RISKS OF WOUND CARE

A fact of life for patient care in the United States is the risk of liability. Wounds cared for in EDs are often considered "minor." Yet in a study of closed malpractice claims against emergency physicians in Massachusetts, wounds were the most common source of those claims.[8] Of the 109 claims, 32% involved retained foreign bodies, and another

34% were caused by allegedly undiagnosed injuries to a tendon or a nerve. The four leading causes of mistakes in emergency-care malpractice cases are failure to order tests (such as radiographs for retained glass), inadequate history and physical exam (tendon or nerve injuries), misinterpretation of tests, and failure to obtain a consultation (often necessary in hand wounds).[9]

The most commonly retained foreign body is glass.[10] Patients who receive injuries from glass cannot report accurately whether the glass remains in the wound.[11] Radiographs are recommended for most of these wounds. Under study conditions, more than 95% of glass, of all types, as small as 0.5 mm, can be visualized by radiography.[12] In the clinical setting, however, fragments can be missed. In addition to radiographs, wound exploration is recommended in wounds potentially bearing glass (see Chapter 16).

Tendon injuries of the hand are not always apparent. The patient can appear to have normal hand function but have a laceration of one or more tendons. The most commonly missed injury is to the extensor tendon.[13] Extensor tendons are cross-linked at the level of the metacarpals. An injury to a tendon proximal to the adjacent tendon cross-link can give the appearance of normal extensor function. Tendons also can be partially severed and retain function. A good understanding of the complex functional anatomy of the hand and a thorough testing of each tendon reveal most complete injuries. Only exploration can define accurately the extent of partial injuries, however.

If a claim is made against an emergency physician, the care of the patient is most likely to be compared with what a specialist would have done in a similar circumstance. In other words, physicians who do not practice emergency medicine often define the "standard of care." An example of this dilemma is an infected wound. If an infection results from a sutured laceration, specialists often opine that prophylactic antibiotics should have been administered. Currently, there are no solid, evidenced-based data showing that antibiotics prevent traumatic skin-wound infections. Because antibiotics are administered frequently without firm science, however, it is important for emergency physicians to follow local practice or relevant guidelines that address these circumstances.

References

1. McCaig LF, Ly N: National hospital ambulatory medical care survey: 2000 emergency department summary, *Adv Data* 22:1–37, 2002.
2. Pitts SR, Niska RW, Xu J, Butt CW: National hospital ambulatory medical survey: 2006 emergency department survey, *Natl Health Stat Report* 6:1–38, 2008.
3. Hollander JE, Singer AJ, Valentine S, Henry MC: Wound registry: development and validation, *Ann Emerg Med* 25:675–685, 1995.
4. Gosnold JK: Infection rate of sutured wounds, *Practitioner* 218:584–591, 1977.
5. Rutherford WH, Spence R: Infection in wounds sutured in the accident and emergency department, *Ann Emerg Med* 9:350–352, 1980.
6. Thirlby RC, Blair AJ, Thal ER: The value of prophylactic antibiotics for simple lacerations, *Surg Gynecol Obstet* 156:212–216, 1983.
7. Baker MD, Lanuti M: The management and outcome of lacerations in urban children, *Ann Emerg Med* 19:1001–1005, 1990.
8. Karcz A, Korn R, Burke MC, et al: Malpractice claims against physicians in Massachusetts: 1975-1993, *Am J Emerg Med* 14:341–345, 1996.
9. Kachalia A, Gandhi TK, Puopolo AL, et al: Missed and delayed diagnoses in the emergency department: a study of closed malpractice claims from 4 liability insurers, *Ann Emerg Med* 49:196–205, 2007.
10. Kaiser CW, Slowick T, Spurling KP, et al: Retained foreign bodies, *J Trauma* 43:107–111, 1997.
11. Montano JB, Steele MT, Watson WR: Foreign body retention in glass-caused wounds, *Ann Emerg Med* 21:1365–1368, 1992.
12. Tanberg D: Glass in the hand and foot, *JAMA* 248:1872–1874, 1982.
13. Guly HR: Missed tendon injuries, *Arch Emerg Med* 8:87–91, 1991.

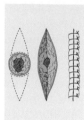

CHAPTER 2
Patient Evaluation and Wound Assessment

Key Practice Points

- To prevent unexpected syncope and to provide for patient comfort during wound care, the patient is placed in the supine position. Parents or friends, who want to stay with the patient, are at risk as well.
- Most bleeding can be stopped with simple pressure. Blind instrument clamping is avoided.
- All rings and jewelry are removed from the wound area to prevent ischemia as a result of swelling.
- All wounds are contaminated with bacteria and should be cleansed and irrigated early after arrival if care is to be delayed beyond 1 to 3 hours.
- Severe soft tissue injury is an emergency and requires rapid and aggressive care.
- Small, innocuous wounds can be caused by more serious problems such as cardiac arrythmias.

INITIAL STEPS
Patient Comfort and Safety
If there is the slightest question about a patient's ability to cope with his or her injury, the patient is placed in a supine position on a stretcher. Loss of blood, deformity, and pain are sufficient to provoke vasovagal syncope (fainting), which can cause further injury from an unexpected fall during evaluation or treatment. The attire of the caregiver should be consistent with universal precautions. Because wound care can be strenuous, the caregiver should be comfortable and relaxed before proceeding. Sitting, when possible, is recommended.

Relatives or friends accompanying the patient also can respond in a similar manner. As a rule, relatives and friends are encouraged to sit in the waiting area unless the physician or nurse determines that staying with the patient would be beneficial (e.g., to comfort an injured child). The parent or friend should be asked if he or she feels comfortable with that arrangement.

Initial Hemostasis
Most bleeding can be stopped with simple pressure and compression dressings. There is no need for dramatic clamping of bleeders. Clamping is reserved for the actual exploration and repair of the wound under controlled, well-lighted conditions. Blind application of hemostats in an actively bleeding wound can lead to the crushing of normal nerves, tendons, or other important structures.

Jewelry Removal

Rings and other jewelry must be removed from injured hands or fingers as quickly as possible. Swelling of the hand or finger can progress rapidly after wounding, causing rings to act as constricting bands. A finger can become ischemic, and the outcome can be disastrous. Most items of jewelry can be removed with soap or lubricating jelly. Occasionally, ring cutters have to be used (Fig. 2-1). The sentimental value of a wedding ring should never be allowed to impede good medical judgment. A jeweler always can restore a ring that has been cut or damaged during removal. Another technique for removing rings (steel, titanium) that cannot be cut is described in Chapter 13.

Pain Relief

Pain relief begins with gentle, empathic, and professional handling of the patient. Occasionally, it is necessary to administer pain-reducing or sedative medications to patients being treated in the emergency wound care setting. Sedation and specific pain relief measures are discussed more completely in Chapter 6.

Wound Care Delay

If there is going to be a delay from initial wound evaluation to repair, the wound is covered with a saline-moistened dressing to prevent drying. The dressing need not be soaked and dripping wet. Delays that extend beyond 1 hour require that the wound be thoroughly cleansed and irrigated before the saline dressing is applied.[1] If extended delays are inevitable, antibiotics occasionally are considered to suppress bacterial growth. If antibiotics are administered, they should be given early to provide the maximal protective benefit.[2,3] Chapter 9 discusses further recommendations for the early administration of antibiotics.

Children with Lacerations

Particular care must be taken with children who have wounds and lacerations. The pain and fear generated by the experience can be reduced significantly by a few simple measures. The child should be allowed to remain in the parent's lap for as long as possible before wound repair. Most of the physical examination can be performed at that time. If hemostasis is required, and if the parent is willing to cooperate, he or she can be allowed to tamponade small, bleeding wounds. Parents also can apply topical anesthetics. Careful judgment has to be used when handling children and their parents. It is common for some parents to be unable to tolerate the sight of their child in pain, and they often do better in the waiting room while care is being delivered. It is remarkable how some children stop crying when the parent has left the treatment area. Pediatric considerations in wound care are discussed in detail in Chapter 5.

Severe Soft Tissue Injuries

Providers of emergency wound care occasionally are confronted with patients who have severe, but not life-threatening, soft tissue injuries, usually of the distal upper or lower extremities. Power tools, industrial machines, farm implements, and mowers commonly cause these injuries. Patients often present with extensive skin lacerations, combined with varying degrees of nerve, tendon, or vascular involvement. On the patient's arrival at the emergency department, several steps, outlined here, are performed to ensure the stability and comfort of the patient and to evaluate and protect the injured limb. These injuries may include an amputated part; guidelines for the management of that part are described in Chapter 13.

- *ABCs (airway, breathing, circulation):* Because of the severity of these injuries, the airway and vital signs are assessed to ensure the stability of the patient. A brief history and general system survey are carried out to rule out any secondary injuries or modifying conditions.

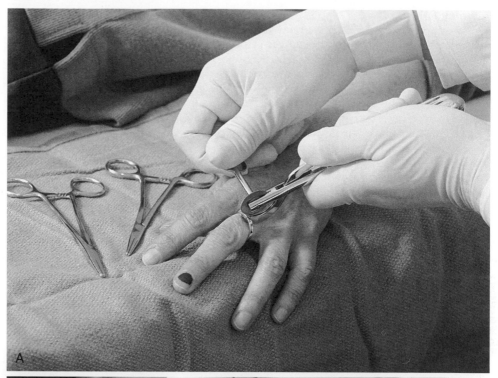

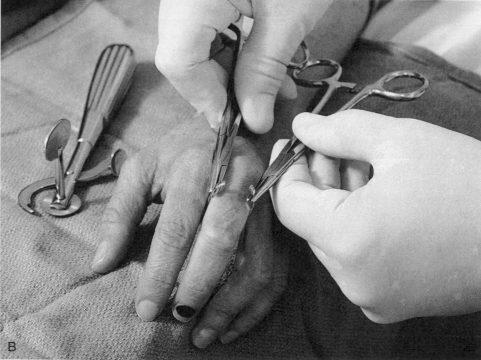

Figure 2-1. **A,** Ring removal. Rings can be removed with a ring-cutting device. A through-and-through cut is made at the thinnest portion of the ring. **B,** Large hemostats are clamped to each side of the cut portion. Taking care not to harm the finger, the ring is gently pried open.

- *Hemorrhage:* Any bleeding, as described earlier, is controlled by direct pressure. Tourniquets are indicated only for severe bleeding of an extremity that cannot be controlled by direct pressure, which is a rare occurrence. Should a tourniquet be necessary, proper technique must be observed. Edlich et al. recommend that "after elevating the injured extremity for 1 minute, the blood pressure cuff is inflated to the lowest pressure that will arrest the bleeding. This measured level of inflation can be maintained for at least 2 hours without injury to the underlying vessels and nerves."[4]
- *Pain relief:* The most effective pain relief for severe hand or foot injuries is nerve blockade with local anesthetics. Nerve blocks are performed only after sensory and motor function is evaluated and documented (see Chapter 6 for nerve block techniques). Pain relief for adults also can be accomplished with parenteral (intravenous or intramuscular) medications, meperidine (Demerol), 25 to 50 mg, or morphine, 2 to 5 mg. These medications can be supplemented with promethazine (Phenergan), 12 to 25 mg to reduce the possibility of vomiting. See Chapter 5 for pain relief in children.
- *Tetanus immunization:* Because patients with severe soft tissue wounds are more likely to be at risk for tetanus, tetanus immunization status has to be determined. See Chapter 21 for immunization recommendations.
- *Antibiotic prophylaxis:* Because of the severe nature of these wounds, they are susceptible to infection. The most common organisms cultured from these wounds are *Staphylococcus aureus* and β-hemolytic streptococci.[5] Coliforms and anaerobes are cultured in smaller numbers. The most feared organisms are the soil-borne *Clostridium* species, but these rarely cause infection. Wounds caused by tools and industrial machines are predominantly contaminated with gram-positive organisms.[6] Farm implements and gardening tools that come in contact with soil have a higher proportion of coliforms. These differences have implications in the selection of antibiotics. For clean, non–soil-laden wounds, a first-generation cephalosporin provides adequate coverage. In patients with severe allergies to penicillin or cephalosporins, vancomycin can be given. In soil-laden wounds, the addition of an aminoglycoside provides good coverage. It cannot be overemphasized that antibiotics are no substitute for aggressive wound cleansing, irrigation, and débridement.
- *Wound evaluation:* A functional examination is performed and documented. Loss of pulse or circulation is a serious finding and requires emergent intervention. Sensory and motor function is evaluated and documented. Tendon function is tested by individual or group action when possible. All severe soft tissue wounds are radiographed to assess bone integrity and the presence of foreign bodies.
- *Wound management:* For the most part, little can be done for these wounds in the emergency department. Loose, gross contaminants can be removed. After evaluation, the wound is covered with sterile gauze pads and a wrap is moistened with sterile saline. Appropriate splints are applied as indicated.
- *Consultation:* These wounds require definitive care by consultants with expertise in managing severe extremity and soft tissue injuries. Most commonly, plastic or hand specialists are consulted early after the arrival of the patient. The operating team is notified early as well to prepare for the definitive care of the patient in the operative room.

WOUND EVALUATION AND DOCUMENTATION

Basic History

The historical items collected and recorded in the wound care patient's medical record need not be lengthy and excruciatingly detailed. Key facts, such as mechanism, age of wound, allergies, and tetanus immunization status, are virtually always pertinent.

The patient's current and past medical history and present medications are frequently elements of the wound care assessment. Diseases such as diabetes and peripheral vascular disease can increase the risk of wound infection and cause delayed or poor wound healing.[7,8] Corticosteroids are known to affect the normal healing process adversely.[9] Finally, a careful detailing of allergies is necessary to prevent an untoward reaction to local anesthetics or antibiotics that might be administered to the patient. Box 2-1 presents the basic history and physical examination elements of a wound care charting document.[10]

Screening Examination

The examination of every patient with a laceration or injury includes assessing the basic vital signs. Each vital sign can provide information pertinent to the management of the patient. Hypotension and tachycardia are the classic signs of hypovolemia. Innocuous-looking scalp wounds can bleed profusely, causing clinically significant blood loss with concomitant hypotension. Because alcohol is a cutaneous vasodilator, this complication is common in intoxicated patients.

Wounds and lacerations are often the result of or the cause of systemic problems and illnesses. Patients who fall and sustain minor injuries may need to be questioned

---

BOX 2-1	**Elements Recommended for Documentation of Wound Evaluation and Care***

Wound History
Mechanism of injury—what happened, possible foreign body
Age of wound—when it happened
Associated symptoms—systemic, numbness, loss of function

Past/Social History
Underlying disorders—diabetes, seizures
Allergies—drugs, anesthetics
Date of last tetanus
Medications—anticoagulants, corticosteroids
Vocation/avocation
Handedness

Physical Examination
Vital signs
General/system findings as appropriate
Wound description
Location
Length/extent
Depth
Condition—clean, contaminated, sharp, irregular
Functional examination—as appropriate

Procedure
Anesthesia—type, amount
Wound cleansing—agent, irrigation
Exploration/débridement
Suture type, size, number
Dressing type

Disposition
Wound care instructions (see Chapter 22)
Interval for suture removal

*Elements vary by patient and circumstances.

and examined for causes of syncope. When caused by blunt trauma, a scalp laceration has the possibility of being associated with a serious intracranial injury. In addition to the wound assessment, a trauma-oriented neurologic examination is often necessary.

A rapid general survey of the patient can reveal other injuries not reported. Because of the nature of a traumatic occurrence, patients often cannot report accurately all that has happened to them. A man who falls on an outstretched hand may be aware only of a bleeding hand laceration on arrival at the emergency department. An underlying radial head fracture might be revealed only when the caregiver examines the elbow and provokes pain.

Wound Assessment

When the wound is examined, several features and findings must be noted and recorded in the medical record (see Box 2-1). Each wound characteristic and examination finding becomes a significant variable that influences repair decisions and all aspects of care, including wound preparation, anesthesia, closure strategy, and dressing choice.

Procedure Documentation

After performing the wound care intervention, whether suturing, foreign body removal, or burn care, a succinct but detailed procedure note is entered into the record. The elements of the procedure note for suturing are outlined in Box 2-1.

Patient Disposition and Follow-up

When care is completed, instructions for wound care, return for suture removal, and follow-up care are provided to the patient and are documented. Details of follow-up care are discussed in Chapter 22.

References

1. Robson MC, Duke WF, Krizek TJ: Rapid bacterial screening in the treatment of civilian wounds, *J Surg Res* 14:426–430, 1973.
2. Burke JF: The effective period of preventive antibiotic action in experimental incisions and dermal lesions, *Surgery* 50:161–168, 1961.
3. Morgan WJ, Hutchinson D, Johnson HM: The delayed treatment of wounds of the hand and forearm under antibiotic cover, *Br J Surg* 67:140–141, 1980.
4. Edlich RF, Rodeheaver GT, Thacker JG, et al: Revolutionary advances in the management of traumatic wounds in the emergency department during the last 40 years: part 1, *J Emerg Med* 20:1–11, 2008.
5. Charalambous CP, Zipitis CS, Kumar R, et al: Soft tissue infections of the extremities in an orthopaedic center, *J Infect* 46:106–110, 2003.
6. Hoffman RD, Adams BD: Antimicrobial management of mutilating hand injuries, *Hand Clin* 19:33–39, 2003.
7. Altemeier W: Principles in the management of traumatic wounds and in infection control, *Bull N Y Acad Med* 55:123–138, 1979.
8. Hunt T: Disorders of wound healing, *World J Surg* 4:271–277, 1980.
9. Pollack S: Systemic medications and wound healing, *Int J Dermatol* 21:489–496, 1982.
10. American College of Emergency Physicians: Clinical policy for the initial approach to patients presenting with penetrating extremity trauma, *Ann Emerg Med* 23:1147–1156, 1994.

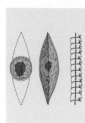

CHAPTER 3
Anatomy of Wound Repair

Key Practice Points

- The most important layer of skin for wound closure is the tough dermis. It is the "anchor" for sutures.
- Proper and careful apposition of the wounded dermis will bring the lacerated outer layer of skin, the thin epidermis, together for the best cosmetic result.
- The superficial fascia, or subcutaneous fatty tissue, lies just below the dermis. Because nerve fibers travel in the subcutaneous layer below and into the dermis, this fatty layer is the preferred site for delivery of local anesthetics.
- Débridement of dermis should be judicious and limited, whereas for subcutaneous fat it can be liberal.
- Lacerations and incisions parallel to skin tension lines leave thinner and less visible scars than those that cross these lines.
- Age and use of corticosteroids weaken skin and make it thinner. Repairing lacerations and wounds to this skin is a challenge.

The primary anatomic focus in surface wound care is the skin. Underlying the skin are two equally important structures, the superficial (subcutaneous) fascia and the deep fascia. The fasciae not only act as a supportive base to the skin but also carry nerves and vessels that eventually branch into the fasciae. All the layers of the skin and fascia are present in every body site, but they vary considerably in thickness. Most skin is 1 to 2 mm thick, but thickness can increase to 4 mm over the back. This variability often dictates the choice of suture needles. Larger, stronger needles are required to penetrate the skin on the palms of the hands and the soles of the feet. Small, delicate needles should be used on the thin skin of the eyelids.

ANATOMY OF THE SKIN AND FASCIA

Although the skin and fascia comprise a complex system of organs and anatomic features, it is the layer arrangement that is most important for wound closure (Fig. 3-1). These layers include the epidermis, dermis, superficial fascia (commonly referred to as the subcutaneous or subcuticular layer), and deep fascia. These layers should be thought of as planes that need to be carefully and accurately reapproximated when disrupted by trauma. Each one has its own set of characteristics that are important to proper wound closure and healing.

Epidermis and Dermis (Skin or Cutaneous Layer)

The epidermis is the outermost layer of the skin. The epidermis consists entirely of squamous epithelial cells and contains no organs, nerve endings, or vessels. Its primary function is to provide protection against the ingress of bacteria and toxic chemicals and

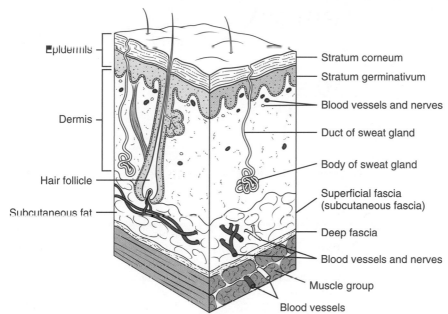

Figure 3-1. Anatomy of the skin illustrating structures pertinent to wound repair.

the inappropriate egress of water and electrolytes. This is the outermost, visible layer and gives skin its final cosmetic appearance.

Although the epidermis is an anatomically separate layer, it is only a few cell layers thick. During wound repair, it cannot be seen by the naked eye as separate from the dermis. Correct approximation of the epidermis naturally results from careful apposition of the lacerated edges of the dermis.

The dermis lies immediately beneath the epidermis. It is much thicker than the epidermis and is composed primarily of connective tissue. The main cell type in the dermis is the fibroblast, which elaborates collagen, the basic structural component of skin. The deeper dermis contains the bulk of adnexal structures of the skin. These include the hair follicles and vascular plexus. Nerve fibers branch and differentiate into specialized nerve endings that reside in the dermis.

The dermis is the key layer for achieving proper wound repair. It is easily identifiable and provides the anchoring site for percutaneous and deep sutures (Fig. 3-2). Every effort is made to cleanse, remove debris, and accurately approximate the dermal edges to allow for optimal wound healing with minimal scar formation. If dermis is devitalized or severely damaged, sharp débridement often is necessary to remove it. Tissue excision and trimming must include only that which is truly unsalvageable, however. Because dermal defects are replaced by scar tissue, any unnecessary dermis removal increases the size and prominence of that scar.

Superficial Fascia (Subcutaneous Layer)

Deep to the dermis is a layer of loose connective tissue that encloses a varying amount of fat. Fat makes the superficial fascia easily recognizable in a laceration. There are several consequences of injury to this layer. Devitalized fat can promote bacterial growth and infection.[1] In contrast to dermis, the superficial fascia can be liberally débrided so that any devitalized portion can be excised completely. Injuries to the superficial fascia

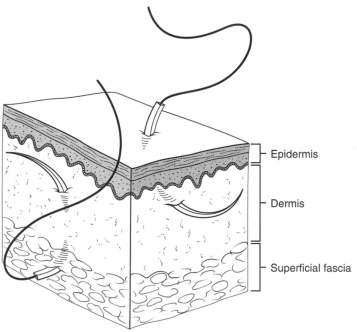

Figure 3-2. Demonstration of either percutaneous or deep suture closure. The needle is anchored in the dermis for each suture placement.

also have the potential for creating "dead" space. Failure to evacuate contaminants and clots in this space can lead to an increased risk of infection.

The sensory nerve branches to the skin travel in the superficial fascia just deep to the dermis. When injecting a local anesthetic, the needle is directed along the plane between the dermis and superficial fascia (see Fig. 6-1). Anesthetic spreads easily along the "floor" of the dermal layer and quickly abolishes sensation from the skin.

Deep Fascia

Deep fascia is a relatively thick, dense, and discrete fibrous tissue layer. It acts as a base for the superficial fascia and as an enclosure for muscle groups. This layer is recognized as an off-white sheath for the underlying muscles. The main function of the deep fascia is to support and protect muscles and other soft tissue structures. It also provides a barrier against the spread of infection from the skin and superficial fascia into muscle compartments. Lacerations of the deep fascia are easily recognized and should be closed, if possible, to reestablish the protective and supportive functions of this layer. Sometimes deep fascia lacerations require too much tension to close with sutures and can be left to heal without them.

SKIN TENSION LINES

There are two types of skin tension—static and dynamic—that have an important impact on the final scar structure of healed lacerations. Because *all* wounds scar, knowledge of skin tension is required when considering repair strategy or when educating the patient about eventual healing outcome.

Because it clings tautly to the body framework, skin is under constant static tension.[2] Static tension lines are commonly called *Langer's lines*. The arrangement, orientation,

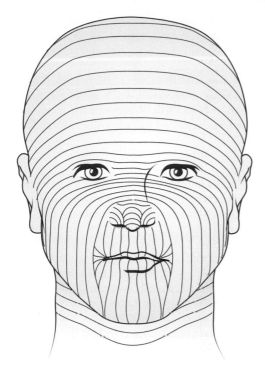

Figure 3-3. Skin tension lines of the face. Incisions or lacerations parallel to these lines are less likely to create widened scars than incisions that are perpendicular to these lines. (Adapted from Simon R, Brenner B: *Procedures and techniques in emergency medicine,* Baltimore, 1982, Williams & Wilkins.)

and distensibility of collagen fibers cause most wounds to retract open. The degree to which wound edge retraction, or "gaping," takes place is an indicator of how wide the resulting scar might be. Gaping of 5 mm or greater indicates significant tension and increased risk for wide scar formation.[3] In a study of poor outcomes of laceration repair, wound width was found to be a significant factor.[4] Lacerations of the lower extremity, particularly over the anterior tibia, tend to retract under great tension and scar conspicuously. A horizontal laceration of the skin of the eyelid is under little tension with little gaping. These lacerations become virtually unnoticeable with time.

Static skin tension plays an important role in wound edge débridement and revision. It is tempting to excise jagged wound edges to convert an irregular laceration into a straight one. If the wound is already gaping because of static tension, débridement of tissue might increase the force necessary to pull the new straight edges together. Scar width is increased, and the purpose of the edge excision is defeated. An irregular laceration under little tension often heals with a less noticeable scar than a straight wound under greater tension. As a rule, a ragged wound with viable tissue edges is repaired best by putting the "puzzle pieces" back together to preserve as much tissue as possible. If the wound needs later revision, the "extra" tissue will be welcomed by the plastic surgeon.

Different from static forces but equally important are dynamic forces on the skin, illustrated by Kraissl's lines in Figure 3-3.[5] These forces are created by the underlying pull of muscles in any given body area and correspond to wrinkles created by compression of the skin during muscle contraction.[6] These forces are most dramatically visible in the face during the various changes in facial expression. Lacerations that are perpendicular to these lines tend to heal with wider scars than do lacerations that are parallel. In choosing elective incisions of the face, surgeons apply the scalpel to correspond with these lines.

Ultimately, the final appearance of a scar is determined in part by static and dynamic forces, and the patient should be counseled accordingly. The patient is advised that it takes at least 6 months for scar contraction and collagen remodeling to diminish and 1 year for these forces to stabilize before a wound takes on its final shape.[7] During this time, the wound undergoes many visible changes. If the scar is still worrisome to the patient after this time elapses, tension-relieving procedures, such as W-plasty or Z-plasty, can be applied to improve the appearance of the scar. Whenever the cosmetic outcome is in doubt at the time of injury or the issue is raised by the patient, consultation with a plastic surgeon can be considered.

ALTERATIONS OF SKIN ANATOMY

Often, there are clinical situations in which the anatomic structure of the skin is altered so much that it requires special wound care. The most common skin changes in this setting are changes caused by aging and long-term corticosteroid administration.[8,9]

In aging, there is a flattening of the dermoepidermal junction with an accompanying decrease in the prominence of the dermal papillae. This effacement seems to result in a reduction of vascularity and nutrient supply to the epidermis. The dermis itself loses its thickness and becomes increasingly acellular and avascular. The net result is that the tensile strength of the dermis decreases significantly, which makes it less resistant to injury. More important to wound care is that the dermis does not support sutures well: They tend to "tear" the skin or cause ischemia, because the dermis has a low resistance to suture tension. Although sutures can be effective in younger patients, wound tapes are more appropriate for many lacerations that occur in older people (see Chapter 19).

Corticosteroids have a profound effect on collagen deposition through inhibition of collagen fiber synthesis and accelerated collagen degradation. The dermis becomes atrophic, thin, and poorly resistant to trauma. Small vessels seem to become increasingly fragile and readily cause ecchymoses in response to even the most trivial trauma. As in aging, the poor quality of the skin makes it less able to support sutures. Skin tapes or simple bandages are often preferable for managing these wounds.

References

1. Haury B, Rodeheaver G, Vensko J, et al: Debridement: an essential component of traumatic wound care, *Am J Surg* 135:238–242, 1978.
2. Thacker IG, Iachetta FA, Allaire PE, et al: Biomechanical properties: their influence on planning surgical excisions. In Krizek TI, Hoopes PE, editors: *Symposium on basic science in plastic surgery*, St Louis, 1975, Mosby.
3. Edlich RF, Rodeheaver GT, Morgan RF, et al: Principles of emergency wound management, *Ann Emerg Med* 17:1284–1302, 1988.
4. Singer AJ, Quinn JV, Thode HC Jr: Determinants of poor outcome after laceration and surgical incision repair, *Plast Reconstr Surg* 110:429–435, 2002.
5. Kraissl C: The selection of lines for elective surgical incisions, *Plast Reconstr Surg* 8:1–28, 1951.
6. Borges A, Alexander J: Relaxed skin tension lines, Z-plasties on scars and fusiform excision of lesions, *Br J Plast Surg* 15:242–254, 1962.
7. Hollander JE, Blaski B, Singer AJ, et al: Poor correlation of short- and long-term cosmetic appearance of repaired lacerations, *Acad Emerg Med* 2:983–987, 1995.
8. Qun T, Shao Y, He T, et al: Reduced expression of connective tissue growth factor (CTGF/CCN2) mediates collagen loss in chronically aged human skin, *J Invest Dermatol* 130:415–424, 2009.
9. Gans EH, Sadiq I, Stoudemayer T, et al: In vivo determination of the skin atrophy potential of the super-high potency topical corticosteroid fluocinonide 0.1% cream compared to clobetasol proprionate 0.05% cream and foam, and a vehicle, *J Drugs Dermatol* 7:28–32, 2008.

CHAPTER 4
Wound Healing and Cosmetic Outcome

Many of the elements of scar formation are beyond the control of the operator repairing a traumatic wound. In contrast to surgical incisions, wounds and lacerations are not planned with regard to location, length, depth, or cosmetic concerns. Wounds caused at random present a variety of biologic and technical problems that need to be solved to produce the best cosmetic outcome. Age, race, body region, skin tension lines, associated conditions and diseases, drugs, type of wound, and technical considerations all affect scar formation. The choice of repair strategy depends on these and other factors. Finally, knowledge of the spectrum of wound healing ensures that patients with traumatically induced wounds receive the proper advice and counseling. A key biologic reality in wound healing is that the wounded tissue is replaced by collagen scar tissue. By definition, the scar will look different than uninjured skin. Only recently has tissue regeneration research, studied in the lab, been tried with some success on animals.[1] True scar reduction, or even elimination, may become a valid therapy for lacerations and wounds.

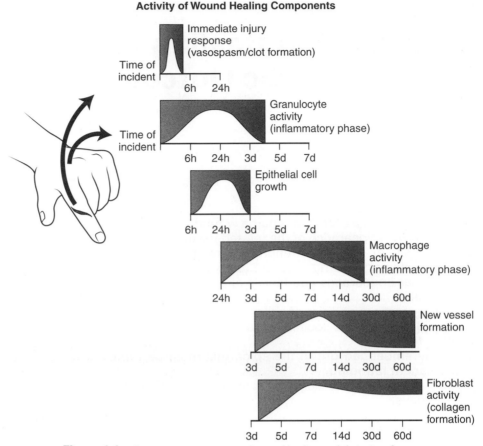

Figure 4-1. The various components of wound healing and their time frames.

NORMAL WOUND HEALING

Although wound healing is commonly described as a discrete event, it is actually a continuum of overlapping phases. For the sake of clarity, these phases are described separately and their interrelationships are graphically depicted in Figure 4-1.

Hemostasis

At the moment of injury, several events take place that culminate in rapid hemostasis. The traumatic insult causes changes in skin architecture that result in wound edge retraction and tissue contraction, which lead to compression of small venules and arterioles. Vessels also undergo intense reflex vasoconstriction for 10 minutes. Platelets begin to aggregate in the lumens of the severed vessels and on the exposed wound surfaces. The clotting cascade is activated by tissue clotting factors, and within minutes, the wound begins to fill with a hemostatic coagulum.

Inflammatory Phase

When hemostasis has been achieved and exudation begins, the inflammatory response rapidly follows. The complement system is activated, and chemotactic factors, which attract granulocytes to the wound area, are released. These cells are followed shortly by lymphocytes. Peak granulocyte numbers can be found 12 to 24 hours after the injury is sustained. The chief function of granulocytes and lymphocytes seems to be the control of bacterial growth and the suppression of infection. These cells are aided by immuno-globulins that are included in the wound exudate. In most simple wounds, granulocyte counts diminish markedly after 3 days.

After 24 to 48 hours, macrophages can be detected in large numbers, and by day 5, they are the predominant inflammatory cells in the wound area. These cells play a major role in the inflammatory responses and in the early fibroblast and collagen formation.

Epithelialization

While the inflammatory response proceeds, epithelial cells undergo morphologic and functional changes. Within 12 hours, intact cells at the wound edge begin to form pseu-dopod-like structures that facilitate cell migration. Replication takes place, and the cells begin to move over the wound surface. An advancing layer can be seen traveling over the damaged dermis and under the hemostatic coagulum. When these cells reach the inner wound area, they begin to meet other advancing epithelial extensions. The origi-nal cuboidal shape of the epithelial cells is regained, and desmosomal attachments to other cells are made. Continued replication eventually reestablishes the normal layers of epidermis. After repair of lacerations, initial epithelialization can take place within 24 to 48 hours, but the architecture and thickness of this layer continually change over the months of the wound maturation process.

Neovascularization

The phenomenon of new vessel formation is crucial to wound repair. These vessels replace the old injured network and bring oxygen and nutrients to the healing wound. Neovas-cularization is evident by day 3 and is most active by day 7; this explains the marked ery-thematous appearance of the wound at the time of suture removal. Vascularity decreases rapidly by day 21, with continued regression as the wound matures. New vessels form loops of capillaries that are surrounded by actively growing fibroblasts. These two com-ponents on the wound surface give it the classic appearance referred to as granulation.

Collagen Synthesis

With the establishment of a vascular supply and stimulation by macrophages, fibro-blasts rapidly undergo mitosis. They begin to produce new collagen fibrils by day 2. Peak synthesis occurs between days 5 and 7, and the wound has its greatest collagen mass by 3 weeks. By then, the wound is devoid of inflammatory infiltrate and edema.

New collagen is laid down in a random, amorphous pattern. It is a gel with little tensile strength. Over the months, however, this gel continually remodels itself, creat-ing an organized basket-weave pattern that is achieved by the cross-linking of collagen fibers. The balance between synthesis and lysis of collagen creates a vulnerable period approximately 7 to 10 days after injury, when the wound is most prone to unwanted opening or dehiscence. The wound has only 5% of its original tensile strength at 2 weeks and 35% at 1 month (Fig. 4-2). Final tensile strength is not achieved for several months.

Wound Contraction and Remodeling

Every wound undergoes scar remodeling over several months. With this remodeling comes some degree of wound contraction. It is most pronounced in full-thickness skin losses. The scar that forms gradually contracts centripetally over the wound defect through the action of specialized fibroblasts called myofibroblasts. Contraction pulls normal surrounding skin over the defect. Practically speaking, a properly everted suture line contracts to a flat, cosmetically acceptable scar, whereas a wound closed with the

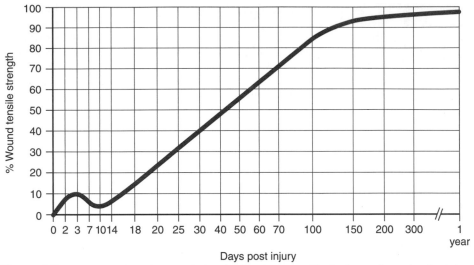

Figure 4-2. Percentage of tensile strength that develops in a wound in the days and months after injury.

edges already inverted forms an unsightly depression in the epidermis that stands out because of shadow formation from incident light (see Chapter 10).

As scars remodel, they change in appearance as well. In a study of scar appearance at suture removal versus appearance 6 to 9 months later, there was little correlation in appearance.[2] Patients need to be advised that the final appearance may not be evident for 6 months to 1 year after suture removal.

FACTORS AFFECTING COSMETIC OUTCOME (BOX 4-1)

There are numerous biologic and nonbiologic causes of scar and cosmetic outcome. In a study of 800 patients, followed for 3 months, who sustained traumatic lacerations or were surgically incised, several factors were found to be associated with a suboptimal wound appearance.[3] These included extremity wounds, wide wounds, incompletely apposed wound edges, significant tissue injury, and infection.[3] Below is a more complete discussion of the mechanisms and factors that ultimately can affect the cosmetic result.

Mechanism of Injury

The mechanism of injury is important because it is a significant determinant in the choice of management technique and in estimating the probability of wound infection. The injury mechanism also plays a role in scar formation and in the eventual cosmetic outcome. The mechanism of injury can be described as three forces that are applied to the skin under injury conditions: shearing, tension, and compression forces.[4,5] Table 4-1 lists the various causes of emergency department wounds and their frequency.

Shearing

Shearing injuries, which result in a simple dividing of tissues, are caused by sharp objects, such as knives or glass (Fig. 4-3). This mechanism accounts for most lacerations seen in the emergency department.[6] The skin is divided traumatically, but little energy is imparted to the tissues and minimal cell destruction occurs. These lacerations can be repaired primarily (primary intention), and they have a low incidence of wound infection. The resulting scar usually is thin and cosmetically acceptable.

BOX 4-1	Interference with Wound Healing

Technical Factors
Inadequate wound preparation
Excessive suture tension
Reactive suture materials
Local anesthetics

Anatomic Factors
Static skin tension
Dynamic skin tension
Pigmented skin
Oily skin
Body region

Associated Conditions and Diseases
Advanced age
Severe alcoholism
Acute uremia
Diabetes
Ehlers-Danlos syndrome
Hypoxia
Severe anemia
Peripheral vascular disease
Malnutrition

Drugs
Corticosteroids
Nonsteroidal antiinflammatory drugs
Penicillamine
Colchicine
Anticoagulants
Antineoplastic agents

TABLE 4-1	Etiology of Traumatic Wounds

Cause of Wound	No. of Cases (%)*
Blunt object	417 (42)
Sharp (nonglass)	338 (34)
Glass	133 (13)
Wood	35 (4)
Bites:	
Human	5 (1)
Dog	29 (3)
Other	15 (2)
Totals	972 (99)

*Taken from a study of 1000 wounds. The etiology of the wound was not described in 28 cases.
From Hollander JE, Singer AJ, Valentine S, Henry MC: Wound registry: development and validation, *Ann Emerg Med* 25:675–685, 1995.

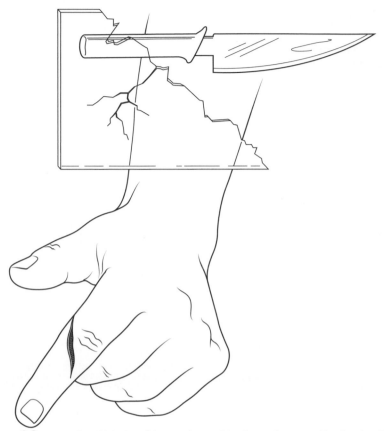

Figure 4-3. Examples of injuring objects and a resulting laceration caused by shearing forces.

Tension

Tension injuries occur as a result of a blunt or semiblunt object striking the skin at a glancing angle (Fig. 4-4). Under these conditions, a triangular flap, a partial avulsion, of skin often is created. Because the blood supply is interrupted on two sides of the flap, ischemia can occur, leading to devitalization and necrosis. The remaining blood vessels entering the flap from the base have to be preserved by careful handling and special suturing techniques, which are described in Chapter 11. If the flap base is distally based (i.e., the flap tip points back against the regional arterial flow), the compromise is even greater. The energy necessary to create this type of wound is greater than that caused by shearing forces. The combination of potential ischemia and greater cell destruction can increase the risk of wound infection. These wounds also tend to lead to greater scar formation.

Compression

Crushing or compression injuries occur when a blunt object strikes the skin at right angles (Fig. 4-5). These lacerations often have ragged or shredded edges and are accompanied by significant devitalization of skin and superficial fascia (subcutaneous tissue). Under these conditions, there is increased susceptibility to infection.[7] These wounds require extensive cleansing, irrigation, and débridement. Despite a meticulous primary repair, the resulting scars can be cosmetically poor in appearance.

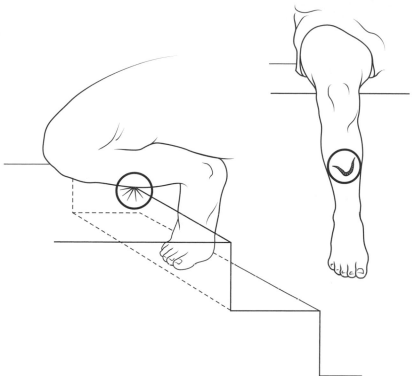

Figure 4-4. Example of the mechanism of injury and the resulting flaplike laceration caused by tension forces.

Wound Infection

The most common and serious complication of wound and laceration repair is infection. Because all accidentally induced wounds occur in unsterile conditions, they have to be considered contaminated with bacteria and debris on arrival to the emergency department. The epidermis normally acts as an effective barrier against the penetration of bacteria into the deeper layers of the skin and superficial fascia. Any violation of the epidermis provides a pathway for bacterial invasion. Not only do environmental microorganisms find their way into wounds, but also the skin, which is populated with a variety of indigenous microflora, can harbor a potentially infective inoculum of pathogenic bacteria.[8] Areas of the body with high concentrations of bacteria include scalp, perineum, axillae, mouth, feet, and nail folds. The trunk and proximal extremities are sparsely populated with bacteria.

A crucial factor in determining whether contaminating bacteria go on to cause an established wound infection is the time elapsed from injury to cleansing and repair. It has been established that 100,000 (10^5) bacteria per gram of tissue constitute an infective inoculum.[6] Wounds with counts less than that number heal without event. If bacterial counts are greater than that number, the risk of infection increases manyfold.[9] In a series of patients studied in an emergency department, it was observed that wounds less than 2.2 hours old contained 100 (10^2) bacteria per gram of tissue.[10] Wounds that were 3 hours old harbored 10^2 to 10^6 bacteria per gram of tissue. Wounds more than 5 hours old consistently grew more than 10^6 bacteria per gram of tissue. Despite experimental support for bacterial growth and invasion early after injury, the true clinical significance has not been established. It remains prudent, however, to cleanse and irrigate wounds in a timely manner. If antibiotics are considered necessary, early administration is appropriate.

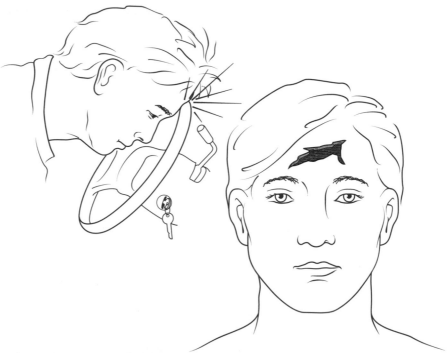

Figure 4-5. Example of the mechanism and result of an injury caused by compression forces.

Technical Factors

Soil, in particular clay, can impair healing in two ways.[11] First, the threshold infective inoculum is reduced to 10^2 bacteria, even in the presence of a small amount of dirt.[12] Second, soil and grit of any kind can lead to permanent tattooing if not aggressively removed. Consultation with a plastic surgeon may be indicated if wound cleansing and débridement cannot eliminate grit that is visibly embedded in the epidermis and superficial dermis.

Excessive tension when tying the suture knot created by improper suture technique can cause unnecessary wound ischemia.[13] Ischemia promotes cellular necrosis with greater inflammatory and scarring responses. Deep sutures, undermining, and increasing the number of sutures per laceration are methods that can reduce the danger of excessive tension.

Because tissue reactivity and inflammation vary with different suture materials, these materials can have differing effects on the healing process.[14] Although silk has excellent mechanical properties, it has a propensity for causing marked tissue reactivity. Nylon and polypropylene are the least reactive of the nonabsorbable materials. Absorbable sutures act as foreign material, and excessive numbers can increase the risk of infection and may provoke a greater scarring response.[15,16] Wound tapes and staples are the least reactive of wound closure alternatives and are associated with low infection rates even in contaminated wounds.

Experiments have shown that local anesthetics can cause retardation of wound healing.[17] This negative effect is enhanced by increasing concentrations of local anesthetics and the use of epinephrine in anesthetic solutions.[12] There is no question, however, that local anesthetics need to be used in wound care. Judicious amounts at the lowest concentrations possible are recommended.

Anatomic Factors

Body region and skin tension lines have a significant effect on wound healing, specifically on final scar morphology (see Chapter 3). Wounds over the anterior thorax or the extremities heal with the most evident scars, whereas wounds of the eyelid heal with the least obvious scars. Pigmented and oily skin also tends to heal with greater scar formation than fairer, less oily skin.

Associated Conditions and Diseases

Several conditions and diseases cause an alteration in wound healing. Advanced age has been implicated in slower healing of wounds.[18] If an older patient is basically healthy, however, normal healing and scar formation ultimately take place.[19] Wound healing can be retarded in a patient with chronic alcoholism who has advanced liver disease and impaired protein synthesis. Acute uremia has long been thought to impede healing.[20] In patients with uremia, there is an inhibition of fibroblast growth and a decrease in tensile strength during wound healing. Patients with diabetes also have numerous problems with wound healing.[21] Not only do they have an increased chance of wound infection, but also there is retardation of neovascularization and collagen synthesis. A rare disease that causes problems with collagen formation and wound healing is Ehlers-Danlos syndrome.[22]

Any condition that leads to failure of oxygen and nutrient delivery to the wound profoundly affects wound healing.[23] Shock, severe anemia, peripheral vascular disease, and malnutrition all fall into this category. Patients with severe underlying diseases, such as advanced cancer, hepatic failure, and severe cardiovascular disease, are subject to poor wound healing. Victims of major trauma, particularly individuals who have undergone prolonged shock and complicated resuscitations, also are at risk for poor wound healing.

Drugs

Numerous drugs and pharmacologic preparations alter wound healing.[24] Drugs that seem to have negative effects include corticosteroids, nonsteroidal antiinflammatory drugs (aspirin, phenylbutazone), penicillamine, colchicine, anticoagulants, and antineoplastic agents. Of these drugs, corticosteroids have the most profound effect on healing and interfere with the process at many points. They adversely alter the inflammatory response, fibroblast activity, neovascularization, and epithelialization. Nonsteroidal antiinflammatory drugs depress the normal inflammatory response and can decrease overall wound tensile strength. Anticoagulants and aspirin increase the possibility of wound hematoma formation with subsequent delays in healing time. Although in theory antineoplastic agents would be expected to inhibit wound healing, in actual practice it is not clear that they do so in a clinically significant manner.

Vitamins C and A, zinc sulfate, and anabolic steroids have a generally positive effect on wound repair.[25] Vitamin C deficiency profoundly impairs collagen formation, but normal synthesis can be restored with administration of ascorbic acid. Vitamin A and anabolic steroids are able to reverse corticosteroid-induced suppression of the inflammatory response. Zinc deficiency seems to play a role in slowing the healing process. Correction of the deficiency reverses that effect. Use of zinc ointments in non–zinc-deficient patients can cause a cross-linking failure during collagen maturation.[25] Experimental evidence that zinc sulfate can retard wound contraction supports this observation.[25]

SUTURE MARKS

Skin suture marks can be an unsightly and unnecessary complication of laceration repair. There are several causes of suture marks, some within and some out of the control of the operator.[26] The causes are as follows:

- *Skin type:* Some areas of the skin, including the skin of the back, chest, upper arms, and lower extremities, are more prone to retaining suture marks than others. On the face, skin of the lower third of the nose and cheeks adjacent to the nasal alae also is vulnerable. Suture marks are unusual on the eyelids, palms of the hands, and soles of the feet.
- *Keloid tendency:* Keloid formers have a higher risk of suture mark formation.
- *Suture tension:* Excessive suture tension during knot tying can cause tissue constriction, which increases the risk for larger, more obvious suture marks.
- *Stitch abscess:* Occasionally a small abscess forms adjacent to the suture itself. Because suture material is a foreign body, the risk of abscess formation, although small, is inherent. Silk and braided sutures are more likely to provoke an inflammatory response at the suture site than monofilament nylon or metallic staples.[13]
- *Duration sutures left in place:* Sutures remaining in place for 14 days or longer uniformly leave behind suture marks.[26] By 14 days, epithelialization of the suture track occurs, and a permanent epithelial "plug" is left behind. Conversely, no suture marks remain if sutures are removed before 7 days. The period between 7 and 14 days is less predictable with regard to retention and permanency of suture marks. These findings are independent of needle type or suture size.

KELOID AND HYPERTROPHIC SCARS

A keloid is an inappropriate accumulation of scar tissue that originates from a wound and extends beyond its original boundaries (Fig. 4-6). Keloids are more common in blacks but can occur in darkly pigmented skin areas of people of different races. These scars more commonly tend to be located on the ears, upper extremities, lower abdomen, and sternum. Eventual outcome and treatment depend on early recognition of keloid formation and prompt therapy.

Hypertrophic scars also have excessive bulk, but in contrast to keloids, they are confined to the original borders of the wound (Fig. 4-7). They tend to occur in areas of tissue stress, such as flexion creases across joints. The cause of this excessive scar response is not known. Physical therapy and splinting can be used during healing in patients who have a history of hypertrophic scarring. Interventions to minimize these abnormal scar formations are discussed in the next section on scar management and revision.

SCAR MANAGEMENT AND REVISION

Currently, there is no chemical or surgical intervention that can eliminate scars. There are many ointments, dressings, vitamins, and herbal preparations that have been used to reduce scar size, color, and symptoms such as itching.[27] To date, the small number of clinical trials to compare these products has not shown a clear advantage of one product over another.[27] In the small but significant number of cases where the scar is unsightly after several months, there are many surgical and nonsurgical techniques to modify that result. Z-plasty and dermabrasion are surgical interventions that have been shown to alter scar appearance effectively and favorably.[28,29]

At the time of wounding, it is important to identify patients who have a history of keloid or hypertrophic scar formation. For these patients, interventions need to be started shortly after the initial repair. Nonsurgical techniques include cryotherapy, pressure dressings, radiation therapy, and antimitotics.[30] Other techniques shown to be effective for these patients are laser therapy and intralesional corticosteroids.[30,31]

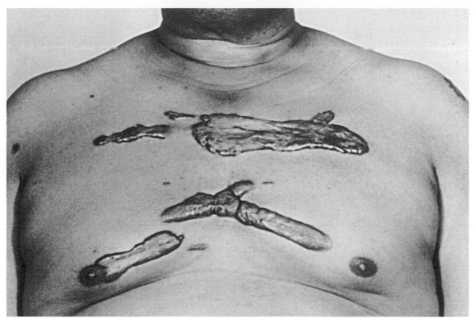

Figure 4-6. Example of a keloid scar. The scar extends beyond the margins of the original wound.

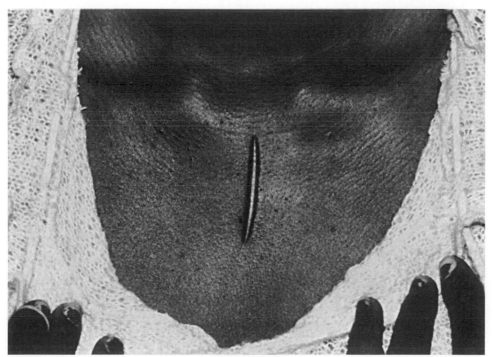

Figure 4-7. Example of a hypertrophic scar. The scar remains confined to the original borders of the wound.

These patients need to be referred to specialists skilled in these therapies during the initial phases of wound healing.

In the future, regenerative therapy may replace traditional scar formation as a true advance in wound healing and cosmetic outcome.

References

1. Rhett MJ, Ghatnekar GS, Palatinus, et al: Novel therapies for scar reduction and regenerative healing of skin wounds, *Trends Biotech* 26:173-180, 2008.
2. Hollander JE, Blasko B, Singer AJ, et al: Poor correlation of short- and long-term cosmetic appearance of repaired lacerations, *Acad Emerg Med* 2:983-987, 1995.
3. Singer AJ, Quinn JV, Thode HC, et al: Determinanats of poor surgical outcome after laceration and surgical incision repair, *Plast Reconstr Surg* 110:429-435, 2002.
4. Edlich R, Rodeheaver G, Thacker J: Technical factors in the prevention of disease. In Simmons RL, Howard RJ, Henriksen AI, editors: *Surgical infectious diseases*, New York, 1982, Appleton-Century-Crofts.
5. Trott AT: Mechanisms of surface soft tissue trauma, *Ann Emerg Med* 17:1279-1283, 1988.
6. Edlich RF, Rodeheaver GT, Morgan RF, et al: Principles of emergency wound management, *Ann Emerg Med* 17:1284-1302, 1988.
7. Cardany R, Rodeheaver GT, Thacker TG, et al: The crush injury: a high risk wound, *J Am Coll Emerg Physicians* 5:965-970, 1976.
8. Marples M: Life on the human skin, *Sci Am* 220:108-115, 1969.
9. Krizek TJ, Robson MC, Kho E: Bacterial growth and skin graft survival, *Surg Forum* 18:518-520, 1967.
10. Robson MC, Duke WF, Krizek TJ: Rapid bacterial screening in the treatment of civilian wounds, *J Surg Res* 16:299-306, 1974.
11. Rodeheaver GT, Pettry D, Turnbull V: Identification of the wound infection-potentiating factors in soil, *Am J Surg* 128:8-14, 1974.
12. Haury BB, Rodeheaver GT, Pettry D, et al: Inhibition of nonspecific defenses by soil infection-potentiating factors, *Surg Gynecol Obstet* 144:19-24, 1977.
13. Price P: Stress, strain, and sutures, *Ann Surg* 128:408-421, 1948.
14. Swanson N, Tromovitch T: Suture materials: properties, uses and abuses, *Int J Dermatol* 21:373-378, 1982.
15. Edlich RF, Rodeheaver G, Kuphal J, et al: Technique of closure: contaminated wounds, *J Am Coll Emerg Physicians* 3:375-381, 1974.
16. Losken HW, Auchincloss JA: Human bites of the lip, *Clin Plast Surg* 11:773-775, 1984.
17. Morris T, Appleby R: Retardation of wound healing by procaine, *Br J Surg* 67:391-392, 1980.
18. Grove G: Age-related differences in healing of superficial skin wounds in humans, *Arch Dermatol Res* 272:381-385, 1982.
19. Goodson W, Hunt T: Wound healing and aging, *J Invest Dermatol* 73:88-91, 1979.
20. Colin J, Elliot P, Ellis H: The effect of uraemia upon wound healing: an experimental study, *Br J Surg* 60:793-797, 1979.
21. Hunt T: Disorders of wound healing, *World J Surg* 4:271-277, 1980.
22. Cohen I, McCoy B, Biegelmann R: An update on wound healing, *Ann Plast Surg* 3:264-272, 1979.
23. Hotter A: Physiologic aspects and clinical implications of wound healing, *Heart Lung* 11:522-530, 1982.
24. Pollack S: Systemic medications and wound healing, *Int J Dermatol* 21:491-496, 1982.
25. Soderberg T, Hallmans G: Wound contractions and zinc absorption during treatment with zinc tape, *Scand J Reconstr Surg* 16:255-259, 1982.
26. Crikelair GF: Skin suture marks, *Am J Surg* 66:631-639, 1958.
27. Shih R, Waltzman J, Evans GRD, et al: Review of over the counter topical scar treatment products, *Plast Reconstr Surg* 119:1091-1095, 2007.
28. Hove CR, Williams EF 3rd, Rodgers BJ: Z-plasty: a concise review, *Facial Plast Surg* 17:289-294, 2001.
29. Poulos E, Taylor C, Solish N: Effectiveness of dermasanding (manual dermabrasion) on the appearance of surgical scars: a prospective, randomized, blinded study, *Am Acad Dermatol* 48:897-900, 2003.
30. Chang CW, Ries WR: Nonoperative techniques for scar mangement and revision, *Facial Plast Surg* 17:283-288, 2001.
31. Alster T: Laser scar revision: comparison study of 585-nm pulsed dye laser with and without intra-lesional steroids, *Dermatol Surg* 29:25-29, 2003.

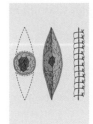

CHAPTER 5
Wound Care and the Pediatric Patient

Carolyn K. Holland, MD, MEd; Gregg A. DiGiulio, MD; and Javier A. Gonzalez del Rey, MD, MEd

―――――――――――――― Key Practice Points ――――――――――――――

- Addressing the emotional needs of children and parents is as important as wound care.
- If the history is inconsistent with the wounds, physical abuse of the child should be considered.
- Examination of the child should begin at a site away from the wound so that the child can become accustomed to the examiner.
- Physical restraints are more commonly used in the preverbal child. A gentle, empathetic approach can help avoid the need for restraints in older children.
- Use of topical anesthetics and a gentle approach reduces the need for oral or intravenous sedation.
- Topical anesthetics can be safely applied by parents.
- Absorbable suture materials have the same cosmetic outcome as nonabsorbable sutures for superficial skin closure of the scalp, face, and hand. Absorbable sutures eliminate the need for a return visit for suture removal.
- Because young children cannot accurately report loss of function in hand injuries, simple observation and special techniques are necessary to detect tendon and nerve injuries.
- Fingertip amputations can heal with regeneration alone without surgical intervention.
- Uncomplicated puncture wounds of the foot do not need prophylactic antibiotics.
- Lidocaine 4% cream applied to a superficial skin abscess with an occlusive dressing can cause spontaneous drainage.
- A dressing can be secured with Coban (3M, St. Paul, Minn.) to help prevent a young child from removing it.

Children commonly present to emergency departments (EDs) with lacerations, representing approximately 30% to 40% of all injuries seen in a pediatric ED.[1,2] Estimates of the annual rate of lacerations are 50 to 60 per 1000 children.[3,4] Lacerations often involve younger children who lack the experience, common sense, and motor coordination of older children. Boys are involved twice as often as girls. Lacerations frequently result from falls from stairways, bicycles, and furniture.[5] In children, lacerations occur most often on the head (60% of the time), followed by the upper and lower extremities.[5] Overall, lacerations are a common type of pediatric injury requiring functional and cosmetic evaluation by a physician.

GENERAL APPROACH AND CALMING TECHNIQUES

Assessing the Child

Lacerations in pediatric patients represent not only a technical challenge for the provider, but also an emotional challenge for the clinician, the child, and the parent or caregiver. Thus, it is important to take time to explain the procedure, the approach, and the possible discomforts to the child and the parents. Time spent up front preparing the child for the procedure is gained back in the end.

Assuming that there are no life-threatening or limb-threatening injuries, the clinician first should obtain the history while gaining the child's confidence. The clinician should not undress the child or examine the wound immediately. A rapport should be established by talking directly to the child using age-appropriate terms. The clinician can involve toddlers by asking them how they got their "boo-boo," but one should not expect to obtain an adequate history from the child alone; the specifics are better obtained from the parent. Children 4 years old and older frequently can provide some of the history, which allows them a sense of control. Information recommended for wound care documentation can be found in Chapter 2, Box 2-1.

Distraction can be effective at any age, such as asking about toys, cartoon characters, friends, siblings, or favorite colors or activities at an age-appropriate level. Table 5-1 summarizes the developmental abilities and distraction techniques for children of different ages.[6] Toys, interactive books, bubbles, videos, music, and sparkle wands can all be used to engage a child and divert their attention from the procedure at hand. Mental imagery is most effectively used with children who are 4 years old and older. Children younger than 4 years of age are distracted best by visual and auditory stimulation such as songs, books, or toys, as well as personal comfort items such as pacifiers, blankets, and stuffed animals. The outcome frequently relates to the verbal abilities of the individual child. Often a parent can be an ally and help distract the child if he or she is permitted and wants to be at the bedside. A general understanding of developmental milestones is invaluable in enabling the physician to interact appropriately with children.

Child life specialists have been used successfully in inpatient settings for distraction during painful procedures. More and more pediatric EDs are employing child life specialists.[7] These professionals can provide all of the following support to staff before and during procedures: coaching children through coping techniques such as deep breathing, imagery, or story telling; distraction with bubbles, toys, and games; and parent and child preparation before procedures.[8] Studies have found that child life specialists have a positive effect in reducing fears and improving satisfaction in children requiring repair for facial lacerations and angiocatheter placement.[7,9] A general ED with as few as 15,000 pediatric visits annually can financially support the presence of a child life specialist.[8]

As in all trauma situations, the history should focus on the events of the injury and the potential for injury to other areas of the body. If the history is not consistent with the injury pattern, then the possibility of intentional injury is raised. Physical abuse should be considered when the history and the injury are not consistent with one another, or when the event cannot be explained by the developmental age of the patient (e.g., a 6-month-old climbing onto and falling from a counter). There are some specific injury patterns that should raise suspicion of abuse, including burns in an immersion pattern, linear marks or lacerations consistent with a belt or hanger, or an unusual injury location not usually prone to injury. A social services referral is necessary for any case in which abuse is suspected.

TABLE 5-1	Childhood Developmental Abilities by Age			
Age (yr)	**Development Issues**	**Fears**	**Techniques**	**Distraction/Comfort Items**
Infant	Minimal language Feel like an extension of parents Sensitive to physical environment	Stranger anxiety	Keep parents in sight Address possible hunger Use warm hands Keep room warm	Lullabies sung by parents Pictures, cartoons Nonnutritive sucking (pacifier) Skin-to-skin contact Swaddling
Toddler (1-3)	Receptive language more advanced than expressive See themselves as individuals Assertive will	Brief separation Pain	Maintain verbal communication Examine in parent's lap Allow some choices (if possible)	Pop-up books Suspension wands Puppets Water toys Bubbles Light-up toys
Preschool (3-5)	Excellent expressive skills Rich fantasy life Magical thinking	Long separation Pain Disfigurement	Allow expression Encourage fantasy and play Encourage participation in care	Pop-up books Suspension wands Puppets Water toys Bubbles Distracting conversations Deep breathing methods
School age (5-10)	Fully developed language Understanding of body structure and function Able to reason and compromise Experience with self-control	Disfigurement Loss of function Death	Explain procedures Explain pathophysiology and treatment Project positive outcome Stress child's ability to master situation Respect physical modesty	Blowing bubbles Singing songs Squeeze balls Relaxation breathing Playing electronic devices Music on headphones Reading book Imagery Self-hypnosis
Adolescent (10-19)	Self-determination Decision making Realistic view of death	Loss of autonomy Loss of peer acceptance Death	Allow choices and control Stress acceptance by peers Respect autonomy	Video games

Adapted from Stein MT: Interviewing in a pediatric setting. In Dixon SD, Stein MT, editors: *Encounters with children,* ed 4, St Louis, 2006, Mosby.

Immunization Status

Special attention should be paid to the immunization status. Simply asking the parent if the child's shots are up to date most often elicits a positive response whether or not this is actually true. It is better to inquire about the number of "shots" and the age when the last one was given. Children should receive a total of 5 doses of diptheria/tetanus/pertussis (DTaP) at pediatrician visits at 2, 4, 6, and 15 to 18 months and at 4 to 6 years of age. For routine tetanus prophylaxis in children 6 years old or less who have not completed their primary immunization series, DTaP should be used instead of single-antigen tetanus toxoid (Td). The final booster for children should be around 11 years of age.[10,11] In the event a child is completely unimmunized and parents refuse administration of tetanus prophylaxis, involvement of your local risk management department and local/state department of immunization may be necessary to facilitate appropriate treatment for the minor patient. Unfortunately, there are no alternatives to immunization for the prevention of tetanus because administration of antibiotics is "neither practical nor useful in managing wounds."[12] An in-depth discussion of tetanus prophylaxis is presented in Chapter 21.

Assessing the Wound

Next, the wound is assessed. Allowing the child to remain with the parent for as long as possible facilitates the examination. The physician can gain the child's confidence by telling him or her that initially the physician is just going to "look." However, it is important to avoid a "promise not to touch," thus misleading the child about your plans for an examination. The physician should continue to involve the parent in the evaluation process so that the child knows that the physician is there to help. Generally, kindness and patience should be accompanied by a thorough and directed approach. The examination should begin away from the injury, especially in a toddler or younger child. If the injury is on the hand or face, the physician should start by playing gently with a foot. This provides the child time to become comfortable with the exam and to develop confidence that the physician is not going to hurt him or her. After this development of trust, the provider can slowly advance to the site of the injury. Direct probing of the wound is painful and should not be done until after anesthesia is achieved. In cases in which hemostasis is necessary, pressure should be applied; this often can be done safely by the parent.

Parents can be of great help in calming and distracting their children, so they should be offered the opportunity to participate to the degree that their level of comfort allows. When asked, more than 80% of parents indicate that they would like to stay with their children through invasive procedures such as IV placement or laceration repair in EDs, and 90% of physicians and nurses support this parental presence.[13-15] Some parents, however, cannot tolerate being present during the invasive treatment of their children, and these parents should also be given the option of going to the waiting area, if close by.

RESTRAINT FOR WOUND CARE

Physical restraints (Fig. 5-1) should be considered in a preverbal child if imagery and verbal calming techniques are ineffective. Limited language and limited ability to comprehend the situation make it difficult for preverbal children to cooperate with caregivers. Velcro restraint boards (Papoose Boards [Olympic Medical, San Carlos, Calif.]) are usually well tolerated, especially if used in conjunction with pharmacologic anxiolysis such as oral midazolam. It is our experience that, once in place on a board, an infant or toddler frequently becomes less agitated after infiltration is performed. Parents understand the need for restraints to protect the child from harming himself or herself and generally think that the child is comfortable in restraint and would be willing to have a Papoose Board used in a future visit.[16]

Regardless of the method used, the caregiver always must take the time to explain the need for restraints to the parents. Restraints protect the child and caregiver during the procedure and ensure the best result. Their use is not without complication, however. Restraints limit the child's protective reflexes should he or she vomit. Excessive crying increases gastric pressure, and, together with a full stomach, the possibility of emesis increases. Suction should be readily available, and the child should be turned to a lateral decubitus position while in the papoose if emesis occurs.

PEDIATRIC PATIENT SEDATION

Despite caregivers' best efforts, occasionally there are children who are not able to cooperate. When the child's inability to cooperate interferes with the physician's ability to

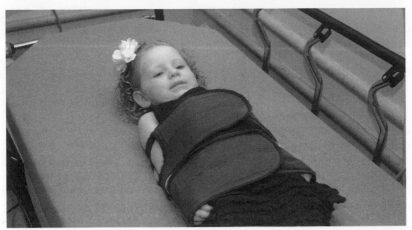

Figure 5-1. Example of a restraining device to immobilize a child during a wound care procedure of the face and scalp. When placing the device, ensure that it is not too tight to impair breathing.

perform an adequate repair, or poses a danger to the caregivers or to the child himself or herself, the physician can consider the use of pharmacologic sedation. The type, location, and complexity of the laceration, and the emotional state of the child, help to determine the type of sedative to use. In small, simple lacerations, the risk of sedation may outweigh the benefits. In our experience, by using the previously described techniques and a topical anesthetic such as LET (lidocaine 1%, epinephrine 0.1%, and tetracaine 0.5% solution or gel), rather than an injected anesthetic, we are able to repair most small lacerations, including facial lacerations, without the use of sedatives.

For repair of a laceration, the physician usually induces moderate sedation, where the child retains protective reflexes, maintains his or her own airway, and is able to respond to a directed command. All sedation techniques can inadvertently evolve into deep sedation, which is a more depressed state of consciousness in which the child is not easily aroused and cannot maintain protective reflexes or an open airway, or even into general anesthesia, which is a drug-induced complete loss of consciousness with impaired ventilatory function. Titrating the sedative dose to the desired level of sedation may help prevent the evolution of consciousness into deep sedation; however, practitioners must be prepared to intervene during any airway emergency. In the office or ED, conscious sedation should be limited to children with American Society of Anesthesiologists (ASA) classifications I and II (class I is a normally healthy patient; class II is a patient with mild systemic disease).[17] Additionally, the time of the last meal must be considered when deciding whether or not to sedate a child. ASA and American Academy of Pediatrics guidelines for fasting are 2 hours for clear liquids, 4 hours for breast milk, and 6 hours for formula, cow's milk, and food.[18] However, there is controversy regarding the applicability of these guidelines in the ED setting. The American College of Emergency Physicians Clinical Policy concerning sedation of pediatric patients in the ED specifically states that "procedural sedation may be safely administered to pediatric patients in the ED who have had recent oral intake."[19] Overall, as with any area in medicine in which there are conflicting recommendations, the relative risk of providing sedation must be weighed against the risk of delaying the procedure.

The room where sedation is performed must have equipment available for airway and cardiovascular interventions for children of all ages and sizes. The physician must have the ability to handle a sudden change in the child's status. Whenever sedatives are used, there should be one practitioner present whose sole job is to monitor the patient and to assist in any resuscitative measures that become necessary.[20] Continuous monitoring of pulse oximetry, pulse, and intermittent documentation of respiratory rate and blood pressure are necessary in all of these patients. The monitoring of any child who has received a sedative continues until discharge criteria are met. Discharge criteria include an ability to converse at an age-appropriate level, maintenance of a clear airway, stable cardiovascular function, and the ability to sit unaided. Regardless of the agent used, parents should be informed of the type of sedative to be used and the potential side effects. Consent should be documented in accordance with hospital, local, and state requirements.

Medications for Sedation

For pain control during moderate sedation, fentanyl is an excellent choice (Table 5-2). It is a synthetic opioid agonist that is 100 times more potent than morphine. It is commonly used in combination with a sedative (e.g., midazolam) for conscious sedation.[21] The benefits of this agent are rapid onset of pain control, short duration, and predictability. Fentanyl must be used with caution, especially when combined with another sedative agent, because of an increased risk of respiratory depression. If administered intravenously, it should be titrated in 1 μg/kg increments with a maximal dose of 5 μg/kg over 1 hour. Higher doses administered rapidly can induce chest wall rigidity with impaired ventilation.

Midazolam is a short-acting benzodiazepine frequently used both for anxiolysis and as a sedative in children.[22] The main attributes of this drug are the provision of effective anxiety reduction and anterograde amnesia, combined with a favorable overall safety profile.[23] To help calm a mildly anxious child, multiple routes of midazolam administration are available. The intravenous route provides the quickest onset of action, and it is easiest to titrate dosing using this method.

The intranasal route can be limited by discomfort of application because of the volume of midazolam necessary and because of a burning sensation. If this route is chosen, the operator uses the intravenous solution and draws it into a tuberculin syringe; the needle is removed, and, with the child supine, the dose is administered in aliquots of two drops per nostril over 2 to 5 minutes. Because the solution can be irritating to the mucosa, it is prudent to warn the child and the parent of a stinging sensation.

Alternatively, a Mucosal Atomization Device (Wolfe Tory Medical, Salt Lake City, Utah) can be used to anesthetize the nasal passages with lidocaine before administration of the midazolam, and the device can also be used to administer the midazolam itself.[24] Sedation usually occurs within 5 to 10 minutes. Because of a significant and variable first-pass effect, there is considerable variation in the dose required to induce sedation. Another option is midazolam oral syrup (2 mg/mL), which is given at a dose of 0.25 to 0.5 mg/kg. In children 6 months to 6 years old, as much as 1 mg/kg is sometimes necessary, but the maximal dose should not exceed 20 mg. Onset of action is usually between 10 and 30 minutes.

Nitrous oxide in concentrations less than 50% has been used commonly in pediatric dentistry. It is completely painless and has anxiolytic, sedative, and mild analgesic properties. Nitrous oxide has been used as an adjunct to local infiltration or nerve block in wound repair and has been shown to reduce suturing-related distress in pediatric patients in EDs.[19,25] Portable devices have made this modality more available to EDs than previously; however, there are still some drawbacks to the use of nitrous. The delivery and scavenging systems are expensive, and because of the need for cooperation, nitrous oxide should be used only in children older than 4 years.[26]

Ketamine (4 mg/kg intramuscularly or 0.5-2 mg/kg intravenously) is a dissociative agent that provides effective sedation without loss of airway reflexes. Its effectiveness and safety have been demonstrated in children in a variety of painful ED procedures.[27,28] Its use in pediatric sedations for these painful procedures is associated with high parental satisfaction.[29] IV dosing is associated with shorter recovery times and

TABLE 5-2	Selected Drugs for Sedation and Analgesia[18]		
Medication	**Recommended Dose**	**Route of Administration**	**Additional Information**
Fentanyl	1-3 µg/kg	IV or IM	Immediate effect with IV. Effect within 7-10 min with IM. Titrate slowly (1 µg/kg/min). Maximal dose 5 µg/kg/hr.
	2-3 µg/kg	IN	Effect within 5 min. Use in children age 1 yr and older. Repeat in 10 min if no effect. Best if used with atomizer.
Morphine	0.08-0.1 mg/kg	IV or IM	Effect within 10-20 min. Maximal dose: infants 2 mg, children (1-6) 4 mg, children (7-12) 8 mg.
Midazolam	0.025-0.1 mg/kg	IV	Effect in 1-5 min. Titrate over 3 min to desired effect. Maximal initial dose 5 mg. Higher dose/wt in patients younger than 6 yr.
	0.25-0.5 mg/kg	PO	Effect in 10-20 min. Maximal initial dose 20 mg; may repeat in 45-60 min if patient not sedated well. May need up to 1 mg/kg in children 6 yr or less.
	0.2-0.5 mg/kg	IN	Effect within 5 min. Slowly drip into nostrils. May repeat in 5-15 min. Maximal initial dose 10 mg. Can cause stinging sensation in nose.
	0.1-0.15 mg/kg	IM	Effect within 5-10 min. Maximal dose 10 mg.
Diazepam	0.05-0.1 mg/kg	IV	Effect within 1-3 min. Titrate over 3 min to desired effect. Maximal dose 0.25 mg/kg.
	0.2-0.3 mg/kg	PO	Effect in 45-60 min. Maximal dose 10 mg.
Ketamine	0.5-1 mg/kg	IV	Effect in 1 min. Administer slowly; do not exceed 0.5 mg/kg/min.
	4 mg/kg	IM	Effect in 3-5 min. May cause vomiting.
Propofol	0.5-1 mg/kg	IV	Effect in 30 sec. Very short acting.
Reversal Agents			
Naloxone	0.1 mg/kg	IV or IM	Effect in 1-2 min. For reversal of opiates. May repeat in 5 min if no effect.
Flumazenil	0.01 mg/kg	IV	Effect in 1-3 min. Maximal single dose 0.2 mg/kg, 1 mg total.

decreased length of stay as compared with IM dosing.[30] However, IM administration may be an appropriate choice in a distressed child in whom establishing an IV would be exceedingly difficult. Ketamine's disadvantages include increased incidence of post-sedation vomiting, which is even worse with IM administration, high doses, and older children (i.e., adolescents).[30,31] Emergence reactions, including vivid dreams, hallucinations, and/or frank delirium, can occur up to 24 hours after use. Although present in up to 12% of patients, they are much less common in the pediatric population. Severe reactions can be treated with a small dose of a short-acting benzodiazepine or barbiturate.[32]

Propofol is another agent that is gaining popularity for procedural sedation in children in the ED. This drug is classified as a nonopioid, nonbarbiturate, sedative-hypnotic agent.[33] The drug has a rapid onset and offset, antiemetic properties, and a smooth recovery profile. Its main drawbacks are the potential for respiratory depression and hypotension, both of which are dependent on the dose and speed of administration. Propofol is more commonly used in the management of fracture reduction, abscess drainage, wound exploration, and ocular examination after ocular burn, but propofol can also be used for procedural sedation in children with lacerations.[33]

LOCAL ANESTHETIC TECHNIQUES

The area of a wound or abscess should always be anesthetized before cleansing and irrigation. Wound cleansing is painful, and often the adequacy of anesthesia can be assessed during irrigation. Cleansing and irrigation techniques are the same for children and adults and are described fully in Chapter 7.

Topical anesthetics such as LET are being used more frequently and are as effective as other local anesthetics[34] (see Chapter 6). This preparation provides anesthesia without causing the discomfort associated with an injection, and it does not distort the local anatomy. Another potential advantage that we have noted is that we need to use physical restraints less often when we use LET. As LET contains epinephrine, there is always concern that areas of end artery flow, such as fingers, toes, and ears, could be at risk of ischemia. However, studies have demonstrated no harm from the use of LET in digital anesthesia in pediatric patients.[35,36] Studies have shown that the application of LET at triage significantly reduces total treatment time for children with simple lacerations.[37] These topical anesthetics should be used before wound cleansing and repair. If the gel formulation is unavailable, the caregiver saturates with the solution a small pledget of cotton or a piece of gauze that is of similar size to the wound. The maximal dose is 0.1 mL/kg (average dose 2 to 3 mL). Any blood coagulum is removed from the wound. The pledget is placed directly into the wound and can be held in place by an adhesive bandage or by tape, or it can be held directly by the parent. If held in place by hand, caregivers should wear gloves to prevent absorption through their own fingers. The pledget is left in place for 20 to 25 minutes. The pharmacy also can compound LET with methylcellulose to form a gel preparation. This gel preparation can be placed directly in the wound and can be covered with a Band-Aid or occlusive dressing. Effective application usually blanches the skin around the wound. The caregiver should show the parents the blanched skin and should explain its significance to the parent and the child. Topical and local anesthetic techniques are discussed further in Chapter 6.

Regional blocks are another useful method of providing anesthesia for children. Blocks do not distort the anatomy at the site of the injury and may be less traumatic than local infiltration because they often require only one or two injections, as opposed to the multiple injections sometimes required for local anesthesia. Digital, infraorbital, mental, and supraorbital blocks are probably the most commonly used, although all of the blocks described in Chapter 6 may be used in children.

CHOICE OF CLOSURE MATERIALS

A wide array of suture materials and sizes is available to the practitioner (see Chapter 8). Personal preferences often determine which material is used. In general, the choice of material to use is the same as described for adults, but there are particular situations in which children may benefit from other means of closure. Because suture removal often is fraught with the same anxiety and difficulties as suture application, the use of absorbable sutures sometimes is the best option in wounds that would be closed with nonabsorbable material in adult patients. For nail bed and scalp lacerations, we often use chromic gut or Vicryl Rapide (Ethicon, Somerville, NJ), which has been shown to have cosmetic results and an infection risk profile similar to those of nylon for repair of simple noncontaminated lacerations.[38,39] If the sutures still remain at 5 to 7 days on the face or 8 to 10 days at other sites, the parent is instructed to remove the sutures by gently rubbing the materials with gauze. This technique should be done parallel to the wound to minimize the potential for wound dehiscence. Removal is necessary to prevent the formation of suture marks.

Skin staples are a fast, effective method of closing scalp lacerations, especially in an uncooperative child, and staples provide the same cosmetic outcome as standard sutures.

Skin tapes are an alternative method of repair for simple lacerations. The advantages are that they are easy to apply, leave no marks, and no follow-up is necessary. The tapes are not reliable, however, for infants and young children, who may remove them prematurely. Tissue adhesives are fully described in Chapter 14. They have many advantages over sutures and staples, including ease of use, decreased pain, decreased procedure/application time, and lack of the need for follow up.[40] There is, however, a small but statistically significant increase in the risk of wound dehiscence; thus our recommendation is to use adhesives only for sites where there is minimal skin tension. Additionally, as previously discussed, children often have a difficult time sitting still and following directions during procedures. Initial use of tissue adhesives near and around the eye had some documented adverse events, specifically, eyelids glued together.[41] In view of this risk, careful application with precautions against accidental runoff into the eyes is warranted.

SPECIAL CONSIDERATIONS FOR DIFFERENT ANATOMIC SITES

Scalp

There are several closure options for scalp lacerations. Nonabsorbable sutures, such as 4-0 or 5-0 nylon, is widely used. Staples have become increasingly common because of their ease of use and speed of application. More recently, absorbable sutures—chromic gut, Vicryl Rapide—are being used because suture removal is unnecessary, thereby decreasing the expense and inconvenience to the child and parent. Before closure, the wound has to be anesthetized and cleansed (see Chapter 7 for Wound Cleansing). If hair interferes with closure, it can be flattened away from the wound with a petroleum-based ointment. Trimming hair with scissors can also uncover a wound, but shaving is not recommended because of the possibility of skin injury with an increased rate of infection.

Rapid repair of a linear scalp laceration can be accomplished with staples. Stapling is less expensive, less time consuming, and provides similar cosmetic outcomes when compared with sutures; however, assistance may be required to bring wound edges close together to facilitate wound edge eversion in large gaping wounds.[42] When using sutures, the simple interrupted technique or horizontal mattress can be applied. Staples and nonabsorbable sutures are removed at 6 to 7 days.

Simple, small scalp lacerations that are not grossly contaminated, are not actively bleeding, and have not interrupted the galea aponeurotica may be closed using the hair-tie technique. An adequate length of hair from opposite sides of the wound is necessary. The caregiver twists the hair strands on both sides of the suture line, pulls them across the wound, and knots them (the number of knots should be equal to the number of stitches that normally would have been used in the care of this wound), or merely twists the hairs together and applies a drop of tissue adhesive.[43] Postclosure wound care is similar to that of a routine scalp closure with sutures. The knot or glued area is allowed to grow away from the wound edge and can be cut free in 1 to 2 weeks.

Face

An assistant is invaluable and necessary when closing facial wounds in children. The assistant is needed to maintain immobilization, and this is best accomplished if he or she uses firm, consistent pressure, being careful to use the flat surfaces of his or her hands or forearms to immobilize the head. Use of fingertips alone, which can cause localized pressure and pain, should be avoided. When closing chin lacerations, firm, consistent pressure can be applied to keep the jaw closed and minimize "quivering" of the chin.

Face lacerations can be closed with numerous materials. In low tension, uncomplicated, straight lacerations, wound adhesives are a good choice. Absorbable sutures—6-0 Vicryl Rapide, fast-absorbing gut—can be used on the face with the same cosmetic result as nonabsorbable sutures.[38,39] It is important to note that absorbable sutures need to be removed to prevent suture marks if they have not dissolved within 5 to 7 days. Absorbable sutures can be gently "rubbed off" by the parent with a moistened gauze sponge.

Hand

In the treatment of pediatric hand lacerations, difficulties most commonly arise during the evaluation of the wound. Cooperation for formal nerve and tendon function tests is difficult to obtain. Young children are unable to follow commands or verbalize the concepts of numbness and paresthesia. Often the practitioner must rely on observation rather than formal testing. The resting position of the extremity should be observed. Is there consistency in the amount of resting flexion between digits? A finger extended or flexed while the others are not raises the suspicion of a tendon injury and should prompt further investigation. The clinician should watch for spontaneous movement of the injured part. Does the child withdraw from touch or noxious stimuli? When anesthesia is obtained, does the depth of the wound suggest tendon or nerve involvement?

In children younger than 5 years old, the classic sensory examination is modified. Two methods are available to determine the sensory innervation in the area distal to the wound. The first method is based on the principle that denervated fingers do not sweat. If one runs the body of a clean plastic pen along an area with normal innervation, the sweat creates a slight drag, whereas in a denervated area, the pen moves more swiftly. Another popular method is the submersion test. Normal skin becomes wrinkled after 20 minutes of being underwater, whereas denervated skin usually remains smooth.[44] Frequently the final answer cannot be determined at the initial encounter. Under such circumstances, only the skin should be closed, and serial examinations over the next few days will help clarify if there is any nerve or tendon involvement. Phone consultation for reevaluation with a hand specialist is indicated at this time to arrange follow-up within 3 to 5 days after the initial injury. Tendon or nerve repair can be performed within the first 3 weeks after the injury with good results.

Uncomplicated hand and finger lacerations can be closed with either nonabsorbable or absorbable sutures. 5-0 nylon or polypropylene is effective and should be removed in 7 to 10 days. 5-0 chromic gut and Vicryl Rapide are the absorbable sutures of choice. They have the same cosmetic outcome as nonabsorbable sutures, and removal is not necessary.

Fingertip avulsions are common pediatric injuries. These injuries occur most often in toddlers when windows or doors close on their fingers. In cases of complete fingertip amputation, several studies have shown superior results when the fingertip is allowed to regenerate on its own.[45,46] The granulation tissue that develops contains neural buds and provides superior sensation compared with a graft. In cases of partial amputation or a flap laceration of the fingertip, the flap may be reattached after blood clots are removed. In most cases an x-ray should be obtained to exclude the presence of a fracture. For a distal tuft fracture, copious irrigation should be followed by the use of prophylactic antibiotics. More proximal open fractures should be managed in direct consultation with a hand specialist. In cases in which the laceration involves the nail bed, the same principles described in Chapter 13 should be applied. Formal splinting of the injury after repair protects the repair and the injury. Children are quite skilled at extricating themselves from dressings and bandages. The prognosis of these injuries depends on how much of the fingertip is involved. These injuries may take weeks for complete healing. It is advisable to arrange follow-up with a plastic or an orthopedic surgeon.

Foot

A foot injury presents problems with the injury itself and with postinjury ambulation difficulties. Unless the child is more than 6 to 8 years old, crutches are not recommended because of insufficient motor coordination. Younger children may need to be carried or encouraged to crawl. Lacerations of the foot should be closed with nonabsorbable suture such as 5-0 nylon or polypropylene. They are removed in 8 to 10 days. Foot dressings are reinforced with Coban to try to prevent premature loosening or removal.

Puncture wounds present some unique controversies. No prospective studies have addressed this common entity. Although some authors recommend routine coring for puncture wounds, we discourage this technique, because it is uncomfortable, increases local pain, makes ambulation difficult, and does not have proven efficacy.[47] Every puncture wound has the potential to harbor foreign material, however, which increases the risk of infection. Most foreign bodies are not radiopaque and are difficult to find on probing. Removal of any organic material or identifiable foreign body is recommended, and opening the wound with a small incision may be necessary in these instances. Because of the thick skin on the plantar aspect of the foot, topical anesthesia is much less effective, and direct injection of local anesthetic is usually required. Chapter 16 discusses plantar puncture wounds further.

Serious complications can occur for puncture wounds through athletic shoes. *Pseudomonas* osteomyelitis has been reported in 4% of these cases.[48] It is our opinion, and most authors agree, that antibiotics are not routinely required after puncture wounds to the feet. If cellulitis develops within the first few days of the injury, antibiotic coverage is needed and is directed toward the most common causes of infection—*Staphylococcus* and *Streptococcus* species.[49] The quinolones that are frequently used in adults are relatively contraindicated in preadolescents because of a concern for inhibition of cartilage growth and development. *Pseudomonas* osteomyelitis should be considered in cases of persistent inflammation despite adequate antistaphylococcal coverage or increasing bone tenderness over time.[48]

Perineum/Straddle Injuries

Careful and complete examination is necessary when evaluating injuries to the perineum or straddle injuries. Blunt straddle injuries occur when the perineum strikes a fixed object, such as the crossbar of a bicycle. This mechanism is associated with trauma to the labia and posterior fourchette in young girls.[50] In young males, blunt injuries are unlikely to sustain any significant lacerations in the scrotum or perineum. With penetrating injury, such as occurs with falling onto a fence post, vaginal injury is more likely.[51] If there is any concern for internal vaginal lacerations, unexplained bleeding, or lacerations involving the rectum, complete visualization is required.[52] Often the use of general anesthesia and consultation with a subspecialist are necessary. Straddle injuries in both male and female patients can be accompanied by trauma to the urethra and concomitant urinary retention.[53] Foley catheterization is sometimes necessary if watchful waiting is unsuccessful. Small superficial labial or penile lacerations can be sutured within the ED. Because children are afraid of a stranger manipulating their genitalia, sedation may be necessary for appropriate repair of even small lacerations.

Chromic gut or any other appropriate absorbable material is recommended to avoid the stress and anxiety of suture removal.

ABSCESS DRAINAGE

Cutaneous and superficial abscess evaluation and treatment are fully covered in Chapter 18; however, there are a few additional tips that can help with this disease process in the pediatric patient. Incision and drainage are painful as is the infiltration of a field block to provide local anesthesia. A normally quick and easy procedure in adult patients can rapidly devolve into a protracted battle with pain control and patient comfort. Use of a topical anesthetic cream, such as lidocaine 4% cream, applied and held in place with an occlusive dressing, has been associated with spontaneous abscess drainage in pediatric patients. Additionally, use of a topical agent significantly decreased the need for procedural sedation in pediatric patients requiring abscess drainage.[54] Because community-acquired methicillin-resistant *Staphylococcus aureus* (CA-MRSA) has become a common cause of skin infections, if antibiotics are necessary, local resistant patterns should be considered when choosing antibiotics. The primary care pediatrician may also be able to provide guidance in these situations.

WOUND AFTERCARE

Wound care after laceration repair in a pediatric patient is the same as described in Chapter 22. Bandages and dressings should be applied, but they need to be secured adequately because of the child's curiosity. Materials such as Coban may be used, but the clinician should be careful to avoid creating a tourniquet effect. In general, sutures can be removed earlier than is done for the adult. Oral and written discharge instructions must be clear and concise, indicating possible complications, follow-up care, and the timing of suture removal. Written instructions are invaluable because parents often may not recall the details of the instructions after discharge from the ED.

Other important issues are related to the psychological well-being of the child. The clinician should always give a reward when the procedure is complete, such as a sticker. The parents should be encouraged to minimize the stress of the accident by making the event a positive experience and not a punishment. Throughout the encounter, the clinician should try to engage the child, gain his or her confidence, and possibly become a friend. In the end, the attentive clinician is rewarded with a satisfying experience for all involved.

References

1. Wallace HMGE, Liss EF, editors: *Maternal and child health practices*, Springfield, Ill, 1973, Charles C Thomas.
2. Izant RJ Jr, Hubay CA: The annual injury of 15,000,000 children: a limited study of childhood accidental injury and death, *J Trauma* 6:65–74, 1966.
3. Manheimer DI, Dewey J, Mellinger GD, Corsa L Jr: 50,000 child-years of accidental injuries, *Public Health Rep* 81:519–533, 1966.
4. Rivara FP, Bergman AB, LoGerfo JP, Weiss NS: Epidemiology of childhood injuries. II. Sex differences in injury rates, *Am J Dis Child* 136:502–506, 1982.
5. Baker MD, Selbst SM, Lanuti M: Lacerations in urban children. A prospective 12-January study, *Am J Dis Child* 144:87–92, 1990.
6. Dixon SD: *Encounters with children: pediatric behavior and development*, St Louis, 1992, Mosby.
7. Krebel MS, Clayton C, Graham C: Child life programs in the pediatric emergency department, *Pediatr Emerg Care* 12:13–15, 1996.
8. Child life services can provide competitive edge, *ED Manag* 16:115–117, 2004.
9. Alcock DS, Feldman W, Goodman JT, et al: Evaluation of child life intervention in emergency department suturing, *Pediatr Emerg Care* 1:111–115, 1985.
10. Centers for Disease Control and Prevention: *Vaccines for children program: vaccines to prevent diptheria, tetanus and pertussis* (PDF file). www.cdc.gov/vaccines/programs/vfc/downloads/resolutions/1010dtap-508.pdf. Accessed February 4, 2011.

11. Diphtheria, tetanus, and pertussis: recommendations for vaccine use and other preventive measures. Recommendations of the Immunization Practices Advisory committee (ACIP), *MMWR Recomm Rep* 40:1–28, 1991.

12. Centers for Disease Control and Prevention: In Adkinson W, Wolfe S, Hamborsky J, McIntyre L, editors: *Epidemiology and prevention of vaccine-preventable diseases*, ed 11, Washington, DC, 2009, Public Health Foundation.

13. Bauchner H, Waring C, Vinci R: Parental presence during procedures in an emergency room: results from 50 observations, *Pediatrics* 87:544–548, 1991.

14. Beckman AW, Sloan BK, Moore GP, et al: Should parents be present during emergency department procedures on children, and who should make that decision? A survey of emergency physician and nurse attitudes, *Acad Emerg Med* 9:154–158, 2002.

15. Boie ET, Moore GP, Brummett C, Nelson DR: Do parents want to be present during invasive procedures performed on their children in the emergency department? A survey of 400 parents, *Ann Emerg Med* 34:70–74, 1999.

16. Frankel RI: The Papoose Board and mothers' attitudes following its use, *Pediatr Dent* 13:284–288, 1991.

17. American Academy of Pediatrics Committee on Drugs: Guidelines for monitoring and management of pediatric patients during and after sedation for diagnostic and therapeutic procedures, *Pediatrics* 89:1110–1115, 1992.

18. Cote CJ, Wilson S: Guidelines for monitoring and management of pediatric patients during and after sedation for diagnostic and therapeutic procedures: an update, *Pediatrics* 118:2587–2602, 2006.

19. Mace SE, Brown LA, Francis L, et al: Clinical policy: critical issues in the sedation of pediatric patients in the emergency department, *Ann Emerg Med* 51:378–399, 2008.

20. Practice guidelines for sedation and analgesia by non-anesthesiologists: A report by the American Society of Anesthesiologists Task Force on Sedation and Analgesia by Non-Anesthesiologists, *Anesthesiology* 84:459–471, 1996.

21. Billmire DA, Neale HW, Gregory RO: Use of i.v. fentanyl in the outpatient treatment of pediatric facial trauma, *J Trauma* 25:1079–1080, 1985.

22. Feld LH, Negus JB, White PF: Oral midazolam preanesthetic medication in pediatric outpatients, *Anesthesiology* 73:831–834, 1990.

23. Diament MJ, Stanley P: The use of midazolam for sedation of infants and children, *AJR Am J Roentgenol* 150:377–378, 1988.

24. Chiaretti A, Barone G, Rigante D, et al: Intranasal lidocaine and midazolam for procedural sedation in children, *Arch Dis Child* 96:160–163, 2011.

25. Gamis AS, Knapp JF, Glenski JA: Nitrous oxide analgesia in a pediatric emergency department, *Ann Emerg Med* 18:177–181, 1989.

26. Dula DJ, Skiendzielewski JJ, Snover SW: The scavenger device for nitrous oxide administration, *Ann Emerg Med* 12:759–761, 1983.

27. Green SM, Rothrock SG, Harris T, et al: Intravenous ketamine for pediatric sedation in the emergency department: safety profile with 156 cases, *Acad Emerg Med* 5:971–976, 1998.

28. Green SM, Rothrock SG, Lynch EL, et al: Intramuscular ketamine for pediatric sedation in the emergency department: safety profile in 1,022 cases, *Ann Emerg Med* 31:688–697, 1998.

29. Holloway VJ, Husain HM, Saetta JP, Gautam V: Accident and emergency department led implementation of ketamine sedation in paediatric practice and parental response, *J Accid Emerg Med* 17:25–28, 2000.

30. Deasy C, Babl FE: Intravenous vs intramuscular ketamine for pediatric procedural sedation by emergency medicine specialists: a review, *Paediatr Anaesth* 20:787–796, 2010.

31. Green SM, Roback MG, Krauss B, et al: Predictors of emesis and recovery agitation with emergency department ketamine sedation: an individual-patient data meta-analysis of 8,282 children, *Ann Emerg Med* 54:171–180.e1-4, 2009.

32. Lexi-Comp Online: *Pediatric Lexi-Drugs Online*, Hudson, Ohio, 2011, Lexi-Comp, Inc.

33. Pershad J, Godambe SA: Propofol for procedural sedation in the pediatric emergency department, *J Emerg Med* 27:11–14, 2004.

34. Schilling CG, Bank DE, Borchert BA, et al: Tetracaine, epinephrine (adrenalin), and cocaine (TAC) versus lidocaine, epinephrine, and tetracaine (LET) for anesthesia of lacerations in children, *Ann Emerg Med* 25:203–208, 1995.

35. White NJ, Kim MK, Brousseau DC, et al: The anesthetic effectiveness of lidocaine-adrenaline-tetracaine gel on finger lacerations, *Pediatr Emerg Care* 20:812–815, 2004.

36. Chale S, Singer AJ, Marchini S, et al: Digital versus local anesthesia for finger lacerations: a randomized controlled trial, *Acad Emerg Med* 13:1046–1050, 2006.

37. Priestley S, Kelly AM, Chow L, et al: Application of topical local anesthetic at triage reduces treatment time for children with lacerations: a randomized controlled trial, *Ann Emerg Med* 42:34–40, 2003.

38. Luck RP, Flood R, Eyal D, S, et al: Cosmetic outcomes of absorbable versus nonabsorbable sutures in pediatric facial lacerations, *Pediatr Emerg Care* 24:137–142, 2008.

39. Karounis H, Gouin S, Eisman H, et al: A randomized, controlled trial comparing long-term cosmetic outcomes of traumatic pediatric lacerations repaired with absorbable plain gut versus nonabsorbable nylon sutures, *Acad Emerg Med* 11:730–735, 2004.

40. Beam JW: Tissue adhesives for simple traumatic lacerations, *J Athl Train* 43:222–224, 2008.

41. Resch KL, Hick JL: Preliminary experience with 2-octylcyanoacrylate in a pediatric emergency department, *Pediatr Emerg Care* 16:328–331, 2000.

42. Kanegaye JT, Vance CW, Chan L, Schonfeld N: Comparison of skin stapling devices and standard sutures for pediatric scalp lacerations: a randomized study of cost and time benefits, *J Pediatr* 130:808–813, 1997.

43. Karaduman S, Yuruktumen A, Guryay SM, et al: Modified hair apposition technique as the primary closure method for scalp lacerations, *Am J Emerg Med* 27:1050–1055, 2009.

44. Tindall A, Dawood R, Povlsen B: Case of the month: the skin wrinkle test: a simple nerve injury test for paediatric and uncooperative patients, *Emerg Med J* 23:883–886, 2006.

45. Allen MJ: Conservative management of finger tip injuries in adults, *Hand* 12:257–265, 1980.

46. Ashbell TS, Kleinert HE, Putcha SM, Kutz JE: The deformed finger nail, a frequent result of failure to repair nail bed injuries, *J Trauma* 7:177–190, 1967.

47. Fitzgerald RH Jr, Cowan JD: Puncture wounds of the foot, *Orthop Clin North Am* 6:965–972, 1975.

48. Fisher MC, Goldsmith JF, Gilligan PH: Sneakers as a source of *Pseudomonas aeruginosa* in children with osteomyelitis following puncture wounds, *J Pediatr* 106:607–609, 1985.

49. Eidelman M, Bialik V, Miller Y, Kassis I: Plantar puncture wounds in children: analysis of 80 hospitalized patients and late sequelae, *Isr Med Assoc J* 5:268–271, 2003.

50. Bond GR, Dowd MD, Landsman I, Rimsza M: Unintentional perineal injury in prepubescent girls: a multicenter, prospective report of 56 girls, *Pediatrics* 95:628–631, 1995.

51. Dowd MD, Fitzmaurice L, Knapp JF, Mooney D: The interpretation of urogenital findings in children with straddle injuries, *J Pediatr Surg* 29:7–10, 1994.

52. Muram D: Genital tract injuries in the prepubertal child, *Pediatr Ann* 15:616–620, 1986.

53. Livne PM, Gonzales ET Jr: Genitourinary trauma in children, *Urol Clin North Am* 12:53–65, 1985.

54. Cassidy-Smith T, Mistry RD, Russo CJ, et al: Topical anesthetic cream is associated with spontaneous cutaneous abscess drainage in children, *Am J Emerg Med* 30:104–109, 2012.

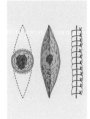

CHAPTER 6
Infiltration and Nerve Block Anesthesia

Key Practice Points

- A gentle and empathetic approach to patients is necessary when administering local anesthesia because of the near universal fear of injections and needles.
- The onset of action of lidocaine is almost immediate when giving the anesthetic around the wound. For nerve blocks, onset of action is 5 to 10 minutes.
- The addition of epinephrine reduces bleeding and extends the duration of local anesthesia.
- Toxicity of local anesthetics can cause hypotension, bradycardia, and (rarely) seizures that are most often caused by inadvertent injection into a blood vessel. To avoid complications, aspirate before injecting.
- Allergies to local anesthetics are uncommon and are often due to the preservative, methylparaben, in the solution.
- Buffering local anesthetics with bicarbonate can reduce, in some patients, the pain of infiltration.
- Moderate sedation with midazolam and fentanyl can effectively reduce pain in a procedure such as abscess drainage.
- Topical anesthesia is most effective for small lacerations in pediatric patients.
- Through-the-wound direct infiltration is the most common form of local anesthesia for lacerations repaired in emergency settings.
- Nerve blocks create larger areas of anesthesia and do not cause tissue distortion with unwanted swelling of the wound.

Effective anesthesia is essential for successful patient intervention and wound repair. As with any procedure, success depends on a thorough understanding of the properties of anesthetic solutions and injection techniques. The choice of anesthetics and techniques must be individualized for every patient. The type, location, and extent of the wound and estimated length of time for repair are variables that make each patient unique. Besides technical considerations, patients have differing emotional characteristics and responses. Almost all patients often fear that injections and needles will cause excessive pain. A clear explanation of the procedure and gentle handling gain the confidence of the patient and ease any apprehension.

LOCAL ANESTHETICS: PRACTICAL POINTS
- *Onset of action:* Local wound infiltration of a laceration with lidocaine 1% brings on rapid anesthesia. If the anesthetic is delivered at the interface of the superficial fascia and dermis, nerve fibers are vulnerable to immediate blockade (Fig. 6-1). Wound

41

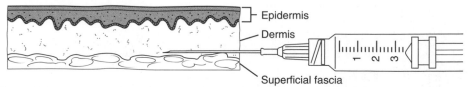

Figure 6-1. The plane of anesthesia for local skin infiltration is just below the dermis at the junction of the superficial fascia (subcutaneous tissue).

cleansing and suturing can begin almost immediately. A slightly shorter onset of action is yielded by lidocaine 2% solutions than by 1% solutions, but clinically speaking, this effect is negligible.[1] The addition of epinephrine and the buffering of local anesthetics also can shorten the onset of action and are discussed later in this chapter. When blocking larger nerve trunks, such as digital nerves, onset of action is significantly slower. Technique of delivery is crucial, and knowledge of anatomy can mean the difference between a successful and an unsuccessful blockade. A bolus of local anesthetic delivered immediately adjacent to a digital nerve can lead to complete digital anesthesia within 1 to 2 minutes. Poor technique and delivery of that bolus even 2 or 3 mm from the nerve trunk can delay onset of action or lead to inadequate blockade and the need for repeat injection.

- *Duration of anesthesia:* Duration of action is significantly affected by vasoactivity of the anesthetic, blood supply of the anesthetized region, addition of epinephrine to anesthetic solutions, and formulation (bupivacaine lasts longer than lidocaine). Of the commonly used anesthetics, lidocaine produces the most vasodilation. The duration of action can be significantly shortened in areas such as the face, which is highly vascular. In addition, vasodilation can cause excessive bleeding in a wound during repair. The addition of epinephrine to lidocaine eliminates unwanted bleeding and extends the action of lidocaine by 1 hour for facial lacerations and 5 hours for extremity injuries.[2] Bupivacaine without epinephrine also extends the duration of action 2 to 4 hours compared with lidocaine alone.

- *Differential blockade:* Myelin sheath coverings of nerve fibers within axons vary in diameter and thickness. Fibers that carry stimuli from pain receptors in the skin have no myelin sheath and have the smallest diameter. The sensations of pressure and touch and motor impulses are transmitted by larger, myelinated fibers. The thin pain fibers are blocked more rapidly and more easily by local anesthetic solutions. This fact is significant in wound care because a solution of 1% lidocaine might block pain stimuli only and not the sensation of touch and pressure. An overly anxious patient may react to touch and pressure as if in pain. A higher concentration of lidocaine (e.g., 2%) abolishes all awareness of stimuli and allows for unimpeded repair. Adding epinephrine to these solutions achieves the same effect.

- *Addition of epinephrine:* Adding epinephrine to local anesthetic solutions increases the duration of action and the amount of drug that can be used. Epinephrine not only extends the duration of action of lidocaine, but it also increases the intensity of the block without an increase in concentration of the anesthetic in the neuron.[3] The extended action lasts 1.3 times to 10 times longer than the action of lidocaine alone.[2] The extension of time is shorter on the face than on other body locales. The most useful property of epinephrine is to decrease the amount of bleeding in a wound during laceration repair. There are potential but infrequent complications to its use. The most serious side effect, ischemia, can occur if epinephrine-containing anesthetics are improperly injected into fingers, toes, tip of the nose, pinna of the ear, or penis. Caution in the use of vasoconstrictors has been expressed because of the potential

TABLE 6-1	Local Anesthetics for Wound Care					
			Onset of Action			
Agent	**Concentration**	**Infiltration**	**Block (min)**	**Duration of Action for Blocks (min)**	**Maximal Allowable Single Dose**	
Lidocaine (Xylocaine)	1%, 2%	Immediate	4-10	30-120	4.5 mg/kg of 1% (30 mL per average adult)	
Lidocaine (with epinephrine)	1%	Immediate	4-10	60-240	7 mg/kg of 1% (50 mL per average adult)	
Mepivacaine (Carbocaine)	1%, 2%	Immediate	6-10	90-180	5 mg/kg or 1% (40 mL per average adult)	
Bupivacaine (Marcaine, Sensorcaine)	0.25%, 0.5%	Slower	8-12	240-480	3 mg/kg of 0.25% (70 mL per average adult)	
Articaine	4%	1-6 min	6-10	60	7 mg/kg of 4% (12.5 mL per average adult)	
Topical anesthesia	See text	5-15 min	—	20-30	2-5 mL of mixture	

for tissue damage and increased rate of infection.[4] However, lidocaine mixed with epinephrine continues to be used successfully for laceration repair.[5,6]

ANESTHETIC SOLUTIONS

Three anesthetic solutions are commonly used for local infiltration and simple nerve block (Table 6-1): lidocaine, mepivacaine, and bupivacaine. The amide derivatives have largely replaced the older ester compounds such as procaine.

Lidocaine

Lidocaine is the most commonly used anesthetic solution. The drug has a rapid onset of action that is almost immediate in local infiltration. Lidocaine's tissue-spreading properties are good, and it readily penetrates nerve sheaths. Duration of action for nerve blocks is approximately 75 minutes (range 60 to 120 minutes). Although there is no clear information in the literature concerning the duration of action for direct wound infiltration, the anesthetic effect wears off in approximately 20 to 30 minutes, which is much sooner than with a full nerve block. A small percentage of patients appear to metabolize lidocaine rapidly and require repeated local injections. Finally, it is important to note that the low pH environment of abscesses markedly reduces the anesthetic effect of lidocaine. Field blocks, sometimes supplemented by conscious sedation, might be necessary to achieve adequate pain control when draining abscesses.

Lidocaine with Epinephrine

With the addition of epinephrine 1:100,000, the duration of action is increased, and local hemostasis is better achieved. The maximal allowable doses of lidocaine and the other local anesthetics are summarized in Table 6-1. The addition of epinephrine increases the duration of action and reduces bleeding. It is effective for most laceration repairs and foreign-body retrievals. I have found it the most useful anesthetic combination for common wound care problems requiring a local anesthetic. Anesthetics with epinephrine are contraindicated in anatomic areas with terminal circulation, such as the fingers, toes, ears, and nose. In a study comparing lidocaine 2% with and without epinephrine for digital blocks, there were no ill effects of vasoconstriction, and the anesthesia was more effective in the epinephrine group.[7] Although one study should not lead to the elimination of a time-honored caution against the use of epinephrine in digital blocks, it does open the question to further investigation.

Mepivacaine

Mepivacaine is widely used as an emergency wound anesthetic but has some properties that are different from lidocaine. The drug has a slightly slower onset of action: 6 to 10 minutes for a simple block. The duration of action is 30 to 60 minutes, which is longer than lidocaine. Mepivacaine has a less vasodilatory effect than lidocaine and usually does not require the use of epinephrine for local wound area hemostasis.

Bupivacaine

Bupivacaine is an amide that is widely used in emergency wound care. It is an effective anesthetic, but its chief drawback is that it has slow onset of action, approximately 8 to 12 minutes for simple blocks of small nerves. The main advantage of bupivacaine is its duration of action, which is considerably longer than lidocaine and mepivacaine. In a study comparing lidocaine with bupivacaine, no significant difference was noted in the pain of local infiltration, onset of action, and level of satisfactory anesthesia.[8] Because the anesthetic effects of bupivacaine lasted four times longer than those of lidocaine, and significantly extended the period of pain relief, bupivacaine was recommended by Fariss et al[8] to be considered for anesthesia of lacerations sutured in the emergency department.

Articaine

Articaine hydrochloride 4% (Septocaine) is an amide local anesthetic that has been used in Europe and other parts of the world for years and has now been approved for use in the United States. The only preparation available contains 1:100,000 epinephrine. Articaine is particularly effective in dental procedures because of its ability to penetrate hard tissues such as bone. It has yet to be studied for nondental procedures but can be used for facial and oral blocks. Onset of action is 1 to 6 minutes, and the duration of action is approximately 1 hour. Its safety profile is similar to other local "caine" anesthetics.[9]

TOXICITY OF LOCAL ANESTHETICS

The injection of local anesthetics can cause three toxic, but uncommon, reactions. Cardiovascular reactions include hypotension and bradycardia and are caused by a myocardial inhibitory effect of the anesthetic.[10] Local anesthetic solutions can cause excitatory phenomena in the central nervous system that ultimately can culminate in seizure activity. The cardiovascular and central nervous system effects commonly are caused by an inadvertent injection of a solution directly into a vessel, causing a bolus effect on the heart or brain. A key principle in the use of local anesthetics is always aspiration of the syringe before injection to check for blood return. If blood is aspirated, the needle has to be moved to avoid injecting the solution into a vein or artery.

The most common reaction to local anesthetics is vasovagal syncope (fainting). The anxiety and pain of injection can cause dizziness, pallor, bradycardia, and hypotension. This reaction can largely be avoided with gentle handling of the patient, proper counseling, and slow and careful injection technique. No anesthetic infiltration is ever performed on a patient who is not in the supine position. Preferably the patient should be placed so that he or she cannot see the injection being administered.

Treatment of toxic reactions is largely supportive. The airway is appropriately protected, and ventilations are maintained. Hypotension and bradycardia usually are self-limited and can be reversed by placing the patient in the Trendelenburg position. An intravenous line is started with normal saline, and a bolus of 250 to 500 mL is infused to counteract hypotension in any patient who does not respond to that maneuver. Cardiac monitoring with frequent vital signs is instituted. Seizures also are self-limited but may need to be controlled by intravenous lorezapam (Ativan) or diazepam (Valium).

ALLERGY TO LOCAL ANESTHETICS

Allergic reactions are uncommon with the newer amide local anesthetics, such as lidocaine, mepivacaine, and bupivacaine. Reactions were more frequent with the older ester solutions, procaine (Novocain) and tetracaine.[11] Multiple-dose vials still contain the preservative methylparaben, which has been implicated as a possible mediator of allergic responses.[1] Allergic reactions are characterized by either delayed appearances of skin rashes or the acute onset of localized or general urticaria. Rarely, outright anaphylactic shock can occur. True allergic responses occur in fewer than 1% of patients receiving local anesthetics.[11] This observation was confirmed in a study of 59 patients who reported previous reactions to local anesthetic agents. None responded adversely to skin testing and provocative drug challenge.[12]

Management of Allergic Responses

Allergic responses are managed in the standard manner with airway control; establishment of intravenous access; and administration of epinephrine, diphenhydramine, and steroids as needed.

Alternatives for Allergic Patients

Because patients cannot always describe accurately a prior adverse reaction to a local anesthetic, and it is usually impossible to perform skin testing in an emergency department setting, the clinician may be faced with a patient who is truly allergic to local anesthetics. The following strategies are suggested:

- For calm patients who have small lacerations, no anesthetic should be used. Often the pain of injection exceeds the pain of placing two or three sutures.
- Ice placed directly over the wound can provide a short period of decreased pain sensation.
- Because the preservative methylparaben has been implicated in allergic reactions, local anesthetic preparations for spinal, epidural, and intravenous anesthesia should be used. They are preservative-free. They can be obtained from the operating room of the hospital.
- If the allergy-causing drug can be identified as an ester (tetracaine, benzocaine, chloroprocaine, cocaine, procaine), it can be substituted with an amide (lidocaine, mepivacaine, bupivacaine, diphenhydramine [Benadryl]).
- Diphenhydramine has properties similar to standard local anesthetics.[13,14] Compared with lidocaine, it provides adequate anesthesia for laceration repair for at least 30 minutes.[15] Compared with lidocaine, it is not as effective for procedures lasting longer than 30 minutes. A 50-mg (1-mL) vial is diluted in a syringe with 4 mL of normal saline to produce a 1% solution. Local infiltration is carried out in the usual manner. Diphenhydramine is more painful to inject than lidocaine, and this pain is not reduced by buffering.[16,17]

REDUCING THE PAIN OF LOCAL ANESTHESIA

Anesthetic Buffering

It has been demonstrated that buffering of lidocaine can reduce the pain of injection.[18-20] In addition, buffering can reduce the time to onset of anesthesia and increases the intensity of the blockade. However, more recent studies, although showing a positive effect of buffering, do not reach significance when compared with nonbuffered solutions.[6,15] In addition, buffering can reduce the shelf life of local anesthetics. It seems that lidocaine alone, when buffered with bicarbonate, has a shelf life of at least 7 days.[21] Buffering also has been shown to degrade epinephrine, up to 20% of the total, within 24 hours in open containers exposed to light.[22,23] Buffered solutions containing epinephrine do not show any significant epinephrine degradation in a 72-hour period if kept in a closed container that is stored in the dark. Shelf life studies of buffered mepivacaine and bupivacaine have not been performed.

Because they have shown some positive effect, the following techniques are included for the buffering of local anesthetics:

- *Lidocaine:* 1 mL of bicarbonate per 9 mL of 1% lidocaine; buffering of 2% solutions may cause precipitates; shelf life 7 days
- *Mepivacaine:* 0.5 to 1 mL of bicarbonate per 9 mL of mepivacaine; shelf life unknown after 24 hours
- *Bupivacaine:* 0.1 mL of bicarbonate per 20 mL of bupivacaine; shelf life unknown after 24 hours

When mixing a 20-mL lidocaine or mepivacaine vial, 2 mL of anesthetic is removed and is replaced with 2 mL of bicarbonate. This technique not only ensures the correct buffering mixture, but also maintains the original volume of solution in the vial. Because shelf life is shortened, the vial should be marked or labeled with the date of preparation. Bicarbonate is available in solutions of 8.4% sodium bicarbonate stored as 50 mEq/50 mL (1 mEq/mL).

Choice of Needles

Experienced operators caring for wounds often limit themselves to 27-G or 30-G needles. Not only is a small gauge likely to reduce the pain of needle insertion, but also it reduces the rate of injection. Rapid injection and tissue expansion are significantly more painful than slow injection.[22]

Considerable experience is necessary in handling small-diameter needles. They bend easily, and it can be difficult to judge the amount of anesthetic injected without observing plunger movement past the syringe hatch marks. It is recommended that inexperienced operators become familiar with the properties of a 25-G needle before proceeding to smaller 27-G and 30-G needles. A 25-G, 1½-inch needle can be used for most local infiltration procedures and for facial and digital blocks.

ADULT PATIENT SEDATION

Patient sedation for emergency wound care (see Chapter 5 for pediatric sedation) has become a common procedure, most commonly used for abscess drainage. Wound care can cause significant anxiety and discomfort, and patients can benefit by the administration of anxiolytics or pain relievers that supplement local anesthesia. Opiates, such as fentanyl, morphine, and meperidine (Demerol), and the benzodiazepines, midazolam and diazepam, can be delivered orally or parenterally for this purpose. Other sedative agents used for painful procedures are ketamine and nitrous oxide. Commonly used sedative and pain-reducing agents are summarized in Table 6-2.

TABLE 6-2	Agents for Adult Sedation in Wound Care Procedures	
Agent(s)	**Initial Dose***	**Route**
Midazolam[†]	0.02-0.1 mg/kg	IV
	0.3-0.5 mg/kg	Oral
Diazepam	0.05-0.10 mg/kg	IV
Fentanyl[†]	1-2 mg/kg	IV
Meperidine	0.5-1 mg/kg	IV, IM
Morphine	0.05-0.2 mg/kg	IV, IM

*Often two doses are needed to obtain adequate sedation in many patients. The use of additional doses should be based on individual responses. In the elderly, smaller doses should be used in an incremental fashion.
†Midazolam and Fentanyl are commonly used in combination for moderate sedation.

Midazolam is an effective anxiolytic that comes in oral, intranasal, parenteral, and rectal forms but is most commonly administered parenterally in adults.[24-26] Intravenously, it achieves sedation in 3 to 5 minutes and has an elimination half-life of 1 hour. Alone or in combination with fentanyl, it has become commonly used for moderate sedation (Box 6-1). Hypoxia and oversedation are the most significant, but uncommon, side effects of midazolam. Administration must be in a controlled setting with readily available airway and resuscitation equipment. The reversal agent, flumazenil, is effective if needed to reverse the actions of this benzodiazepine. Caution must be used, however, in patients on chronic benzodiazepines, because reversal might cause seizures.

Fentanyl is a synthetic opioid with properties that make it an excellent agent for immediate pain relief and support during invasive procedures.[27] Peak effect after intravenous administration is 2 minutes with a duration of action of 30 to 90 minutes. In contrast to other opioids, fentanyl does not commonly cause nausea and vomiting (<1% of patients). Its most serious side effect is respiratory depression, which can be reversed readily with naloxone. See Chapter 5 for sedation techniques for children.

When full moderate sedation in an adult is unecessary, but pain or anxiety relief are anticipated, single doses of an IV or IM opiate or benzodiazepine 5 to 10 minutes before the procedure can be administered. Several choices are available as delineated in Table 6-2. Ventilation support, intravenous fluids, and reversal agents should be immediately available if needed.

Although ketamine has been in use worldwide for children, there is less experience in its use in the United States and in using it for adults.[28,29] Most experience with ketamine use is in the intravenous or intramuscular form. Its onset of action intravenously is 1 minute, with a duration of action 10 to 15 minutes. This drug can cause a dissociative reaction in the patient during administration and an emergence reaction in 30% of adults in which there is misperception of visual and auditory stimuli by the patient.[30] However, when administered with midazolam in adults, the emergence reactions are considerably less.[31] Ketamine can cause vomiting and laryngospasm and should be used with caution in adults with coronary artery disease because of its sympathomimetic properties.[29-32] Parenteral ketamine requires significant experience and operator comfort with its sedation profile. Further studies of its oral use in wound care are needed to delineate fully its appropriate use in that setting.

Nitrous oxide is a sedative and an analgesic substance that can provide effective procedure sedation.[33] It comes in 30% and 50% concentrations in combination with oxygen. Onset of action begins in 30 to 60 seconds with maximum effect in 5 minutes. Side effects include nausea, dizziness, and euphoria with laughter. Equipment

BOX 6-1	Procedure for Moderate Sedation in Painful Wound Care and Abscess Drainage Interventions

1. Establish an intravenous infusion of normal saline (18-G catheter preferred in adults) in the supine patient with the bed rails in the up position.
2. Pulse, respiratory rate, blood pressure, and level of consciousness should be recorded initially, *after every dose of each agent, and every 5 to 10 minutes throughout the procedure.*
3. Continous monitoring of oxygen saturation with a pulse oximeter probe (to maintain at >95% or no less than 3% to 5% less than the initial value) must be performed. Supplemental oxygen via nasal prongs can be administered based on need. ECG monitoring is optional but suggested in the elderly or in patients with a cardiac history.
4. A resuscitation cart with a bag-valve mask, oral and nasal airways, endotracheal tubes, and a functioning laryngoscope must be nearby. Suction equipment and naloxone should be at the bedside.
5. Administer 1 mg of midazolam over 30 to 60 seconds; if after 3 to 5 minutes there is no evidence of mild sedation (subjective relaxation by the patient with mild drowsiness and normal or minimally altered speech), additional 1-mg doses can be administered in a similar fashion, up to a maximum of 0.1 mg/kg.* The goal is *mild* sedation and anxiolysis, achievable in most patients with 1 to 2 mg of midazolam.
6. Reassess clinical status (see Step 2).
7. Administer fentanyl[†] 100 µg (2 mL) over 60 seconds; this may be repeated in 0.5- to 1-µg/kg (50 to 100 µg) increments every 3 to 5 minutes until adequate analgesia and sedation have been obtained (slurred speech, ptosis, drowsy, but responsive to painful and verbal stimuli, and good analgesia with initial stages of procedure). The maximal total dose recommended is 5 to 6 µg/kg.*
8. Administer local anesthesia if indicated (this often helps gauge effectiveness of systemic analgesia).
9. Perform the procedure. Additional doses of fentanyl may be required based on the response and length of the procedure.
10. If hypoxemia, deep sedation, or slowed respirations unresponsive to external stimuli are seen during or after procedure, ventilation should be assisted with a bag-valve mask, and naloxone (0.4- to 0.8-mg increments) should be administered. Naloxone should not be given routinely at the termination of procedures because it abruptly reverses all analgesia.
11. Continue close observation until the patient is awake and alert, and discharge the patient only after a minimum 1 hour of further observation. Instruct the patient not to drive or operate dangerous machinery for at least 6 hours.

*For children, fentanyl alone is suggested in 0.5-µg/kg increments up to a maximal total dose of 2 to 3 µg/kg.
†Sublimaze, 50 µg/mL.
From Yealy DM, Dunmire SM, Paris TML: Pharmacologic adjuncts to painful procedures. In Roberts TR, Hedges TR, editors: *Clinical procedures in emergency medicine*, Philadelphia, 1991, Saunders.

requirements, including a gas scavenging system, and operator experience make this method of sedation of limited usefulness in laceration repair and wound care.

ANESTHESIA TECHNIQUES

Most minor lacerations and wounds can be managed by administering a local anesthetic directly into or around (parallel to) the wound area. Other wounds are best served by the application of a nerve block. The following are descriptions of the techniques for administering local anesthetics most useful in emergency wound and laceration repair.

Topical Anesthesia
Indications
Topical anesthesia is an established method to anesthetize uncomplicated lacerations.[5] Pediatric patients are ideal candidates for this technique. It requires no injection and can be administered by the parent. Because of the profuse vascularity of the face and scalp, lacerations of those areas are more effectively anesthetized than the trunk or proximal extremities. Because of tissue absorption of topical agents, this technique is best limited to lacerations of 5 cm or less. Contraindicated sites include the finger, toe, nose, pinna of the ear, and penis. Care is taken to avoid mucous membranes. The death of a 7½-month-old infant whose nasal mucous membranes and lips were inadvertently exposed to 10 mL of the solution underscores the need for caution.[34]

In emergency departments with triage systems, topical anesthesia can shorten the patient's emergency department length of stay and improve the efficiency of care. Topical anesthetics can be applied at the triage for appropriate wounds. They take approximately 20 minutes to achieve effect.[35] Wounds can be cleansed and repaired in a shortened time frame with good outcomes and improved patient satisfaction. A newer topical preparation, EMLA (eutectic mixture of local anesthetics; see contents of EMLA in the following bulleted list), has been used in this setting with good effect compared with standard topical preparations.[36,37] EMLA has two major drawbacks, however: It is only approved for intact skin (such as for IV needle use) but not open wounds, and it takes 60 minutes to take effect.

Numerous topical anesthetic mixtures have comparable efficacy. Because cocaine was one of the original components of TAC (tetracaine-adrenaline-cocaine), this preparation has proven efficacy, but preparations without cocaine are comparable in their effectiveness.[38] Topical anesthetics are commonly prepared as liquids but can be mixed in gels.[39] Gels can decrease the risk of mucosal exposure and possibly reduce the total dose delivered. The following is a range of topical anesthetic alternatives:
- *LAT (lidocaine-adrenaline-tetracaine):* tetracaine (1%), epinephrine (1:2000), and lidocaine (4%)[40]
- *TLE (topical lidocaine-epinephrine):* lidocaine (5%) and epinephrine (1:2000)[41]

These figures represent the final concentrations and dilutions when calculated amounts of each ingredient are combined and brought to a predetermined volume with saline. Preparation of a topical anesthetic solution should be carried out by or under the supervision of a pharmacist.
- *LET (lidocaine, epinephrine, tetracaine):* lidocaine (2%), epinephrine (1:1000), tetracaine (2%)
- *EMLA:* eutectic cream mixture, lidocaine (2.5%), Prilocaine (2.5%), suspended in oil and water emulsion

Technique
A 2 × 2 inch sponge is saturated but should not be dripping with solution. The sponge is placed in and around the laceration and left for at least 20 minutes. Shorter application times are associated with higher failure rates. When the sponge is fashioned to conform to the wound, it can be secured with tape, and the caregiver or parent should apply gentle manual pressure over the taped sponge. Gloves are recommended to prevent absorption by the caregiver. Common errors include failure to place a sponge fold into the wound, "dabbing" the wound, or releasing the manual pressure prematurely. For small lacerations, cotton swabs soaked with the solution can be used.

Complete anesthesia is reached when a zone of blanching is observed around the wound. Time to anesthesia is 20 to 30 minutes for all preparations previously listed except for EMLA, which is 60 minutes. The maximal dose of the solution is 2 to 5 mL. The average wound requires 2 to 3 mL. In approximately 5% of wounds, supplemental infiltration is required to achieve complete anesthesia.[42]

Direct Wound Infiltration
Indications
Direct infiltration through the wound is indicated for most minimally contaminated lacerations in anatomically uncomplicated areas. Injecting directly into the wound is technically easy to do, and because intact skin is not pierced, needle-stick pain is less. Some patients may express concern, or even alarm, at this prospect. Explaining the advantage of less pain allays those fears.

Anatomy
The proper plane of injection is immediately beneath the dermis at the junction of the superficial fascia (see Fig. 6-1). Tissue resistance is less in this plane, and sensory nerves are reached easily by the spreading solution. Trying to inject directly into the dermis meets with great resistance. Injecting deep down into the fatty fascia unnecessarily delays onset.

Technique
Direct infiltration can be carried out with 25-, 27-, or 30-G needles of varying lengths (½ inch to 1¼ inches). The needle is inserted through the open wound into the superficial fascia (subcutaneous fat) parallel to and just deep to the dermis (Fig. 6-2). A small bolus of anesthetic solution is injected. The needle is removed, and another bolus is injected at an adjacent site just inside the margin of anesthesia of the previous injection. This practice ensures greater patient comfort. This process is repeated until all edges and corners of the wound are anesthetized. A simple laceration approximately 3 to 4 cm in length requires 3 to 5 mL of an anesthetic solution.

Parallel Margin Infiltration (Field Block)
Indications
Parallel margin infiltration is an alternative to direct wound infiltration and has the advantage of requiring fewer needle sticks. It is preferred in wounds that are grossly contaminated so that the needle does not inadvertently carry debris or bacteria into uncontaminated tissues, although this potential complication has not been clearly documented.

Anatomy
The same plane as described earlier for direct wound infiltration is used, but it is approached through intact skin.

Technique
Parallel infiltration requires a 1¼- to 2-inch needle at least 25 G in diameter. The needle is inserted into the skin at one end of the laceration. The needle is advanced to the hub parallel to the dermis–superficial fascia plane (Fig. 6-3). Aspiration is followed by slow injection of a "track" of anesthetic as the needle is withdrawn down the tissue plane to the insertion site. The needle is reinserted at the distal end of the first track, where the skin is beginning to become anesthetized. The second insertion (if needed) is less painful. Reinsertion and injection are repeated on all sides of the wound until complete infiltration has been achieved.

Supraorbital and Supratrochlear Nerve Blocks (Forehead Block)
Indications
Supraorbital and supratrochlear nerve blocks are used for extensive lacerations and wounds of the forehead and anterior scalp.

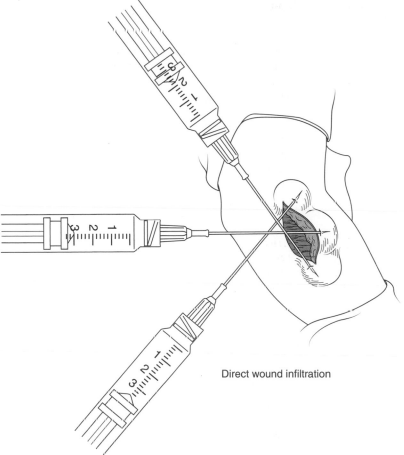

Direct wound infiltration

Figure 6-2. Direct infiltration of the wound is accomplished by multiple adjacent depositions of anesthetic solution to anesthetize the full length of the wound on either side.

Anatomy

The supraorbital and supratrochlear nerves supply sensation to the forehead and anterior scalp and exit from foramina located along the supraorbital ridge.

Technique

The easiest manner to block the nerves and their many branches is to lay a continuous subcutaneous track at brow level as shown in Figure 6-4. The actual injection technique is similar to that discussed earlier in the section on parallel margin infiltration. The plane of injection is just superficial to the bony plane. The needle is inserted to bone, then advanced until the hub is reached. The track laid down floods the nerves as they exit the foramina in the supraorbital rim.

Infraorbital Nerve Block
Indications

Lacerations of the upper lip are common. Local anesthetic infiltration can cause anatomic distortion leading to difficulty with exact wound edge approximation and repair. An infraorbital nerve block can circumvent this problem. This block also can

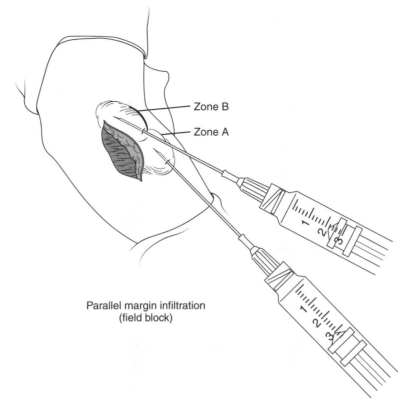

Zone B

Zone A

Parallel margin infiltration
(field block)

Figure 6-3. Parallel margin infiltration is accomplished by laying down adjacent tracks of anesthesia parallel to the wounded edge. Zone A represents the first track. The second track is begun by inserting the needle at the end point of zone A in an area that is anesthetized.

be used to repair lacerations of the lateral-inferior portion of the nose and lower eyelid.

Anatomy
The location and distribution of the infraorbital nerve is illustrated in Figure 6-5C. The infraorbital foramen is located approximately 1.5 cm below the inferior rim of the orbit and 2 cm from the lateral edge of the nose. This foramen can often be palpated (Fig. 6-5A).

Technique
The infraorbital nerve can be approached intraorally and extraorally, although the intraoral route has been shown to be significantly less painful. By the intraoral route, the upper lip is retracted, revealing the maxillary canine tooth. Before actual injection, the site of needle entry into the buccal mucosa can be pretreated with a topical anesthetic such as viscous lidocaine (Xylocaine Viscous). A cotton-tipped applicator soaked in this solution is applied to the gingival-buccal margin for 1 to 2 minutes before the insertion of the needle (Fig. 6-5B). The needle is introduced at the gingival-buccal margin at the anterior margin of the maxillary canine (see Fig. 6-5C). It is advanced parallel and just superficial to the maxillary bone until the infraorbital foramen is reached. If paresthesia results, the needle is pulled back

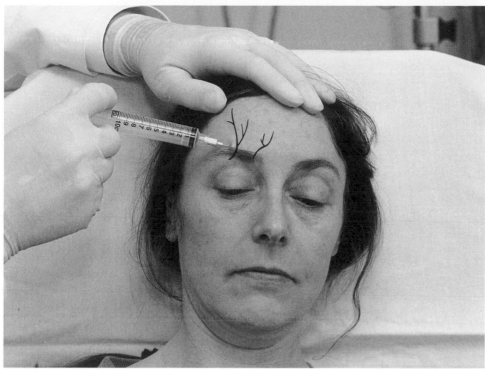

Figure 6-4. Forehead block. Note the path of the supratrochlear and supraorbital nerves that originate from the superior orbital rim. The needle is inserted to its hub at the plane adjacent to the bone itself.

slightly before injection to avoid injecting into the foramen and causing unwanted pressure on the nerve. The operator deposits 1 to 3 mL of anesthetic, and anesthesia results within 4 to 6 minutes. If there is uncertainty about the precise location of the nerve, injection is carried out by depositing multiple small boluses in a "fan" configuration.

Mental Nerve Block
Indications
Mental nerve block is used to repair lower lip lacerations without distorting the anatomy by local infiltration.

Anatomy
The mental nerve foramen lies just inferior to the second mandibular bicuspid, midway between the upper and lower edges of the mandible, and 2.5 cm from the midline of the jaw. This nerve provides sensation to the lower half of the lip but only a portion of the chin. The mental foramen can be palpated as shown in Figure 6-6A.

Technique
The mucosal injection site can be pretreated with viscous lidocaine as described earlier for the infraorbital nerve block (Fig. 6-6B). The lower lip is retracted, and the needle is introduced at the gingival-buccal margin inferior to the second bicuspid (Fig. 6-6C). When the foramen is approximated, 1 to 2 mL of anesthetic is injected after careful

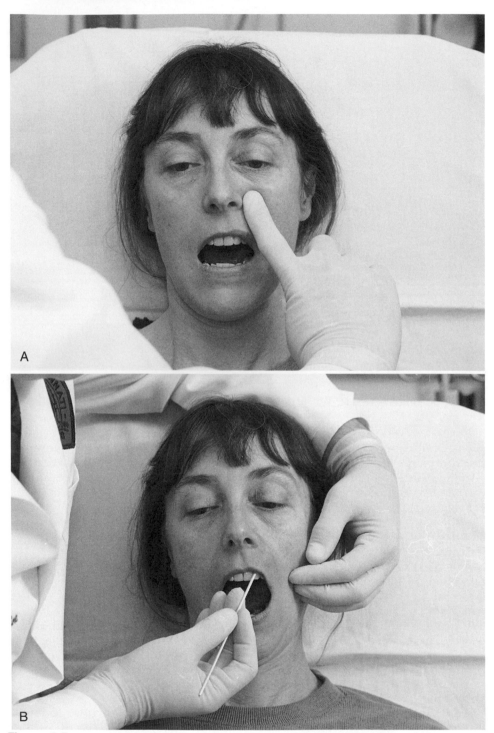

Figure 6-5. Infraorbital nerve block. **A,** The infraorbital foramen can be palpated before injection. **B,** A cotton-tipped applicator soaked in a topical anesthetic, lidocaine gel, is applied to the mucosal site where the needle will be inserted.

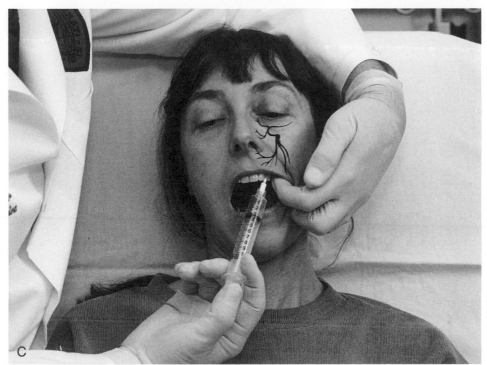

Figure 6-5, cont'd. C, With gentle retraction of the lip, using the maxillary canine as the landmark, the needle is advanced, and anesthetic is deposited at the infraorbital foramen. Note the path of the nerve as it exits the foramen.

aspiration. Full anesthesia is achieved within 4 to 6 minutes. The fanning technique can be applied here as well.

Auricular Block
Indications
Lacerations of the auricle of the ear are common. The skin is tightly adherent to the cartilaginous skeleton, and the deposition of an anesthetic for large or complicated wounds can be difficult or may excessively distort the local tissue relationships. The auricular block is indicated for extensive repairs of the ear.

Anatomy
Sensory innervation of the auricle arises from branches of the auriculotemporal, greater auricular, and lesser occipital nerves. Sensory supply to the meatus derives additionally from the branch of the vagus. For this reason, an auricular block does not always completely block the meatal opening.

Technique
The technical goal of the auricular block is to achieve circumferential anesthesia around the ear. Beginning just below the lobule, the operator fully inserts a 1½- to 2-inch 25-G needle attached to a preloaded syringe with 10 mL of anesthetic (without epinephrine) into the sulcus behind the ear, parallel and just superficial to the bone

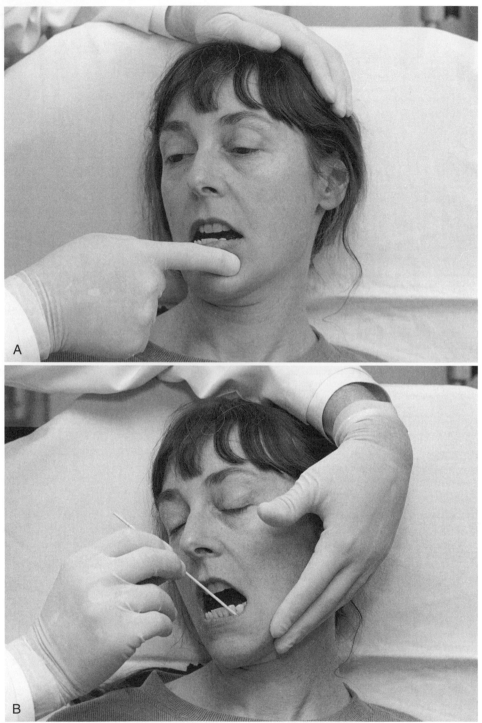

Figure 6-6. Mental nerve block. **A,** The mental nerve foramen can be palpated before injection. **B,** Lidocaine gel is applied to the mucosal injection site.

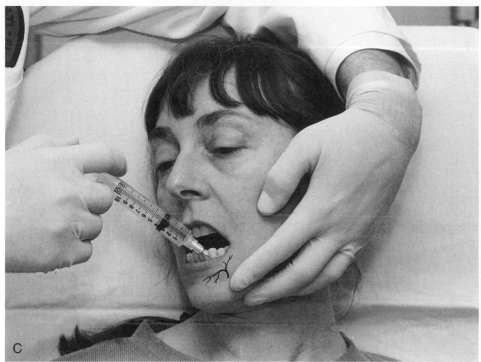

Figure 6-6, cont'd. C, Using the second bicuspid as the landmark, the needle is advanced, and the anesthetic is deposited at the foramen. Note the path of the nerve as it exits the foramen.

(Fig. 6-7). Approximately 2 to 3 mL of anesthetic is left in a track back to the insertion site. Without leaving the insertion site, the needle is redirected anterior to the lobule and tragus. A similar track is left in that area. The syringe is reloaded if necessary. Starting at a point just behind the superior portion of the helix, a similar track is left behind the superior portion of the ear. Without leaving the injection site, a bolus of anesthetic is deposited backward from the tragus. Anesthesia should be complete in 10 to 15 minutes.

Digital Nerve Blocks (Finger and Toe Blocks)

Indications

The most common nerve block in minor wound care is the digital block. The block is the anesthetic method recommended for lacerations distal to the level of the midproximal phalanx of the finger or toe. It is the procedure preferred for nail removal, paronychia drainage, and repair of lacerations of the digits. A study has shown that digital block, as described here, is more effective and less painful than the metacarpal block to achieve finger anesthesia.[43]

One of the most commonly stated cautions about digital blocks is not to use vasoconstrictors, such as epinephrine, with the anesthetic. There is a theoretical concern that the vasoconstrictor can cause digital ischemia and permanent damage. Two studies that compare digital blocks with and without epinephrine have been published.[7,44] No complications were reported in either study.

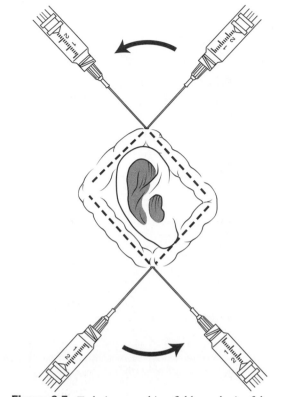

Figure 6-7. Technique to achieve field anesthesia of the ear.

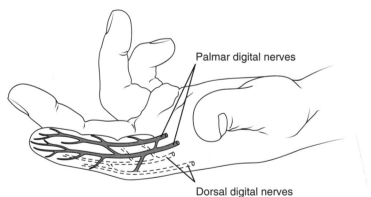

Palmar digital nerves

Dorsal digital nerves

Figure 6-8. Four digital nerves of the digit. The two palmar digital nerves are dominant and provide sensation to the volar surface of the finger and the entirety of the volar pad and nail bed area.

Anatomy

There are four digital nerves for each finger or toe, including the thumb and great toe (Fig. 6-8). The palmar digital nerves have the most extensive sensory distribution and are responsible for distal finger and fingertip sensation, including the nail bed. Although the dorsal nerves have a lesser distribution, there is sufficient overlap with the palmar nerves that all four branches on each finger must be blocked to achieve

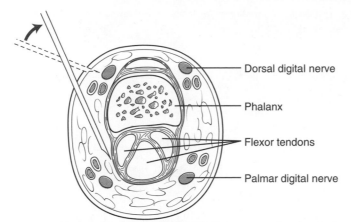

Figure 6-9. Digital nerve block. To block a digit effectively, all four nerves, dorsal and volar, are approached as illustrated. The needle is introduced dorsally to anesthetize the dorsal nerve first. Without reinserting the needle, it is redirected toward the volar nerve, and anesthetic is deposited. The same procedure is done on the opposite side of the same digit to complete the block.

complete digit anesthesia. The digital nerves are immediately adjacent to the phalanges, and these structures act as landmarks for locating the nerves.

Techniques
Technique for Digital Block
Needle size can vary from 25 to 30 G. Small-gauge needles, 27 G and 30 G, require experience and technical comfort of the operator. The technique requires two needle sticks and four small injections of anesthetic. Figure 6-9 illustrates the approach to the dorsal digital nerve followed by redirecting the needle to the palmar nerve. No more than a total of 4 mL of 1% lidocaine without epinephrine or 1% mepivacaine is recommended. The needle is introduced into the dorsolateral aspect of the proximal phalanx in the portion of the web space just distal to the metacarpophalangeal joint (Fig. 6-10). Deposition into the web space prevents buildup of excessive pressure on the digital nerves and blood vessels. The needle is advanced until it touches bone. Approximately 0.5 mL of anesthetic is delivered to the dorsal digital nerve. The needle is withdrawn slightly and redirected adjacent to the bone of the phalanx to the volar surface of the digit, and 1 mL of solution is deposited at the site of the volar or palmar nerve. The procedure is repeated on the opposite side of the digit to achieve full finger or toe anesthesia. A complete block usually is achieved within 4 to 5 minutes. Maintaining close proximity of the nerve to the bone at all times ensures good blockade because the course of the nerve is adjacent to bone. Figure 6-11 illustrates the digital nerve block technique for the thumb.

Alternative Technique for Digital Block
An alternative technique for achieving digital anesthesia is by single injection, using a volar approach.[45] This technique provides anesthesia for the volar, or palmar, surface of the digit and the fingertip, including the nail bed and cuticles. Only the palmar digital nerves are blocked; the dorsal surface, with sensory innervation from the small dorsal digital nerves, remains sensate. In 10% of patients, this technique can cause pain at the injection site for 24 hours after the block.[45] It resolves within 48 hours, however.

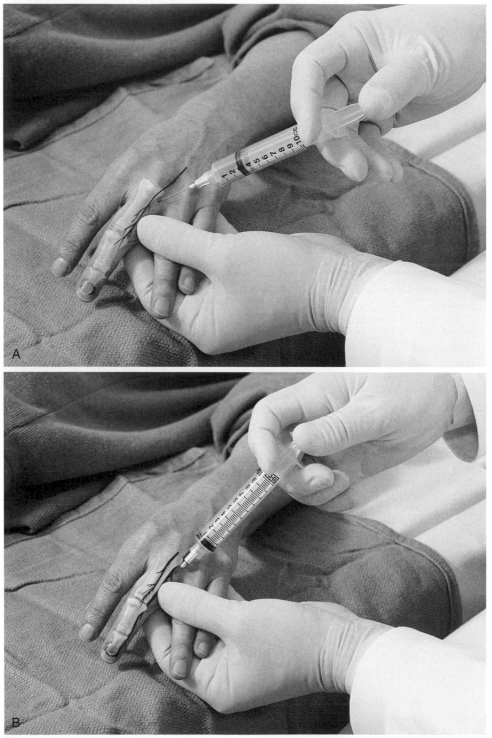

Figure 6-10. Digital nerve block. Note the course of the volar and digital nerves. **A,** Within the web space, the needle is introduced and advanced toward the dorsal digital nerve. **B,** After deposition of the anesthetic, the needle is redirected, without withdrawing it from the skin, toward the volar nerve, and anesthetic is deposited.

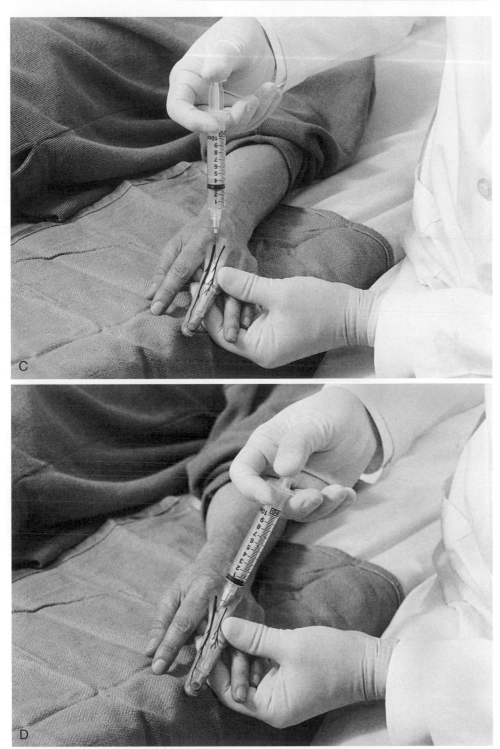

Figure 6-10, cont'd. C and **D,** The same steps are repeated on the opposite side of the same digit.

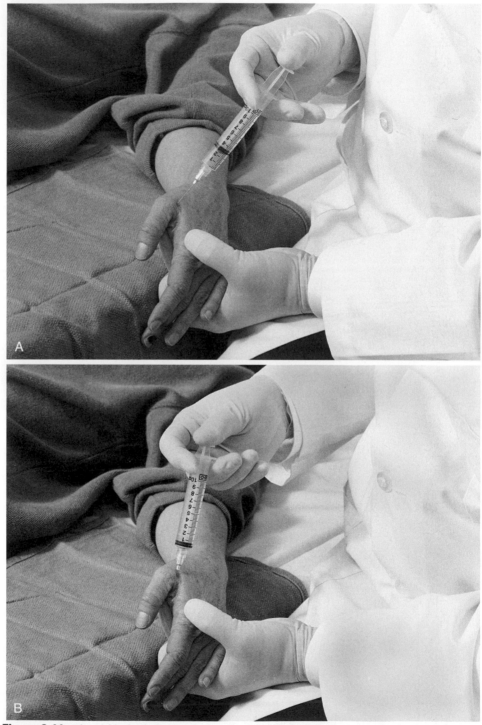

Figure 6-11. Thumb block. The basic procedure for digital block can be carried out for the thumb. Note the nerve pathways as illustrated. **A,** Within the web space, the ulnar dorsal digital nerve to the thumb is blocked. **B,** Through the same injection site, the ulnar volar nerve is blocked after redirection of the needle.

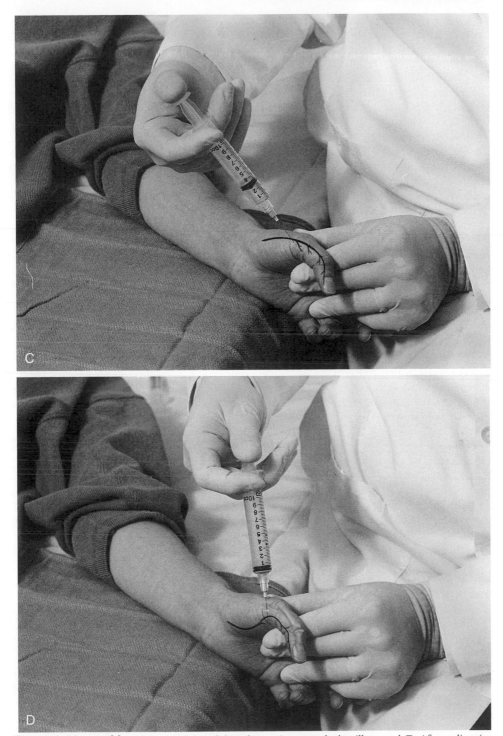

Figure 6-11, cont'd. C, The radial dorsal digital nerve is approached as illustrated. **D,** After redirection, the radial volar nerve is blocked.

A 27-G needle is preferred with approximately 2 to 3 mL of 2% lidocaine or mepivacaine in an appropriate syringe. The skin is prepared carefully with alcohol or povidone-iodine. The needle is inserted at right angles directly into the palmar flexor crease of the digit, through the flexor tendons, to bone. With gentle but insistent pressure applied to the plunger of the syringe, the needle is withdrawn gradually until fluid flows easily into the tendon sheath. Anesthetic quickly flows out of the tendon sheath along the vincular vessels until it surrounds the main digital nerves.

Toe Block Technique

Because the second to fifth toes are relatively thin at the proximal phalanx, a single midline dorsal needle stick can be used to anesthetize both sides of the toe. After depositing the anesthetic on one side, the needle is withdrawn and passed down the opposite side without leaving the original puncture site (Fig. 6-12). The standard digital technique described earlier is best for the great toe.

Median Nerve Block
Indications

Median nerve block is used for lacerations and wounds of the palmar aspect of the thumb, index, and middle fingers and the radial half of the palm.

Anatomy

The median nerve can be found at the proximal flexor crease of the wrist between the palmaris longus and the flexor carpi radialis tendon (Fig. 6-13). The two tendons can be identified by having the patient voluntarily close the fingers into a fist and slightly flex the wrist. Some patients do not have a palmaris longus tendon, in which case the nerve is just radial to the flexor sublimis tendons of the fingers, which usually lie below the palmaris longus tendon. The nerve also can be located 1 cm to the ulnar side of the flexor carpi radialis.

Technique

On identifying the palmaris longus tendon, a 25-G needle is introduced immediately radial to it (Fig. 6-14). The needle is passed just deep to the flexor retinaculum. A "popping" sensation can be felt as the needle traverses the dense retinaculum. An attempt is made to elicit paresthesias by passing the needle slowly deeper into the wrist. If paresthesias are elicited, 2 mL of solution is deposited adjacent to but not into the nerve. If none are elicited, 3 to 5 mL of solution is injected, from deep to superficial as a track. Anesthesia might not be complete for at least 20 minutes.

Ulnar Nerve Block
Indications

Ulnar nerve block is used for repair of wounds to the ulnar dorsal and palmar aspects of the hand, fifth finger, and ulnar side of the fourth finger.

Anatomy

The ulnar nerve has two branches that provide sensory innervation to the ulnar side of the hand. The palmar branch of the ulnar nerve is found immediately radial to the flexor carpi ulnaris tendon at the proximal wrist crease. It accompanies the ulnar artery. The dorsal branch of the ulnar nerve divides from the palmar branch approximately 4 to 5 cm proximal from the wrist and courses under the flexor carpi ulnaris tendon to the dorsal-ulnar side of the hand. Because of this division, both branches must be blocked to achieve successful anesthesia.

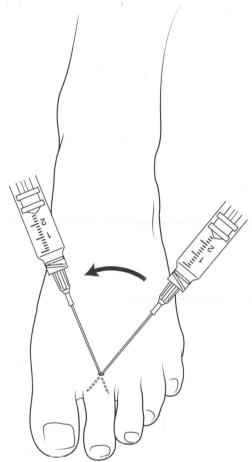

Figure 6-12. Technique to provide anesthetic to toes other than the great toe (see text).

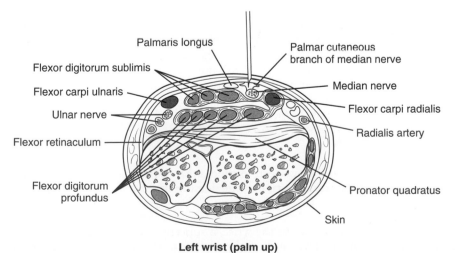

Palmaris longus

Palmar cutaneous
branch of median nerve

Flexor digitorum sublimis

Flexor carpi ulnaris

Median nerve

Ulnar nerve

Flexor carpi radialis

Radialis artery

Flexor retinaculum

Flexor digitorum
profundus

Pronator quadratus

Skin

Left wrist (palm up)

Figure 6-13. Cross-sectional anatomy of the wrist. Note the positions of the palmaris longus, flexor digitorum sublimus, and median nerve.

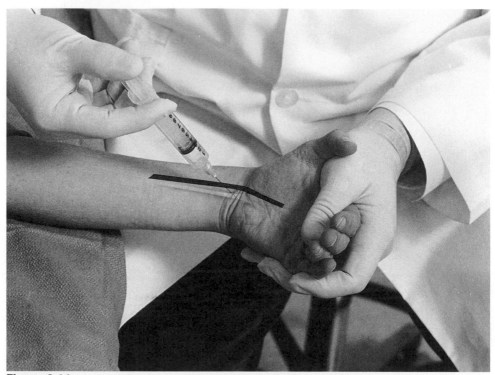

Figure 6-14. Median nerve block. Note the position and path of the palmaris longus and median nerves. Immediately radial to the palmaris longus tendon, the needle is inserted throughout the flexor retinaculum toward the median nerve as described in the text.

Technique

Using a 25-G, 1¼- to 2-inch needle, attached to a 10- to 12-mL syringe, the operator enters the wrist at the radial border of the flexor carpi ulnaris tendon (Fig. 6-15). The operator deposits anesthetic carefully and only after aspiration to prevent inadvertent ulnar arterial injection. If a paresthesia is elicited, 3 to 5 mL is deposited. If no paresthesia occurs, in a small fanlike action, the anesthetic is deposited. The nerve also can be approached from the ulnar aspect of the wrist. By inserting the needle lateral to the same tendon and slipping under it, the nerve can be blocked using the same amount of anesthetic. A block is achieved in 8 to 12 minutes. A separate branch, originating proximal to the wrist, of the ulnar nerve innervates the dorsum of the hand. To block that branch, a subcutaneous track of anesthetic is laid down from the dorsal midline of the wrist to the ulnar border of the flexor carpi ulnaris tendon.

Radial Nerve Block
Indications

Radial nerve block is used for wounds located on the dorsum of the thumb, index, and middle fingers and the radial portion of the dorsum of the hand.

Anatomy

Approximately 7 cm proximal to the wrist, a superficial cutaneous branch leaves the main radial nerve. At the level of the wrist, this branch begins to fan out into several rami that provide sensory innervation to the dorsoradial aspect of the hand. These rami lie in the superficial fascia just deep to the skin.

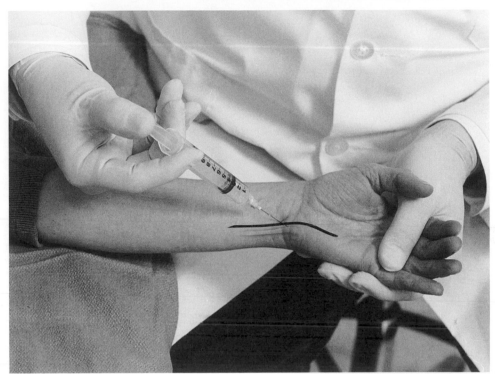

Figure 6-15. Ulnar nerve block. The ulnar nerve lies deep to the flexor carpi ulnaris tendon as shown. The needle is inserted at the radial border of the tendon and directed toward the nerve. Because the nerve lies adjacent to the ulnar artery, great care is taken to aspirate before injection (see text).

Technique

Starting at the dorsoradial aspect of the wrist, a continuous subcutaneous track of anesthetic is laid down to block all the sensory branches (Fig. 6-16). The technique is similar to that described for ulnar nerve blockade. Approximately 10 mL of anesthetic is required. For this block to abolish sensation, 8 to 12 minutes is necessary.

Sural and Tibial Nerve Blocks
(Sole of Foot Blocks)
Indications

One of the most painful areas in which to inject local anesthetic is the sole of the foot. This area is commonly injured and subject to puncture wounds, lacerations, and the embedding of foreign bodies. Sural and tibial nerve blocks are recommended. These blocks are much less painful to the patient than direct infiltration.

Anatomy

The sural nerve courses behind the fibula and lateral malleolus to supply the heel and lateral aspect of the foot. The tibial nerve can be found between the Achilles tendon and the medial malleolus. It can be located easily because it accompanies the posterior tibial artery at that level. This nerve supplies a large portion of the sole and medial side of the foot. As denoted in Figure 6-17, there is some overlap of distribution of these nerves and some overlap of sensation with the anteriorly located saphenous and superficial peroneal nerves. Complete anesthesia is not always achieved by a single block. It can be supplemented by local infiltration

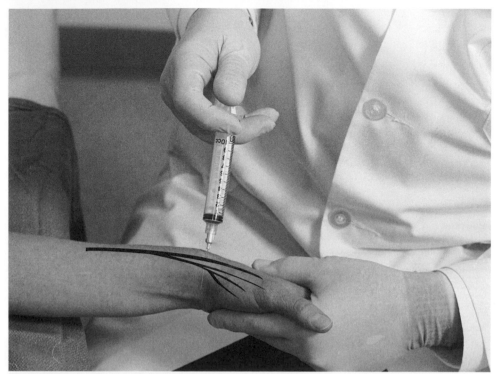

Figure 6-16. Radial nerve block. Note location and branching of the radial nerve. The needle is introduced to its hub. A continuous track of anesthetic is laid down as the needle is withdrawn across the branches of the radial nerve.

with minimal discomfort to the patient because of the preexisting partial anesthesia from the block.

Techniques
Technique for Sural Nerve Block
The needle is introduced just lateral to the Achilles tendon approximately 1 to 2 cm proximal to the level of the distal tip of the lateral malleolus (Fig. 6-18). The needle is directed to the posterior medial aspect of the fibula, and 5 mL of anesthetic is deposited after aspiration of the syringe. To ensure that all the branches of the sural nerve are properly infiltrated, a fan-shaped motion is made with the needle, and multiple small boluses are delivered.

Technique for Posterior Tibial Nerve Block
The posterior tibial artery is palpated as a landmark. The needle is passed adjacent to the Achilles tendon toward the posterior tibial artery behind the medial malleolus (Fig. 6-19). When the area of the artery is approximated, careful aspiration of the syringe is performed. If there is no blood return, 5 mL of anesthetic is injected. Blocks of the posterior tibial and sural nerve take approximately 10 to 15 minutes to achieve appropriate anesthetic levels.

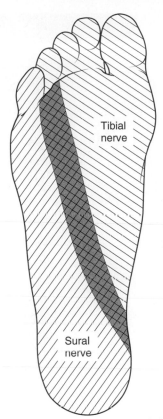

Figure 6-17. Plantar surface of the foot. Distribution of sural and tibial nerve sensory component. There is overlap between the two distributions.

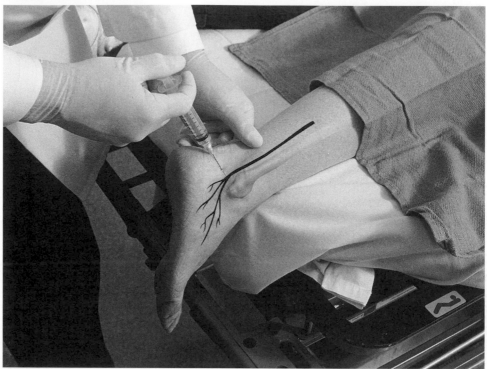

Figure 6-18. Sural nerve block. Note the path of the sural nerve and its relationship to the tip of the fibula. Because of the branching of the nerve, the injection is carried out in a fanlike manner to create an effective block.

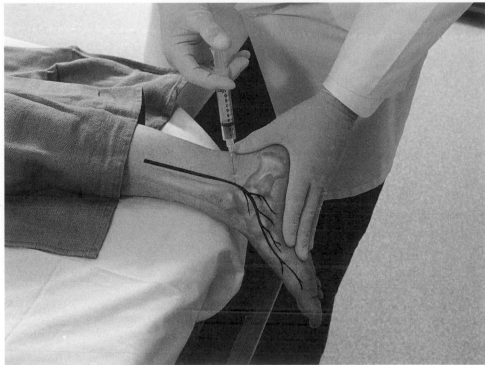

Figure 6-19. Posterior tibial nerve block. Note the path of the nerve and its relationship to the tibial medial malleolus. Because the nerve travels in conjunction with the posterior tibial artery, care is taken to aspirate before injection.

References

1. Mather M, Cousins M: Local anesthetics and their current clinical use, *Drugs* 18:185–205, 1979.
2. Todd K, Berk WA, Huang R: Effect of body locale and addition of epinephrine on the duration of action of a local anesthetic agent, *Ann Emerg Med* 21:723–726, 1992.
3. Sinnott CJ, Cogswell LP III, Johnson A, et al: On the mechanism by which epinephrine potentiates lidocaine's peripheral nerve block, *Anesthesiology* 98:181–188, 2003.
4. Edlich RF, Rodeheaver GT, Thacker JG, et al: Revolutionary advances in the management of traumatic wounds in the Emergency department during the last 40 years: part 1, *J Emerg Med* 20:1–11, 2008.
5. Tarsia V, Singer AJ, Cassara GA, et al: Percutaneous regional compared with local anaesthesia for facial lacerations: a randomised controlled trial, *Emerg Med J* 22:37–40, 2003.
6. Burns CA, Ferris G, Fenc C, et al: Decreasing pain of local anesthesia: a prospective, double-blind comparison of buffered, premixed 1% lidocaine with epinephrine versus 1% lidocaine freshly mixed with epinephrine, *J Am Acad Dermatol* 54:128–131, 2006.
7. Andrades PR, Olguin FA, Calderon W: Digital blocks with and without epinephrine, *Plast Reconstr Surg* 111:1769–1770, 2003.
8. Fariss BL, Foresman PA, Rodeheaver GT, et al: Anesthetic properties of bupivacaine and lidocaine for infiltration anesthesia, *J Emerg Med* 5:275–282, 1987.
9. Malamed SF, Gagnon S, Leblanc D: Articaine hydrochloride: a study of the safety of a new amide local anesthetic, *J Am Dent Assoc* 132:177–185, 2001.
10. de Jong R: Toxic effects of local anesthetics, *JAMA* 239:1166–1168, 1978.
11. Norris RL: Local anesthetics, *Emerg Med Clin North Am* 10:707–718, 1992.
12. Chandler MJ, Grammer LC, Patterson R: Provocative challenge with local anesthetics in patients with a prior history of reaction, *J Allergy Clin Immunol* 79:883–886, 1987.
13. Pollack CV, Swindle GM: Use of diphenhydramine for local anesthesia in "caine"-sensitive patients, *J Emerg Med* 7:611–614, 1989.
14. Pavlidakey PG, Brodell EE, Helms SE: Diphenhydramine as an alternative local anesthetic, *J Clin Aesthet Dermatol* 2:37–40, 2009.

15. Dire DJ, Hogan DE: Double-blinded comparison of diphenhydramine versus lidocaine as a local anesthetic, *Ann Emerg Med* 22:1419-1422, 1993.

16. Ernst AA, Marvez-Valls E, Nick TG, Wahle M: Comparison trial of four injectable anesthetics for laceration repair, *Acad Emerg Med* 3:228-233, 1996.

17. Singer AJ, Hollander JE: Infiltration pain and local anesthetic effects of buffered versus plain 1% diphenhydramine, *Acad Emerg Med* 2:884-888, 1995.

18. Bartfield JM, Crisafulli KM, Raccio-Robak N, Salluzzo RF: The effects of warming and buffering on pain of infiltration of lidocaine, *Acad Emerg Med* 2:254-258, 1995.

19. McKay W, Morris R, Mushlin P: Sodium bicarbonate attenuates pain on skin infiltration with lidocaine, with or without epinephrine, *Anesth Analg* 66:572-574, 1987.

20. Orlinsky M, Hudson C, Chan L, Deslauriers R: Pain comparison of unbuffered versus buffered lidocaine in local wound infiltration, *J Emerg Med* 10:411-415, 1992.

21. Bartfield JM, Homer PJ, Ford DT, Sternklar P: Buffered lidocaine as a local anesthetic: an investigation of shelf life, *Ann Emerg Med* 21:16-19, 1992.

22. Arndt KA, Burton C, Noe JM: Minimizing the pain of local anesthesia, *Plast Reconstr Surg* 72:676-679, 1983.

23. Murakami CS, Odland PB, Ross BR: Buffered local anesthetics and epinephrine degradation, *J Dermatol Surg Oncol* 20:192-195, 1994.

24. Hennes HM, Wagner V, Nonadio WA, et al: The effect of oral midazolam on anxiety of preschool children during laceration repair, *Ann Emerg Med* 19:1006-1009, 1990.

25. Shane SA, Fuchs SM, Khine H: Efficacy of rectal midazolam for the sedation of preschool children undergoing laceration repair, *Ann Emerg Med* 24:1065-1073, 1994.

26. Yealy DM, Ellis JH, Hobbs GD, Moscati RM: Intranasal midazolam as a sedative for children during laceration repair, *Am J Emerg Med* 10:584-587, 1992.

27. Berman D, Graber D: Sedation and analgesia, *Emerg Med Clin North Am* 10:691-705, 1992.

28. Green SM, Clem KJ, Rothrock SG: Ketamine safety profile in the developing world: survey of practitioners, *Acad Emerg Med* 3:598-604, 1996.

29. Green SM, Li J: Ketamine in adults: what emergency physicians need to know about patient selection and emergence reactions, *Acad Emerg Med* 7:278-281, 2000.

30. Green SM, Johnson NE: Ketamine sedation for pediatric procedures: part 2, review and implications, *Ann Emerg Med* 19:1033-1046, 1990.

31. Chudnofsky CR, Weber JE, Stoyanoff PJ, et al: A combination of midazolam and ketamine for procedural sedation and analgesia in adult emergency department patients, *Acad Emerg Med* 7:228-235, 2000.

32. Green SM, Roback MG, Krauss B: Laryngospasm during emergency department sedation: a case-control study, *Pediatr Emerg Care* 26:798-802, 2010.

33. O'Sullivan I, Benger J: Nitrous oxide in emergency medicine, *Emerg Med J* 20:214-217, 2003.

34. Dailey RH: Fatality secondary to misuse of TAC solution, *Ann Emerg Med* 17:159-160, 1988.

35. Priestley S, Kelly AM, Chow L, et al: Application of topical anesthetic at triage reduces treatment time for children with lacerations: a randomized controlled trial, *Ann Emerg Med* 42:34-40, 2003.

36. Singer AJ, Stark MJ: LET versus EMLA for pretreating lacerations: a randomised trial, *Acad Emer Med* 8:223-230, 2001.

37. Zempsky WT, Karasic RB: EMLA versus TAC anesthesia of extremity wounds in children, *Ann Emer Med* 30:163-166, 1997.

38. Pryor G, Kilpatrick W, Opp D: Local anesthesia in minor lacerations: topical TAC versus lidocaine infiltration, *Ann Emerg Med* 9:568-571, 1980.

39. Bonadio WA, Wagner VR: Adrenaline-cocaine gel topical anesthetic for dermal laceration repair in children, *Ann Emerg Med* 21:1435-1438, 1992.

40. Ernst AA, Marvez-Valls E, Nick TG, Weiss SJ: LAT (lidocaine-adrenaline-tetracaine) versus TAC (tetracaine-adrenaline-cocaine) for topical anesthesia in face and scalp lacerations, *Am J Emerg Med* 13:151-154, 1995.

41. Blackburn PA, Butler KH, Hughes MJ, et al: Comparison of tetracaine-adrenaline-cocaine (TAC) with topical lidocaine-epinephrine (TLE): efficacy and cost, *Am J Emerg Med* 13:315-317, 1995.

42. Bonadio WA, Wagner V: Half-strength TAC topical anesthetic, *Clin Pediatr* 27:495-498, 1988.

43. Knoop KJ, Trott AT, Syverud S: Comparison of digital versus metacarpal block for repair of finger injuries, *Ann Emerg Med* 23:1296-1300, 1994.

44. Wilhelmi BJ, Blackwell SJ, Miller JH, et al: Do not use epinephrine in digital blocks: myth or truth? *Plast Reconstr Surg* 107:393-397, 2001.

45. Brutus JP, Baeten Y, Chahidi L, et al: Single injection digital block: comparison between three techniques, *Chir Main* 21:182-187, 2002.

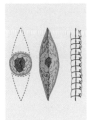

CHAPTER 7
Wound Cleansing and Irrigation

Key Practice Points

- Thorough wound cleansing and irrigation are the most important steps in repairing wounds and lacerations.
- Povidone-iodine solution (not scrub preparation) is the most effective skin, or periphery, cleanser.
- Either water or saline can be used as a wound irrigant to flush debris and bacteria from inside a laceration.
- Hydrogen peroxide has more negative than positive effects on wounds and is not recommended for wound care.
- Shaving hair over wounds can lead to dermal injuries and an increased infection rate. It can be cleaned the same as skin and left alone, clipped with scissors, or flattened away from the wound with lubricants.
- Never shave an eyebrow. It can grow back abnormally or not at all.
- Wound care exposes the caregiver to pathogens such as human immunodeficiency virus (HIV) and hepatitis B and C. Blood and body fluid precautions should be observed.
- Anesthesia should precede wound preparation to minimize the pain of a thorough cleansing and irrigation.

Cleansing and irrigation are the foundations of good wound care. These steps can be time-consuming and tedious. It is essential, however, that all contaminants and devitalized tissue are removed before wound closure. If they are not, the risks of infection and of a cosmetically poor scar are greatly increased. Neither clever suturing technique nor the use of prophylactic antibiotics can replace meticulous cleansing and irrigation and, if needed, judicious débridement.

WOUND CLEANSING SOLUTIONS
Several skin-cleansing preparations are available commercially (Table 7-1). Most of the clinical data that compare the efficacy of these agents come from studies of elective surgery patients or experiments on laboratory animals.[1-3] Only in more recent years have there been reports detailing the use of skin-cleansing preparations for emergency use.[4-7] Based on these studies and the properties of the cleansing solutions, guidelines for use in emergency wound care can be suggested.

Povidone-Iodine
Povidone-iodine (Betadine) is a complex of the potent bactericidal agent iodine and the carrier molecule povidone. On contact with tissues, the carrier complex slowly releases free iodine. Gradual release decreases tissue irritation and reduces potential

TABLE 7-1	Summary of Wound Cleansing Agents			
Skin Cleanser	**Antibacterial Activity**	**Tissue Toxicity**	**Systemic Toxicity**	**Potential Uses**
Povidone-iodine surgical scrub	Strongly bactericidal against gram-positive and gram-negative viruses	Detergent can be toxic to wound tissue	Painful to open wounds	Hand cleanser
Povidone-iodine solution	Same as povidone-iodine scrub	Minimally toxic to wound tissue	Extremely rare	Wound-periphery cleanser
Chlorhexidine	Strongly bactericidal against gram-positives, less strong against gram-negatives	Detergent can be toxic to wound tissue	Extremely rare	Hand cleanser
Poloxamer 188	No antibacterial activity	None known	None known	Wound cleanser (useful on face) Alternative wound periphery cleanser
Saline	None known	None known	None known	Wound irrigant

toxicity while preserving the agent's germicidal activity. Povidone-iodine is effective against gram-positive and gram-negative bacteria, fungi, and viruses.[8] In contrast to chlorhexidine, povidone-iodine has a shorter protective effect against bacterial buildup on the skin after hand washing and seems to be less effective than these agents for that purpose.[9]

Povidone-iodine is manufactured as a solution by itself (povidone-iodine solution) or in conjunction with an ionic detergent (povidone-iodine scrub preparation). The detergent in the scrub preparation seems to be toxic to several normal tissues and to components of an open wound.[1,10] Excessive exposure of open wounds to scrub solutions by wound scrubbing or soaking is not recommended. Scrub solutions were designed for preoperative preparation of intact skin before operative incisions.

Povidone-iodine, without the detergent, is distributed most commonly as a 10% solution. When diluted to a 1% concentration or lower, it can be applied safely to wounds, and it retains its bactericidal activity.[11] It has no inherent negative effect on wound healing.[12] The lack of clinical toxicity of povidone-iodine without detergent was shown with 225 patients undergoing ophthalmologic surgery.[13] Povidone-iodine 10% solution, diluted with saline, was used to prepare the eye and its surrounding structures for surgery. There was no reported corneal, conjunctival, or skin toxicity. Adverse and allergic reactions are extremely rare, even when the solution is used in known iodine-allergic patients.[14]

Chlorhexidine

Chlorhexidine (Hibiclens) is an antibacterial biguanide that is effective against gram-positive bacteria. This agent also is effective against gram-negative bacteria but is less so than povidone -iodine.[15] Its action against viruses is uncertain.[8] Repeated use can lead to buildup on the skin and prolonged suppression of hand bacterial count.[15] For this reason, it is an excellent hand-washing preparation. Under normal conditions of use, chlorhexidine has a low toxicity. The skin cleanser contains an ionic detergent similar to the povidone-iodine scrub preparation, and direct contact with an open wound is discouraged despite its low toxicity.[13,16]

Nonionic Surfactants

Potentially useful wound cleansers are the nonionic surfactants pluronic F-68 (Shur-Clens) and poloxamer 188 (Pharma Clens).[17] These are surface active agents with the cleansing properties of soap but virtually no tissue toxicity, including to the eye and cornea. There are no demonstrable adverse effects in wounds and lacerations. Poloxamer 188 has been used successfully in a trial of more than 3000 patients without serious side effects.[18] The major drawback of the nonionic surfactants is that they have no antibacterial activity.[19] For this reason, alternative cleansing agents, such as povidone-iodine, are preferable for contaminated wounds. Conversely, surfactants are well suited for use on the face because they are nontoxic to the eye, and the face is naturally resistant to infection.

Hydrogen Peroxide

Without a clear scientific basis, as if by tradition alone, hydrogen peroxide is used commonly in emergency wound care. As it comes into contact with blood and tissue peroxidase, hydrogen peroxide makes visible bubbles from liberated oxygen. The reaction causes foaming that is thought to dislodge bacteria, debris, and other contaminants from small crevices in tissues. This effect gives the appearance of cleansing activity, but this agent has many drawbacks. It is naturally hemolytic, and the oxygen bubbles have been shown to separate new epithelial cells from granulation tissue.[20] The germicidal action of hydrogen peroxide is weak and brief at best.[8] In a controlled study of appendectomies, hydrogen peroxide topically applied to the incision site before suture closure did not reduce the infection rate compared with the control.[21] Under experimental wound conditions, it can delay healing.[20] Because of its hemolytic effect, hydrogen peroxide is best limited to a role as an adjunctive agent for wounds encrusted with blood.

PREPARATION FOR WOUND CLEANSING

Before cleansing and irrigating a laceration or wound, several issues, including hand washing, personnel precautions, hair removal, anesthesia, foreign material, wound soaking, wound periphery cleansing, and irrigation, have to be considered.

Hand Washing

Because of the unsterile nature of traumatic wounds, fixed-time hand washing with preoperative scrubbing techniques are not necessary. Although a simple, brief hand washing suffices before each procedure, it is necessary to ensure that the fingernails have been well cleaned because they harbor more bacteria than other parts of the hand.[22,23] Chlorhexidine is a good choice for hand washing. As a skin cleanser, it is well tolerated by users. With repeated washings, it builds up in the skin, with an accompanying prolonged antibacterial effect, and it does not stain clothing the way povidone-iodine does. Compliance with hand washing among emergency personnel has been shown to be poor.[24] Nurses have been observed to comply (hand washing after patient contact before proceeding to the next contact) after 58.2% of patient contacts, residents after 18.6%, and faculty after 17%. Hand washing is just one of the defenses against the risks.

An advance in hand washing has made it much easier to comply with this requirement. Newer alcohol-based products allow for rapid, self-drying application. These agents are equally efficacious as soap-based products are in reducing bacterial counts, and the agents have equivalent cleansing power.[25]

Blood and Body Fluid Precautions

Because preparing and cleansing a wound brings wound care personnel into contact with blood and other secretions, it is recommended that appropriate protective gloves and eyewear are worn at all times. Gowns also are recommended but are not always practical.

The main infective agents that are of concern in the emergency department are hepatitis B and C and HIV. The prevalence of HIV in urban emergency-department patients has been reported to be as high as 4% to 5%.[26] More important, 25% of these patients are unaware of their HIV-positive status on presentation.[27] It is common for practitioners to be diligent about protecting themselves during major trauma resuscitations. The bleeding laceration is no less a threat when suture needles, tissue scissors, and scalpel blades are in use.

Wound Area Hair Removal

It is common practice to shave hair around lacerations and other wounds before repair. Although there are no studies concerning hair removal in the wound care setting, shaving has the potential to increase the wound infection rate. Close shaving of intact skin can cause small dermal wounds that can act as portals of entry for bacterial invasion and possible infection.[23] Two studies of patients, shaved versus not shaved for elective surgery, showed an increase in postoperative wound infection rates in the shaved groups.[28,29] Although hair shafts harbor bacteria, structures such as roots, glands, and follicles do not contain high bacterial counts under normal conditions.[28] Hair can be cleansed easily and successfully using standard techniques for applying antiseptic solutions.[30]

A case for hair removal can be made on technical grounds. In areas such as the scalp, it is much easier to close lacerations without having the suture material become entangled with hair. Hair that is inadvertently buried in wounds can result in wound infection.[31] Clipping hair around the wound with scissors and shaving with a recessed blade razor are techniques for hair removal that avoid dermal damage.

Another technique to expose the wound surrounded by hair is to apply sterile exam lubricant to flatten the hair away from the wound. Antibiotic ointment can be used as well. However, the jelly lubricant is water soluble and easier to remove then the petroleum-based ointment.

The only site from which hair is absolutely not shaved or clipped is the eyebrow (Fig. 7-1). Hair regrowth of the brow is unpredictable in many patients, and return to the original appearance cannot be guaranteed. Eyebrow hair can be cleansed readily, and the brow borders provide excellent landmarks for laceration alignment during wound closure.

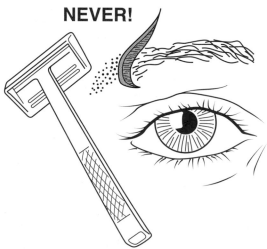

Figure 7-1. Because hair grows inconsistently on the eyebrow, this structure is never shaved.

Anesthesia

Because wound cleansing can be uncomfortable if not outright painful, most wounds should be anesthetized before cleaning. Not only is the patient more comfortable, but also the cleansing can be more vigorous and effective. Techniques for administering anesthetics are discussed fully in Chapter 6.

An issue that often arises concerning the administration of anesthetics before wound cleansing is whether bacteria can be embedded further into a wound if a needle is passed through a contaminated surface. There is no clear scientific evidence that needles can spread bacteria beyond the wound margins.[32] In clean, sharp wounds, this issue is of no concern, and direct wound infiltration can be performed safely. For wounds that are visibly and heavily contaminated, the parallel injection technique or an appropriate nerve block can be used, if necessary, to avoid this hypothetical complication.

Foreign Material

As part of wound preparation, it is important to determine the presence or absence of foreign bodies in the wound. Foreign materials of all types should be considered harmful with the potential for causing infection if left in the tissues. In addition, retained foreign objects are among the most common reasons for malpractice suits brought against emergency physicians.[33] Although irrigation removes most debris, direct visualization and removal by instruments often are required. An alert patient can report the "sensation" of a foreign body still in the wound. Radiographs are particularly useful to find tooth fragments, metallic objects, and glass. It is a popular misconception that glass cannot be visualized by radiographs; 90% of all glass (0.5 mm or larger) can be detected by radiographs.[34] The removal of foreign bodies is discussed in more detail in Chapter 16.

Wound Soaking

Wound soaking is a common practice in wound care. Soaking is believed to loosen debris, to break up blood coagulum, and to help sterilize the wound. Under experimental conditions, however, povidone-iodine solution was unable to penetrate beyond 1.5 mm of tissue despite 20 minutes of wound soaking.[6] Although bacterial counts are lowered with soaking in povidone-iodine solution, significant contamination remains. Wound soaking has some value in loosening, softening, and removing gross contaminants from the skin surrounding the wound, but it is not a substitute for thorough mechanical skin cleansing and wound irrigation.

Wound Periphery Cleansing

The main purpose for periphery wound cleansing or "scrubbing" is to remove any visible contamination and dried blood. Periphery cleansing alone is insufficient for wound preparation without accompanying irrigation. The end point of skin cleansing is when the area surrounding the wound or laceration is visibly clean. There is no fixed scrubbing time. If the skin itself cannot be cleansed of all particulates, the risk for "tattooing" increases. Visible particulate matter "ground" into the skin can become permanently entrapped within the epidermis and dermis of the skin. These particulates need to be removed by sharp débridement. Because tattooing can have serious cosmetic consequences on the face, consultation and referral to a facial plastic surgeon should be considered if routine measures fail.

Scrubbing within the wound itself is controversial. In experimental wounds, scrubbing with surgical sponges has not been shown to decrease the incidence of infection and may produce mechanical trauma to the exposed tissues.[19] The mechanical action of a surgical sponge can be effective in removing gross contaminants and debris from within a wound. Because of the potential for tissue damage, scrubbing within a wound is best reserved for wounds with visible contaminants. The porosity of the surgical sponges used for wound cleansing is also an issue. The standard, common surgical sponge has 45 pores per linear inch. Sponges with 90 pores per linear inch (Optipore) are less irritating to tissues.[22] If handled gently, standard sponges are minimally traumatic, and the increased expense of higher porosity sponges may not justify their use.

Irrigation

"The solution to pollution is dilution" is an old maxim of wound care that still rings true today. Wound irrigation is the most effective way to remove debris and contaminants from within a laceration.[18] Irrigation also is the most effective method of reducing bacterial counts on wound surfaces.[35,36] In comparing methods of irrigation for highly contaminated wounds, high-pressure streams (5 to 70 psi) of saline are clearly superior to low-pressure streams, such as those that might be obtained with a bulb-type syringe (0.5 to 1 psi).[37] Current practice is based on work done with a 35-mL syringe attached to a 19-G catheter.[37] This system develops 7 to 8 psi and is effective in reducing debris and bacterial contamination from the types of wounds and lacerations managed by emergency caregivers. Pulsatile lavage, which develops a psi of 50 to 70, is effective at lowering bacterial counts and wound infection rates.[38] Significant amounts of irrigation fluid can dissect well beyond the wound margins, however.[39] Pulsatile lavage systems are suited for larger, heavily contaminated wounds best managed by surgical specialists in the operating room.

Traditionally, saline has been used as the irrigant of choice. It is sterile and compatible with body tissues. More recently, saline's primacy as the best fluid for this task has been challenged.[40] For example, in a large prospective trial of 530 pediatric patients comparing saline with running tap water, there was no difference in wound infection rates between groups (2.8% versus 2.9%).[40] These were simple wounds with low levels of contamination.

CLEANSING SETUP AND PROCEDURES

The following are suggested guidelines for wound cleansing and preparation:

- *Patient position:* As in any procedure, proper preparation is essential. The patient is placed in a comfortable position, usually supine. It is impossible to predict how the patient will react to the discomfort of wound cleansing, the sight of blood, or the appearance of a wound. Vasovagal reactions (fainting) can occur if the patient is upright. Patients can sustain injuries by falling to the floor during the procedure. It also is prudent to ask relatives to leave the area or at least to monitor their responses to blood and the procedures that are being performed. Onlookers can experience vasovagal syncope as well.
- *Anesthesia:* For the most part, a wound or laceration should be anesthetized before periphery cleansing and irrigation. The pain of cleansing can inhibit the operator and lead to poor cooperation from the patient. The result is an incompletely cleansed wound.
- *Periphery cleansing technique:* Ten percent povidone-iodine solution (not the scrub preparation) diluted 10:1 can also be used as a periphery cleanser as well. If there is significant contamination or debris within the wound itself, the sponges can be used for mechanical, in-the-wound débridement. The technique for scrubbing the wound periphery is illustrated in Figure 7-2. It is essential to be gentle and to start at the wound itself. The cleansing motion is circular, with gradually larger circles away from the wound. The sponge is then discarded. At no time should the chlorhexidine or povidone-iodine sponge be brought from the periphery back toward the wound; this

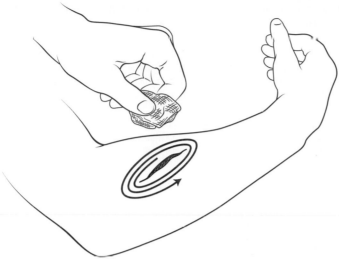

Figure 7-2. Note the spiral technique of scrubbing a wound periphery by beginning at the center and moving away to the periphery without crossing back over the actual wound area.

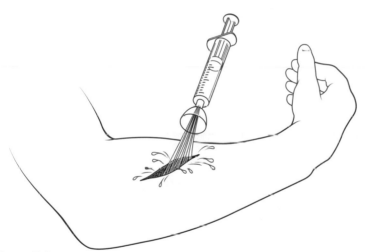

Figure 7-3. Technique for wound irrigation. The shield is held close to the wound.

maneuver carries unwanted organisms from unsterile skin areas back to the area of the cleansed wound site. There is no specified amount of time for periphery cleansing. Scrubbing continues until the skin is visibly free of contaminants and dried blood.

- *Irrigation:* After periphery cleansing, the wound is irrigated with the syringe and splash shield (Fig. 7-3). Periphery cleansing and irrigation can be alternated until there are no visible skin or wound contaminants. The amount of irrigation fluid can vary from 100 to 250 mL or more, depending on the level of contamination of the wound. The 35-mL syringe and splash shield are held close to the wound so that the force of the stream is not dissipated by distance. Whatever cannot be irrigated out of the wound is removed by mechanical scrubbing with a sponge or sharp débridement.
- *Débridement:* If visible contamination remains despite thorough cleansing and irrigation, sharp débridement is performed with tissue scissors or a surgical scalpel with a

no. 15 blade. Ultimately, other strategies, such as wound excision, might be necessary to handle wounds that cannot be managed with these steps. Strategies for the difficult wound are discussed in Chapter 9.

Cleansing is complete and a wound is ready to close when, literally, the wound looks clean to the eye. There should be no visible contaminants, and the tissue should appear pink and viable. Usually there is slight fresh bleeding. A sterile sponge can be laid over the wound until the operator is ready to proceed with repair.

References

1. Berry AR, Watt B, Goldacre MJ: A comparison of the use of povidone-iodine and chlorhexidine in the prophylaxis of postoperative wound infection, *J Hosp Infect* 3:55–63, 1982.
2. Custer J, Edlich RF, Prusak M, et al: Studies in the management of the contaminated wound, *Am J Surg* 121:572–575, 1971.
3. Kaul A, Jewett J: Agents and techniques for disinfection of the skin, *Surg Gynecol Obstet* 152:677–685, 1981.
4. Valente JH, Forti RJ, Freundlich LF, et al: Wound irrigation in children: saline solution or tap water? *Ann Emerg Med* 41:609–616, 2003.
5. Dire DJ, Welch AP: A comparison of wound irrigation solutions used in the emergency department, *Ann Emerg Med* 19:704–708, 1990.
6. Gravett A, Sterner S, Clinton J, et al: A trial of povidone-iodine in the prevention of infection in sutured lacerations, *Ann Emerg Med* 16:167–171, 1987.
7. Howell JM, Stair TO, Howell AM, et al: The effect of scrubbing and irrigation with normal saline, povidone iodine, and cefazolin on wound bacterial counts in a guinea pig model, *Am J Emerg Med* 11:134–138, 1993.
8. Harvey S: Antiseptics and disinfectants; fungicides; ectoparasiticides. In Goodman A, Goodman L, Gilman A, editors: *The pharmacologic basis of therapeutics*, New York, 1980, Macmillan.
9. Koburger T, Hubner NO, Braun M, et al: Standardized comparison of antiseptic efficacy of triclosan, PVP-iodine, octenidine dihydrochloride, polehexanide and chlorhedine digluconate, *J Antimicro Ther* 65:1712–1719, 2010.
10. Faddis D, Daniel D, Boyer J: Tissue toxicity of antiseptic solutions, *J Trauma* 17:895–897, 1977.
11. Berk WA, Welch RD, Bock BF: Controversial issues in clinical management of the simple wound, *Ann Emerg Med* 21:72–80, 1992.
12. Smith RG: A critical discussion of the use of antiseptics in acute traumatic wounds, *J Am Podiat Med Assoc* 95:148–153, 2005.
13. Caldwell DR, Kasti PR, Cook J, et al: Povidone-iodine: its efficacy as a preoperative conjunctival and periocular preparation, *Ann Ophthalmol* 16:577–588, 1984.
14. Shelanski H, Shelanski M: PVP-iodine: history, toxicity, and therapeutic uses, *J Int Coll Surg* 25:727–734, 1956.
15. Dineen P: Hand washing degerming: a comparison of povidone-iodine and chlorhexidine, *Clin Pharmacol Ther* 23:63–67, 1978.
16. Main RC: Should chlorhexidine gluconate be used in wound cleansing? *J Wound Care* 17:112–114, 2008.
17. Bryant CA, Rodeheaver GT, Reem EM, et al: Search for a nontoxic surgical scrub solution of periorbital lacerations, *Ann Emerg Med* 13:317–321, 1984.
18. Edlich RF, Rodeheaver GT, Morgan RF, et al: Principles of emergency wound management, *Ann Emerg Med* 17:1284–1302, 1988.
19. Rodeheaver GT, Smith SL, Thacker JG: Mechanical cleansing of contaminated wounds with a surfactant, *Am J Surg* 129:241–245, 1975.
20. Gruber RP, Vistnes L, Pardoe R: The effect of commonly used antiseptics on wound healing, *Plast Reconstr Surg* 55:472–476, 1975.
21. Lau HY, Wong SH: Randomized, prospective trial of topical hydrogen peroxide in appendectomy wound infection, *Am J Surg* 142:393–397, 1981.
22. Edlich RF, Rodeheaver GT, Thacker JG, et al: *Technical factors in wound management: fundamentals of wound management in surgery*, South Plainfield, NJ, 1977, Chirurgecom, Inc.
23. Pecora D, Landis R, Martin E: Location of cutaneous microorganisms, *Surgery* 64:1114–1117, 1968.
24. Meengs MR, Giles BK, Chisholm CD, et al: Hand washing frequency in an emergency department, *Ann Emerg Med* 23:1307–1312, 1994.
25. Hillburn J, Hammond BS, Fendler EJ: Use of alcohol hand sanitizer as an infection control strategy in an acute care facility, *Am J Infect Control* 31:109–116, 2003.
26. Sloan EP, McGill BA, Zalenski R, et al: Human immunodeficiency virus and hepatitis B virus seroprevalence in an urban trauma population, *J Trauma* 38:736–741, 1995.

27. Jue J, Stevens P, Hedberg K, Modesitt S: HIV seroprevalence in emergency department patients, *Acad Emerg Med* 2:773-783, 1995.

28. Cruse P, Foord R: A five-year prospective study of 23,649 surgical wounds, *Arch Surg* 107:206-209, 1973.

29. Seropian R, Reynolds B: Wound infections after preoperative depilatory versus razor preparation, *Am J Surg* 121:251-254, 1971.

30. Winston KR: Hair and neurosurgery, *Neurosurg* 31:320-329, 1992.

31. Mahlor D, Rosenberg L, Goldstein J: The fate of buried hair, *Ann Plast Surg* 5:131-138, 1980.

32. Kelly AM, Cohen M, Richards D: Minimizing the pain of local infiltration anesthesia for wounds by injection into the wound edges, *J Emerg Med* 12:593-595, 1994.

33. Trautlein JJ, Lambert RL, Miller J: Malpractice in the emergency department—review of 200 cases, *Ann Emerg Med* 13:709-711, 1984.

34. Tandberg D: Glass in the hand and foot, *JAMA* 248:1872-1874, 1982.

35. Madden J, Edlich RF, Schauerhamer R, et al: Application of principles of fluid dynamics to surgical wound irrigation, *Curr Top Surg Res* 3:85-93, 1971.

36. Rodeheaver GT, Pettry D, Thacker JG, et al: Wound cleansing in high pressure irrigation, *Surg Gynecol Obstet* 141:357-362, 1975.

37. Stevenson TR, Thacker JG, Rodeheaver GT, et al: Cleansing the traumatic wound by high pressure syringe irrigation, *J Am Coll Emerg Physicians* 5:17-21, 1976.

38. Pigman EC, Karch DB, Scott JL: Splatter during jet irrigation cleansing of a wound model: a comparison of three inexpensive devices, *Ann Emerg Med* 22:1563-1567, 1993.

39. Wheeler CB, Rodeheaver GT, Thacker JG, et al: Side effects of high pressure irrigation, *Surg Gynecol Obstet* 143:775-778, 1976.

40. Fernandez R, Griffiths R: Water for wound cleansing (review), *The Cochrane Library* 5:1-25, 2010.

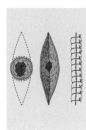

CHAPTER 8

Instruments, Suture Materials, and Closure Choices

Key Practice Points

- Lacerations and wounds can be managed with a few well-chosen instruments: needle holders, tissue forceps, and scissors.
- Each instrument requires special handling (described in this chapter) to close lacerations and repair wounds correctly.
- Proper instrument technique reduces tissue damage and excessive scar formation.
- There two basic suture types: absorbable for deep, subcutaneous closure and nonabsorbable for superficial skin closure.
- In recent years, however, absorbable sutures with rapid absorbing properties have been used for superficial skin closures.
- Studies have shown that there are no cosmetic differences between absorbable and nonabsorbable superficial skin closures.
- Older suture types, such as silk, cause greater tissue reaction than do newer synthetic materials.
- Reverse cutting needles are atraumatic and are recommended more highly than older, tapered needles.

It is not necessary to have large numbers of instruments and suture materials for emergency wound care. Wounds and lacerations can be managed with three or four well-chosen instruments and a few wound closure products. Although the type of instruments remains relatively constant, each wound has differing requirements for wound closure materials. Absorbable and nonabsorbable sutures and a variety of wound tapes, staples, and tissue adhesives can be selected according to the specific patient problem. The following are guidelines for the selection of suture materials and the choice and proper handling of instruments. Tapes, staples, and adhesives are discussed in Chapter 14.

BASIC INSTRUMENTS AND HANDLING

Most wounds can be cared for with the following set of instruments: needle holders, tissue forceps, and suture scissors. For more complex wounds that may require revision or débridement, iris (tissue) scissors, hemostats, a knife handle, and appropriate knife blades might be required. A bewildering array of instruments is currently available through the major suppliers of surgical instruments, but only the types and configurations of instruments necessary to manage wounds and lacerations are discussed here. Also, numerous disposable instrument sets meet the needs of many emergency wound care problems.

Needle Holders

Because most lacerations are closed with relatively small suture materials, the needle holder need not be bulky or large. A 1¼ inch needle holder can accommodate most curved suture needles. Occasionally, large needles are used, and a 6-inch needle holder is necessary.

Technique for Handling Needle Holder

Just as important as the choice of needle holder is the technique used for holding and arming it with the needle. Figure 8-1 shows the right way and the wrong way to hold the instrument during introduction of the needle into tissue for routine emergency

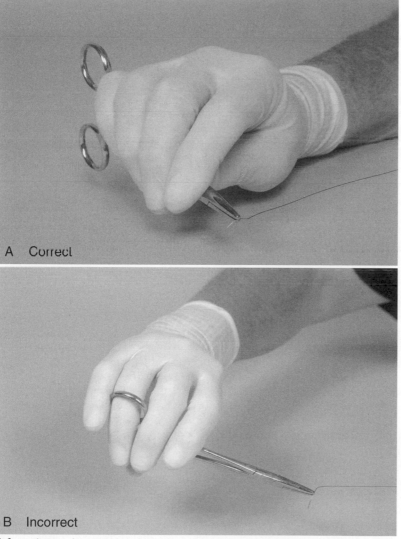

Figure 8-1. Technique for properly holding the needle holder. **A,** The correct way allows for proper needle entry into the skin. **B,** The incorrect way—the finger holes are not used when introducing the needle holder into the skin.

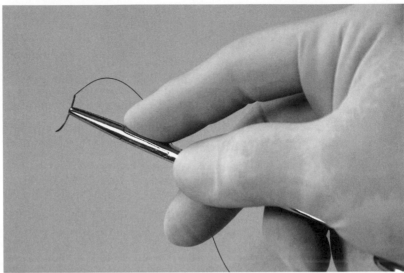

Figure 8-2. Technique for arming a needle holder. The needle is held approximately one third of the way from the swage and is grasped at the tip of the needle holder. The angle of the needle to the holder is exactly 90 degrees.

laceration closure. The rings are used only to clamp and unclamp the jaws by closing and releasing the locking mechanism. When introducing the needle into the skin, better precision can be gained by grasping the needle holder close to the jaws in the manner illustrated. This precision is particularly important when closing lacerations on the face.

The needle holder is armed with the needle by closing the tip of the jaws onto the body of the needle (Fig. 8-2). If the needle is pushed farther back into the jaws of the instrument, the curve is flattened, significantly weakening the needle and making it susceptible to breakage. The needle itself is grasped at right angles, approximately one third of the way down the body shaft from the end to which the suture is attached (the swage).

Forceps

Grasping and controlling tissue with forceps during skin closure is essential to proper suture placement. Whenever force is applied to skin or other tissues, however, inadvertent damage to cells can occur if an improper instrument or technique is used. Forceps still are widely used and are safe when proper technique is applied. The currently recommended forceps are 4¾-inch forceps with small teeth. Teeth decrease the need to apply excessive force to grasp and secure tissue. The use of forceps without teeth is discouraged, because the flat surface of the jaws of the forceps tends to crush tissue more easily.

Technique for Handling Forceps

When handling tissue, the jaws of the forceps are never closed on skin itself. The epidermis and dermis are avoided in favor of the superficial fascia (subcutaneous tissue). By grasping superficial fascia gently, the wound edge is stabilized for needle placement and inadvertent damage to the dermis is avoided (Fig. 8-3). Forceps also can serve as a surrogate skin hook as illustrated. The needle entry point can be immobilized and supported without closing the jaws.

Figure 8-4 illustrates the correct and incorrect methods for grasping forceps. The "pencil grasp" technique allows for better control of the forceps and tends to diminish the amount of force delivered to the tissue.

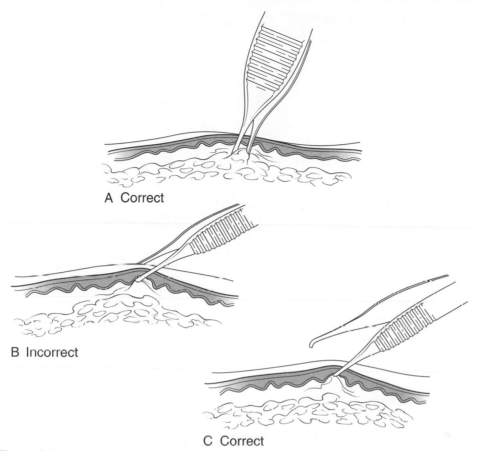

Figure 8-3. The correct and incorrect methods for grasping tissue with a forceps. **A,** The correct way is to grasp the tissue by the superficial fascia (subcutaneous tissue). **B,** The incorrect way to grasp tissue is by crushing the dermis and epidermis between the jaws of the forceps. **C,** Forceps can be used as a skin hook to retract or stabilize the wound edge for exploration or suture needle placement.

Scissors

Standard 6-inch, single blunt-tip, double-sharp suture scissors are most useful for cutting sutures, adhesive tape, sponges, and other dressing materials. Because of their size and bulk, these scissors are durable and practical. Curved and straight, 4-inch iris, or tissue, scissors are used to assist in débridement and wound revision. These scissors are extremely sharp and provide excellent precision in cutting tissue for whatever task. They are delicate, however, and are not recommended for cutting sutures. Occasionally, when small sutures have been used in the face area, iris scissors can be used for suture removal.

Technique for Scissor Tip Control

Whenever scissor tip control is essential, for example, when cutting close to the knots of deep or dermal closures with absorbable sutures, the technique illustrated in Figure 8-5 is recommended. The tips of the scissors are brought gently down to the knot. Just before cutting, the tips are rotated slightly to avoid cutting the knot itself.

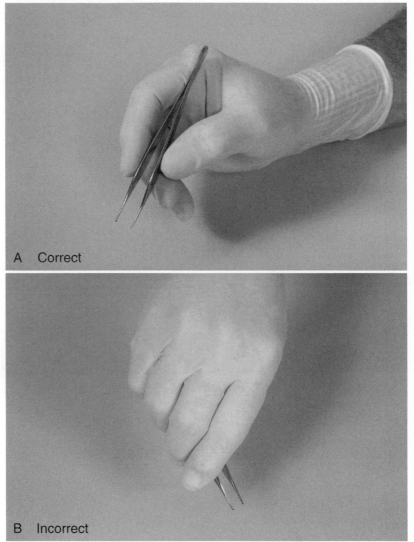

Figure 8-4. The correct and incorrect ways of holding the forceps manually. **A,** The forceps is held in the pencil grasp fashion as the correct technique. **B,** The incorrect technique is to grasp the forceps.

Hemostats

Hemostats have three functions in emergency wound care. Originally, hemostats were designed to clamp small blood vessels for hemorrhage control. Another use is to grasp and secure superficial fascia during undermining and débriding wounds. Finally, this instrument is an excellent tool for exposing, exploring, and visualizing the deeper areas of a wound. Two types of hemostats are commonly used in wound care. For general use, the standard hemostat is recommended. Finer work in small wounds is often best served by the 5-inch curved mosquito hemostat with fine serrated jaws.

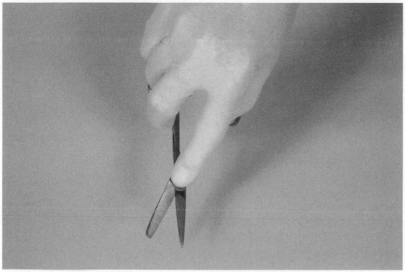

Figure 8-5. Proper technique for tip control for scissors.

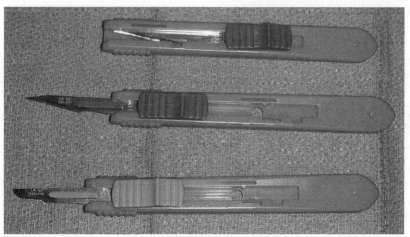

Figure 8-6. Examples of retractable no. 11 and no. 15 scalpels. *Top,* no. 11 in retracted position; *middle,* no. 11 in open position; *bottom,* no. 15 in open position.

Knife Handles and Blades

The choice of scalpels can be limited to three blade configurations, no. 10, no. 15, and no. 11. For safety, the retractable scalpel is recommended (Fig. 8-6). The no. 10 blade is not usually needed in emergency wound care but occasionally is helpful for larger excisions during wound revision. Commonly used and quite versatile is the no. 15 blade, which is small and well suited for precise débridement and wound revision. This blade is also preferred for foreign-body excision and the intricate work necessary around eyes, lips, ears, and fingertips. The no. 11 blade is configured ideally for incision and drainage of superficial abscesses. It also can be used to help remove small sutures such as might be placed in the face.

TABLE 8-1	Absorbable Suture Materials				
Absorbable Suture Materials	Structure	Tissue Reaction	Tensile Strength	Half-Life (Days)	Uses and Comments
Gut	Natural	++++	++	5-7	For mucosal closures, rarely used
Rapid absorbing gut	Natural	+++	++	7-10	Skin closure (face), mucosa
Chromic gut	Natural	++++	++	10-14	For oral mucosa, perineal, and scrotal closures; can be annoying to patients because of stiffness
Polyglycolic acid (Dexon)	Braided	++	+++	25	For subcutaneous closure; coated version easier to use but requires more knots (Dexon Plus)
Polyglactin 910 (Vicryl)	Braided	++	++++	28	For subcutaneous closure; do not use dyed suture on face
Polyglactin 910 (irradiated, Vicryl Rapide)	Braided	++	+++	5-7	Scalp, mucosa, child hand and face
Polyglyconate (Maxon)	Monofilament	+	+++++	28-36	For subcutaneous closure; less reactive and stronger than polyglycolic acid and polyglactin 910
Poliglecaprone 25 (Monocryl)	Monofilament	+	++++	7-10	Deep (subcutaneous) closures
Polydioxanone closures (PDS)	Monofilament	+	++++	36-53	For subcutaneous that need high degree of security; stiffer and more difficult to handle than polyglycolic acid or polyglyconate

SUTURE MATERIALS

Several criteria must be met before a particular suture can be used to close a laceration. A good suture must have appropriate tensile strength to resist breakage, good knot security to prevent unraveling, pliability and workability in handling, low tissue reactivity, and the ability to resist bacterial infection. Currently, there are two main classes of suture materials: absorbable and nonabsorbable. Tables 8-1 and 8-2 summarize the characteristics of suture types. In general, absorbable sutures are placed deep for closure of dead space in large wounds or to reduce closure tension. Nonabsorbable sutures are used most commonly for percutaneous or skin closure. However, there has been a growing trend toward using alternatives for skin, superficial closure (including staples), wound adhesives (see Chapter 14), and absorbable sutures. Table 8-3 lists recommendations for suture and closure materials by anatomic site.

Absorbable sutures have been traditionally used for deep closures to close dead space and to lessen tension of the superficial skin sutures. Numerous studies have demonstrated that absorbable sutures have a cosmetic outcome equal to nonabsorbable sutures when used to close superficial skin layers.[1-6] Vicryl Rapide has been effective in

TABLE 8-2	Nonabsorbable Suture Materials				
Material	Structure	Tissue Reaction	Tensile Strength	Knot Security	Uses and Comments
Silk	Braided	++++	++	++++	Easy to handle but has increased potential for infection
Nylon (Ethilon, Dermalon)	Monofilament	++	+++	++	Commonly used in skin closure but high degree of memory; requires several throws for secure closure
Polypropylene (Prolene)	Monofilament	+	++++	+	High degree of memory, low tissue adhesion; good for subcuticular pull-out technique
Dacron (Mersilene)	Braided	+++	++	++++	Easy to handle, good knot security; similar to silk but less risk to tissue for inflammation and infection
Polybutester (Novafil)	Monofilament	+	++++	++++	Excellent handling, strength, and security; expands and contracts with changes in tissue edema

closing scalp incisions when compared with nonabsorbable sutures.[3] Patients expressed considerable satisfaction with not having to have stitches removed. Fast-absorbing gut and Vicryl Rapide has been successfully used to close adult facial lacerations.[2,5] Much of the experience with absorbable suture superficial skin closure has been in children.[4,6,7] The cosmetic differences between absorbable and nonabsorbable sutures were not significant. One study did show a difference at 6 weeks, but the difference disappeared by 6 months.[1] At 1 month, some Vicryl-sutured wounds, particularly on the hand, were more erythematous compared with nylon-sutured wounds. By 6 months the erythema had disappeared, and the wounds could not be distinguished from one another. An important characteristic of sutures of any type is that they cause suture marks if left in the skin longer than 10 to 14 days. If absorbable sutures on the face have not fallen out by 7 days, the patient or parent can be instructed to gently rub them off with a moistened sponge or cloth.

Absorbable Suture Materials
Polyglactin 910 (Vicryl, Vicryl Rapide)
Polyglactin 910 is a braided synthetic polymer used for deep closures. It has similar dry tensile strength compared with polyglycolic acid (Dexon) but maintains in vivo function and strength somewhat longer. However, polyglycolic acid has greater knot security. Polyglactin 910 can be modified by irradiation (Vicryl Rapide), which greatly increases its tissue absorption.[8] Its half-life is only 5 to 7 days, and the sutures fall off in 10 to 14 days. This quality makes Vicryl Rapide ideal for closure of oral mucosa, face, scalp, scrotal skin, and perineum. The suture can be placed, and because of rapid absorption, no return visit is necessary for removal.

Polyglycolic Acid (PGA) (Dexon, Dexon II)
PGA is a synthetic, braided polymer. When compared with plain or chromic catgut, PGA is much less reactive and is experimentally better able to resist infection from

TABLE 8-3	Wound Closure Type per Anatomic Site		
Anatomic Site	**Layer**	**Closure Type**	**Alternatives**
Scalp	Deep[a]	4-0 Polyglactin 910[b]	4-0 Polyglycolic acid[c]
	Skin	Staples	5-0 Vicryl Rapide
			4-0 Nylon, polypropylene
Face	Deep	5-0 Polyglactin 910	5-0 Polyglycolic acid
	Skin	6-0 Nylon[d]	6-0 Polypropylene[e]
		Wound adhesive (pediatrics)[f]	5-0 Fast-absorbing gut, Vicryl Rapide
Ears	Skin	6-0 Nylon	6-0 Polypropylene
Lip	Muscle/subcutaneous	5-0 Polyglactin 910	5-0 Polyglycolic acid
	Skin	6-0 Nylon	6-0 Polypropylene, Vicryl Rapide
Intraoral	Mucosa	5-0 Chromic gut	4-0 Polyglactin 910
Tongue	Mucosa	4-0 Chromic gut	4-0 Polyglycolic acid
Eyelid	Skin	6-0 Nylon	6-0 Polypropylene
Neck	Deep	5-0 Polyglactin 910	5-0 Polyglycolic acid
	Skin	5-0 Nylon	5-0 Polypropylene
Trunk	Deep	4-0 Polyglactin 910	4-0 Polyglycolic acid
	Skin	4-0 Nylon	4-0 Polypropylene, staples[g]
Arm/forearm	Deep	4-0 Polyglactin 910	4-0 Polyglycolic acid
	Skin	4-0 Nylon	4-0 Polypropylene
Hand	Skin	5-0 Nylon	5-0 Polypropylene, Vicryl Rapide (pediatrics)
Leg	Deep	3-0 Polyglactin 910	3-0 Polyglycolic acid
	Skin	4-0 Nylon	4-0 Polypropylene
			Staples[g]
Foot	Skin	5-0 Nylon	5-0 Polypropylene
Penis	Skin	5-0 Nylon	5-0 Polypropylene
Scrotum	Skin	5-0 Chromic gut	5-0 Polyglactin 910
Introitus	Labia majora	5-0 Nylon	5-0 Polypropylene
	Labia minora	5-0 Chromic gut	5-0 Polyglactin 910
	Vagina	5-0 Chromic gut	5-0 Polyglactin 910

[a]Subcutaneous layer.
[b]Polyglactin 910 (Vicryl).
[c]Polyglycolic acid (Dexon).
[d]Nylon (Ethilon, Dermalon).
[e]Polypropylene (Prolene).
[f]Children.
[g]Avoid weight-bearing surfaces.

contaminating bacteria.[9] PGA has excellent knot security and maintains at least 50% of its tensile strength for 25 days.[10] The main drawback of PGA is that it has a high friction coefficient and "binds and snags" when wet. For this reason, some experience is required to pass this material properly through tissues and to "seat" the throws during knotting. The manufacturer has modified PGA (Dexon Plus) by coating it with poloxamer 188, an agent that significantly reduces the friction and drag through tissues. Although handling has become easier with this modification, more throws (four to six) are required to prevent knot slippage than for plain PGA (three to four). The main uses of PGA are for deep closures of superficial fascia (subcutaneous tissue) in wounds and ligature of small bleeding vessels to effect hemostasis.

Gut (Plain, Chromic, Fast-Absorbing)

An older and less commonly used absorbable suture material is gut. Gut is an organic material manufactured from sheep intestines. A newer form of this suture is gut treated with chromium trioxide (chromic gut) to retard absorption in tissues; however, its holding security is only 14 days. Compared with PGA, plain gut and chromic gut appear to have inferior tensile strength and wound security.[11,12] Because of its relatively rapid absorption, the main use of chromic gut is to close lacerations within the oral mucosa, perineum, and scrotal skin. Wounds within the oral cavity tend to heal rapidly and do not require prolonged suture support. Chromic gut is absorbed more rapidly than PGA on the oral mucosa and does not require suture removal.[13] Fast-absorbing gut is heat treated also to create more rapid absorption than chromic gut. Fast-absorbing gut is useful for wounds that only need 5 to 7 days of holding, such as intraoral mucosa. It also can be used as superficial skin closures in children when suture removal is problematic.

Polyglyconate (Maxon) and Polydioxanone (PDS)

These are two monofilament absorbable suture materials that have some advantages over PGA and polyglactin 910. The main advantage of these suture materials is that they maintain their in vivo tensile strength longer than PGA and the other absorbable suture materials.[10,14] They also appear to have greater knot security and lower friction coefficients. Polyglyconate is less stiff and easier to handle than polydioxanone. Because they are monofilaments, they enjoy the theoretical advantage of creating a lower potential for infection.

Poliglecaprone (Monocryl)

A newer, effective absorbable suture is poliglecaprone (Monocryl).[15] This suture material has high initial tensile strength and low tissue reactivity. It has excellent handling characteristics, with low friction and good knot security. Another intriguing finding is that Monocryl causes less hypertrophic scar formation compared with Vicryl Rapide.[16] Monocryl is a monofilament, whereas Vicryl Rapide is multifilament, and this difference might account for the reduced scar formation. With many patients with this tendency, it is important know that there is a suture material with a lower potential for hypertrophic scar formation. Even though Monocryl is an absorbable suture, it has been recommended for superficial skin closure of surgical incisions in numerous anatomic sites such as face, eyes, ears, neck, abdomen, and other sites.[15] It is also being used in emergency settings.

Nonabsorbable Suture Materials
Nylon (Ethilon, Dermalon)

Of all the nonabsorbable suture materials, monofilament nylon (Ethilon, Dermalon) is used most commonly for superficial closure of skin (see Table 8-2). The monofilament configuration makes it minimally tissue reactive and makes it able to resist infection from experimental wound contamination compared with braided suture material.[10] Nylon has tensile strength that ensures wound security. The main disadvantage of nylon is the difficulty in achieving good knot security. Because monofilaments have greater memory (the tendency to return to their packaged shape) than braided sutures, they tend to unravel if not tied correctly. At least four to five carefully fashioned "throws" or knots are required to achieve a secure final knot.

Polypropylene (Prolene)

The polymer polypropylene (Prolene) is another nonabsorbable monofilament. Polypropylene appears to be stronger than nylon and has better overall wound security.[12] It is also less reactive and is able to resist infection at least as well as nylon.[10] It has greater memory than nylon, however, and is more difficult to manage. The main uses of polypropylene are for percutaneous and subcuticular pull-out closures.

Polybutester (Novafil)

Another monofilament suture material is polybutester (Novafil).[17] Polybutester appears to be stronger than other monofilaments. This material does not have significant memory, nor does it maintain its packaging shape the way nylon and polypropylene do. For this reason, it is reported to be easier to work with, and it has greater knot security. A unique feature of polybutester is that it has the capacity to adapt or "stretch" with increasing wound edema. When the edema subsides, polybutester resumes its original shape. Compared with nylon, this suture material has a lower risk of causing hypertrophic scarring.[18] The ability to adapt to the swelling and changing configuration of a healing wound is credited for this reduction in risk.

Less commonly used for minor wound care problems are braided, nonabsorbable suture materials, including cotton, silk, braided nylon, and multifilament Dacron. Until the advent of synthetic fibers, silk was the mainstay of wound closure. It is the most workable of sutures and has excellent knot security. The usefulness and popularity of silk have declined, however, because of its propensity to cause tissue reactivity and infection.[10,12] Research has shown that, similar to silk, the braided synthetics have a greater tendency to cause wound infection when exposed to contaminating bacteria.[10,19] These materials have excellent workability and knot security, however. Because of the properties just mentioned, braided sutures are useful on the face, where maximal control and precision are needed. The earlier removal time for facial sutures and the natural resistance of the face to infection make the chances of developing inflammation and infection almost negligible.

NEEDLE TYPES

Similar to instruments and suture materials, a bewildering array of needles is manufactured for wound closure. Most wound closures can be accomplished, however, with a few needles. Curved needles have two basic configurations: tapered and cutting (Fig. 8-7). For wound and laceration care, the cutting needle is used almost exclusively. Needles that now are commonly referred to as cutting needles are reverse cutting needles. The needle is made in such a way that the outer edge is sharp so as to allow for smooth and atraumatic penetration of the skin, and the inner portion is flattened so that the needle puncture wound is not inadvertently enlarged when the suture is passed through the hole and the knot is tied.

Needles come in two grades: cuticular and plastic. These grades differ significantly in their usefulness for wound care. Cuticular needles are less expensive but are noticeably less sharp than plastic-grade needles. The increased sharpness of plastic needles allows the operator better to control entry and passage of the needle through tissues. Plastic needles also are less traumatic. Although they are more expensive, these needles are recommended for emergency wound and laceration repair. There is a bewildering number of code designations for needles. Cuticular needles can be

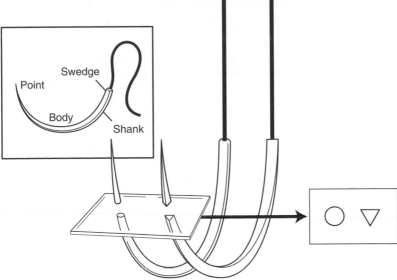

Figure 8-7. Basic needle configurations: The standard round, tapered needle *(left)*; the reverse cutting needle *(right)*. The sharp edge is on the convex portion of the needle.

recognized by the letters *C* (cuticular) or *FS* (for skin). Plastic-grade needle codes usually start with the letter *P*.

References

1. Shetty PC, Dicksheet S, Scalea TM: Emergency department repair of hand lacerations using absorbable vicryl sutures, *J Emerg Med* 15:673–674, 1997.
2. Parell GJ, Becker GD: Comparison of absorbable with nonabsorbable sutures in closure of facial skin wounds, *Arch Facial Plast Surg* 5:488–490, 2003.
3. Missori P, Polli FM, Fontana E, et al: Closure of skin or scalp with absorbable sutures, *Plast Recon Surg* 112:924–925, 2003.
4. Luck RP, Flood R, Eyal D, et al: Cosmetic outcomes of absorbable versus nonabsorbable sutures in pediatric facial lacerations, *Pediatr Emerg Care* 24:137–142, 2008.
5. Holger JS, Wandersee SC, Hale DB: Cosmetic outcomes of facial lacerations repaired with tissue-adhesive, absorbable, and nonabsorbable sutures, *Am J Emerg Med* 22:254–257, 2003.
6. Karounis H, Gouin S, Eisman H, et al: A randomized, controlled trial comparing long-term cosmetic outcomes of traumatic pediatric lacerations repaired with absorbable plain gut versus nonabsorbable nylon sutures, *Acad Emerg Med* 11:730–735, 2004.
7. Collin TW, Blyth K, Hodgkinson PD: Cleft lip repair without suture removal, *J Plast Reconstr Aesthet Surg* 62:1161–1165, 2009.
8. Tandon SC, Kelly J, Turtle M, Irwin ST: Irradiated polyglactin 910: a new synthetic absorbable suture, *J R Coll Surg Edinb* 40:185–187, 1995.
9. Bourne RB, Bitar H, Andreae PR: In vivo comparison of four absorbable sutures: Vicryl, Dexon Plus, Maxon, and PDS, *Can J Surg* 31:43–45, 1988.
10. Edlich R, Panek PH, Rodeheaver GT, et al: Physical and chemical configuration of sutures in the development of surgical infection, *Ann Surg* 177:679–687, 1973.
11. Howes E: Strength studies of polyglycolic acid versus catgut sutures of the same size, *Surg Gynecol Obstet* 137:15–20, 1973.
12. Swanson N, Tromovitch T: Suture materials, 1980s: properties, uses, and abuses, *Int J Dermatol* 21:373–378, 1982.
13. Holt G, Holt J: Suture materials and techniques, *Ear Nose Throat J* 60:23–30, 1981.
14. Rodeheaver GT, Powell TA, Thacker TJ, et al: Mechanical performance of monofilament synthetic absorbable sutures, *Am J Surg* 154:544–547, 1987.

15. Hochberg J, Meyer KM, Marion MD: Suture choice and other methods of skin closure, *Surg Clin North Am* 89:627–641, 2009.
16. Niessen FB, Spauwen PH, Kon M: The role of suture material in hypertrophic scar formation: Monocryl vs. Vicryl-Rapide, *Ann Plast Surg* 39:254–260, 1997.
17. Bernstein G: Polybutester suture, *J Dermatol Surg* 14:615–616, 1988.
18. Trimbos JB, Smeets M, Verdel M, Hermans J: Cosmetic result of lower midline laparotomy wounds: polybutester and nylon skin suture in a randomized clinical trial, *Obstet Gynecol* 82:390–393, 1993.
19. Alexander J, Kaplan J, Altemeier W: Role of suture materials in the development of wound infection, *Ann Surg* 165:192–199, 1967.

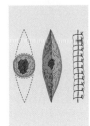

CHAPTER 9

Decisions before Closure: Timing, Débridement, and Consultation

---

Key Practice Points

- Because wounds are often contaminated with bacteria, there is a time limit (the "golden period") between the laceration and closure with sutures. It varies between 6 hours (hand and feet) and 24 hours for the vascular face.
- Wounds outside the "golden period" can heal by secondary intention or by delayed primary closure.
- Whenever suspicion exists that a wound has injured a tendon, nerve, joint, or other important anatomic structure, or has been caused by a foreign body, the wound should be explored before repair.
- Because blood vessels often run in bundles with nerves, the use of "blind" clamping with a hemostat to achieve hemostasis is strongly discouraged. Most hemostasis in wound care can be achieved with pressure alone.
- Some contamination requires sharp débridement and excision of foreign material, to lower the risk of infection, before the wound can be closed.
- If débridement is necessary, it is important to sacrifice as little tissue as possible.
- Wound drains can act as an ingress of bacteria and should be avoided unless there is active drainage, such as in the case of an abscess.

Before proceeding with definitive management, such as suture placement, several issues have to be considered and decisions made that are separate from the choice of closure method. Time from the injury, tissue condition, level of contamination, and potential for foreign material all are factors that affect the total care. Planning the care and closure is as important as the repair itself.

TIMING OF CLOSURE

Determining the time of injury is important for wound repair. The chance of developing a wound infection increases with each hour that elapses from the time of injury.[1] Traditionally, it has been taught that there is a "golden period" within which a wound or laceration can be safely closed primarily (primary intention). The exact length of that period is influenced by factors such as the mechanism of injury, anatomic location, and level of contamination. As a rough guideline, 6 to 8 hours from the time of injury has been considered a safe interval within which to repair the average uncomplicated laceration. This period can range from 6 hours for wounds of the hand and foot to

24 hours or more for clean lacerations of the face. The following is a summary including recommendations for wound closure.

Primary Closure (Primary Intention)

Lacerations that are relatively clean and uncontaminated, with minimal tissue loss or devitalization, are considered for primary closure. These can be caused by sharp-edged objects such as knives (common injury during food preparation) and glass. Repair of these wounds usually is necessary within 6 to 8 hours from the time of injury on most regions of the body. Wounds of the highly vascular face and scalp often can be sutured 24 hours after injury.[2] Because there are no definitive rules that govern every possible situation, the following recommendation is offered: Any injury, less than 24 hours from time from injury, that can be converted with cleansing and débridement to a fresh-appearing, slightly bleeding, nondevitalized wound, with no visible contamination or debris after aggressive cleansing, irrigation, and débridement, can be considered for primary closure.

Secondary Closure (Secondary Intention)

Skin ulcerations, abscess cavities, punctures, small cosmetically unimportant animal bites, and partial-thickness (abrasions, second-degree burns) tissue losses often are better left to heal by secondary intention. Wound care consists of thorough cleansing, irrigation, and débridement of devitalized or contaminant-impregnated tissue. These wounds are not closed with sutures and are allowed to heal gradually by granulation and eventual reepithelialization. They heal best if covered with a sterile, nonadherent dressing that can be changed every 1 to 3 days.

Tertiary Closure (Delayed Primary Closure)

Some wounds are candidates for delayed closure.[3] Bite wounds and lacerations beyond the golden period can be considered for this technique. Although there are no technical contraindications to sutures or staples, these wounds have a high bacterial count and excessive devitalized tissue. In a study of human bites to the face, primary closure led to a 40% wound infection rate.[4] None of the wounds closed after débridement and 48 hours of antibiotics became infected. Delayed wounds can be "converted" to "fresh" ones by cleansing, irrigation, and débridement followed by a 3-day to 5-day period during which the natural host defenses reduce the bacterial load to acceptable minimal levels (Fig. 9-1).[3,5] Antibiotics can aid these defenses.

Technique for Delayed Primary Closure

The clinician cleanses, irrigates, and débrides as much as possible during the initial encounter. The wound is covered with a bulky, absorbent gauze dressing. Oral antibiotics are administered after initial care before delayed closure. Dicloxacillin or a first-generation cephalosporin is appropriate. Erythromycin or clindamycin can be administered to patients who have a significant history of allergy to the penicillins. Amoxicillin/clavulanate can be used for bite wounds.

If no signs of infection or excessive discomfort develop beforehand, the patient should return in 4 to 5 days. If the wound appears clean and uninfected, it can be closed with sutures, tapes, or staples. Dermal (deep) or subcutaneous sutures are avoided in this setting. These wounds can accumulate excessive granulation tissue during the 4-day to 5-day period. This tissue can be excised judiciously to permit better wound edge apposition. The intervals for suture or staple removal are the same as for primary closure starting at the time of closure. Delayed closure is associated with a low (2% to 3%) infection rate.[5,6]

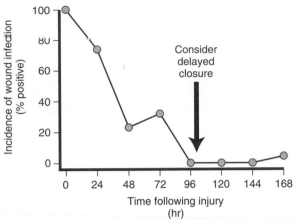

Figure 9-1. Graph showing the incidence of wound infection risk after injury and optimal timing of tertiary or delayed wound closure. (Adapted from Edlich R, Rodeheaver GT, Morgan RF, et al: *A manual for wound closure,* St Paul, Minn, 1979, Surgical Products Division, 3M.)

WOUND EXPLORATION

Some surface wounds and lacerations require thorough inspection and exploration. It is always important to evaluate the functional status of the relevant nerves, tendons, arteries, joints, and other related structures of the wounded area and to remain alert for potentially occult, serious underlying structural damage. Although more specific information is included in other chapters and sections specific to special anatomic sites and problems, the following are general guidelines for wound exploration:

- Suspicion of a foreign body, particularly if it is potentially organic, such as wood or plant material. Radiographs are taken before exploration when glass, gravel, or metallic foreign bodies are suspected.
- Lacerations in the proximity of joint capsules.
- Lacerations over tendons, particularly if functional testing of the hand or foot is "normal." It is common to find serious partial tendon lacerations solely by direct visualization. Unrepaired partially lacerated (≥50%) tendons can undergo delayed rupture within 12 to 48 hours if untreated.
- Scalp lacerations that are large or are caused by a significant force. Unrecognized skull fractures can be found by exploration and palpation of the skull through the wound.
- Lip lacerations, if a tooth or fragment of a tooth cannot be accounted for. A radiograph is another method to reveal missing teeth.

Techniques for Wound Exploration

Often the wound can be exposed adequately with a hemostat by separation of the wound edges. In other cases, the hemostat can be used to grasp the superficial fascia (subcutaneous tissue) of one wound edge while the tissue forceps are applied to the other edge to retract and gain exposure. If available, small self-restraining retractors (mastoid or Wheatlander retractors) are recommended. A second pair of hands is optimal. An assistant can retract the wound with small retractors or skin hooks.

If exposure is still not adequate, a small wound extension incision can be made through the dermis with a knife handle and a no. 15 blade or with iris scissors. The extension begins at one wound end and should proceed carefully to avoid accidental

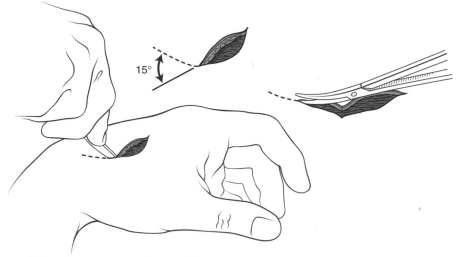

Figure 9-2. Technique to extend a wound for better deep-structure exploration and evaluation. The incision is at a slight angle from the original axis of the wound and is parallel to underlying structures.

injury to underlying structures (Fig. 9-2). On the face, extension incisions are made parallel to the skin tension lines discussed in Chapter 3. When the epidermis and dermis are divided, the superficial fascia (subcutaneous tissue) is not incised but is spread apart gently with forceps or tissue scissors to reveal any suspected foreign body or tendon or joint capsule injury.

HEMOSTASIS

Wounds often bleed actively, particularly during assessment and exploration. In addition to the problem of adequate wound visualization with active bleeding, hematomas can cause an increase in the rate of wound infection and can delay the healing process.[7]

The simplest and most effective way to stop bleeding is to apply direct pressure to the wound with handheld surgical 4 × 4 sponges. Continuous pressure has to be applied for a minimum of 10 minutes. Because of the time involved, sponges secured with an Ace wrap can be substituted if the wound is in an anatomic area that lends itself to wrapping.

An epinephrine-moistened (1:100,000) sponge applied, also with pressure, to the wound for 5 minutes often suffices in cases in which direct pressure fails. Epinephrine is contraindicated, however, for use on the fingers, toes, ears, penis, and tip of the nose. Packing the wound with topical hemostatic agents, such as Gelfoam, Surgicel, and others, is another hemostatic strategy. These agents are useful for persistent oozing or minor capillary bleeding. Arterial "pumpers," even small ones, can wash these agents out of the wound. Use of these agents should be considered only if all other methods fail. These products can have adverse effects such as interference with suture closure and foreign-body reactions.[8]

Direct clamping with a hemostat and a hand-tied ligature with an absorbable suture is reserved for larger, single-bleeding vessels that can be directly visualized under optimal conditions of lighting, instrument preparation, and operator comfort. Because blood vessels often travel with nerves and arteries, "blind" clamping in a bleeding wound, in the hope of grasping the bleeder, is strongly discouraged. Unnecessary tissue damage can occur, particularly in areas where important structures such as nerves and tendons are likely to be found.

Tourniquet Hemostasis

Definitive hemostasis of the extremity can be achieved by the use of tourniquets. Strict observance of proper technique and the time limits of application is imperative. Complications of tourniquets include ischemia of the extremity, compression damage of blood vessels and nerves, and jeopardy to marginally viable tissues.[9]

Technique for Large-Extremity Tourniquet Application

Before placing a single-cuff sphygmomanometer, the extremity is elevated for approximately 1 minute.[10] The cuff is inflated to a pressure higher than the patient's systolic pressure or to a point when the bleeding stops. However, the pressure should not exceed 250 mm Hg. The clinician clamps the cuff tubing with a hemostat instead of closing the air release valve to prevent slow leakage of air and to ensure a rapid release method if needed. Patient discomfort becomes apparent by 30 to 45 minutes of cuff time.[11] The maximal cuff inflation time is 2 hours, although a limit of 30 to 60 minutes is recommended to ensure patient safety.

Technique for Digital Tourniquet Application

A digital tourniquet is often used to repair finger wounds. Lacerated fingers can bleed profusely and visualization is difficult. The clinician unfolds a 4 × 4 gauze sponge to its fullest length and folds it in half so it appears to be an 8-inch band. The band is moistened with saline. The clinician wraps the band firmly around the finger, starting at the tip and proceeding to the base. A Penrose drain is stretched around the base of the finger in a slinglike fashion, and a hemostat is applied to the drain to form a tight "ring" at the base of the finger. The sponge wrapping is removed. A Penrose drain also can be substituted for the gauze sponge wrap. A digital anesthetic block is recommended before applying the tourniquet.

There are preformed disposable tourniquets (Tourni-Cot, T-Ring) that "roll" or slide onto the finger and exsanguinate it before coming to rest at the digit base (Fig. 9-3). After use, they can be easily removed. These tourniquets are easier to apply and are effective in most cases in which the digit circumference can accommodate them. The maximal allowable tourniquet time for a finger is 20 to 30 minutes.

TISSUE DÉBRIDEMENT AND EXCISION

Before actual suturing and knot tying, the wound has to be made free of contaminants and devitalized tissue.[12] Devitalized tissue can be recognized by its shredded, ischemic, or blue-black appearance. Occasionally, these appearances can be misleading, and true demarcation between viable and devitalized skin cannot be made until 24 hours after wounding.[13] One overriding principle of wound débridement is to spare as much skin, epidermis, and dermis as possible immediately after the injury, particularly for the face and hand. Subcutaneous fat can be liberally débrided. Revision of the complex wound can be made at later interventions by consultant surgeons. The surgeons will be grateful if as much preserved skin as possible is left at the wound site.

Static skin tension plays an important role in wound edge débridement and revision. It is tempting to excise jagged wound edges to convert an irregular laceration into a straight one. If the wound is already gaping because of static tension, débridement of tissue increases the tension necessary to pull the new edges together. The resulting scar might be wider and more noticeable than it would have been by piecing together the original irregular edges.

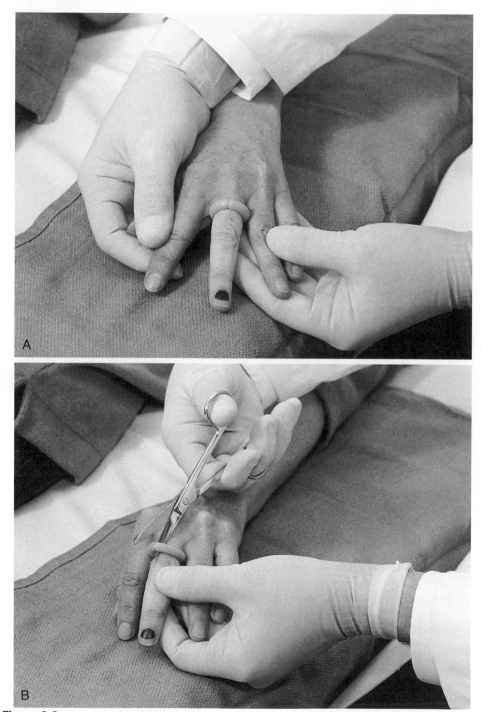

Figure 9-3. Tourniquet hemostasis for finger injuries. **A,** The tourniquet is placed on the finger by rolling it from the nail to the base of the digit. **B,** To avoid disturbing the repaired wound, the tourniquet is removed by cutting it off with scissors.

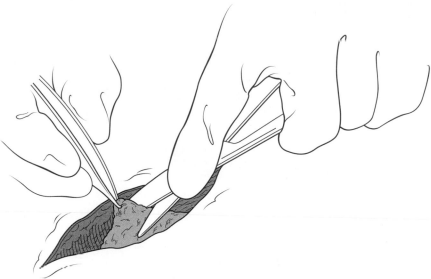

Figure 9-4. Technique to débride deep dermis and superficial fascia (subcutaneous fat).

Technique for Simple Excision and Wound Edge Revision

Most débridement can be performed by simple, minimal excision of debris-laden tissue bits, using tissue forceps and iris scissors (Fig. 9-4). Superficial fascia (subcutaneous fat) under the skin can be freely excised without concern for deleterious cosmetic results. Soiled, devitalized fatty tissue is a fertile substrate for the growth of bacteria with subsequent development of infection.[14] More care has to be taken in débriding and excising epidermis and dermis. The best principle is to trim as little skin as possible, particularly on the face and hand. It is preferable to repair wound edges in a jigsaw-like pattern than to excise the irregular edges only to be left with a wound under excessive tension.

The proper method to trim a dermal wound edge is shown in Figure 9-5. Iris (tissue) scissors or a no. 15 blade can be used. The wound edge is cut or incised at a slight angle so that the epidermal surface of the skin edge juts out slightly farther than the dermal portion. In this manner, when the wound is closed, it naturally everts with the proper suture placement technique and resulting suture loop configuration.

Technique for Full Wound Excision

Full wound excisions are reserved for injuries in which all wound edges are devitalized and are obviously impossible to salvage. There also must be sufficient tissue redundancy in the anatomic location of the wound. If redundancy is inadequate, excision creates a gap or defect that can be closed only under excessive tension. Areas where there is sufficient tissue to accommodate excision include the chest, abdomen, arms, and thighs. Whenever there is doubt about this procedure, it is best to consult a surgical specialist.

The clinician uses the scalpel with a no. 15 blade to outline the tissue to be removed by partially incising or "scoring" the dermis (Fig. 9-6). Generally the excision is lenticular (i.e., shaped like an ellipse). To achieve proper closure without excessive tension or creating tissue "humps" at either end of the wound, the length of the ellipse should exceed the width by at least a 3:1 ratio. When the ellipse is defined, the clinician uses the scalpel or iris scissors, or both in combination, to complete the excision (Fig. 9-7). The

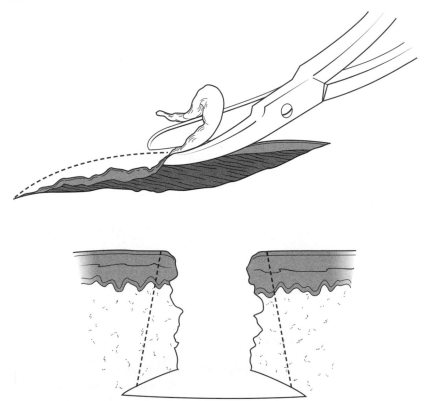

Figure 9-5. Technique for excision by careful tissue scissor trimming of devitalized epidermis and dermis. Note the angle of excision, which facilitates wound edge eversion during percutaneous closure.

wound edges are incised at the same angle as described for dermal edge trimming. Not only do the edges have to be excised, but also the excised tissue has to be released from its base in the superficial fascia (subcutaneous tissue). Considerable bleeding often ensues, and hemostatic measures may have to be used before proceeding to closure. Excisions usually require deep (dermal) and percutaneous sutures for closure.

SURGICAL DRAINS

Surgical drains for emergency wound care are controversial. Drains can act as retrograde conduits for contaminating bacteria from either the wound or the skin. Under experimental wound conditions, subinfective inocula of bacteria have been shown to greatly increase the infection rate in drained versus undrained control wounds.[15] For this reason, they should be used only for wounds in which the benefit clearly outweighs the risk. Drains are indicated to remove large collections of pus or blood or to assist in eliminating large pockets of dead space. As a general rule, wounds that can be managed in an emergency department do not need drains.

IMMEDIATE ANTIBIOTIC THERAPY

For uncomplicated wounds and lacerations, including wounds in key structures such as tendons, there is no good clinical or investigative evidence that systemic antibiotics provide protection against the development of wound infection.[16-18] Occasionally, however, the physician is faced with a wound or laceration that necessitates the

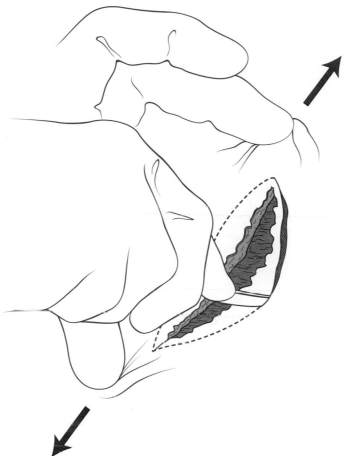

Figure 9-6. Technique for incising or "scoring" the epidermis and dermis before full wound excision. The fingers are used to provide tension to the skin and to the axis of the wound. This tension facilitates easier application of the scalpel to the skin.

consideration of immediate antibiotic coverage during or even before wound management itself. Under these conditions, there is experimental evidence that antibiotic action rapidly decreases in effectiveness if it is not initiated within 3 to 4 hours of the injury.[1] If prophylactic antibiotics are thought necessary by the physician, they need to be administered without delay by the intravenous route. The following are situations in which the immediate administration of intravenous antibiotics should be considered:

- Complex or mutilating wounds, especially of the hand or foot (e.g., lawnmower or chainsaw injuries)
- Grossly contaminated wounds with penetrating debris and "ground-in" foreign material
- Lacerations in areas of lymphatic obstruction and lymphedema
- Extensive lacerations of the ear and its cartilaginous skeleton
- Suspected penetration of bone (open fractures), joints, or tendons
- Amputation injuries, especially where replantation is a consideration
- Extensive or distal extremity animal bite wounds (see Chapter 15)

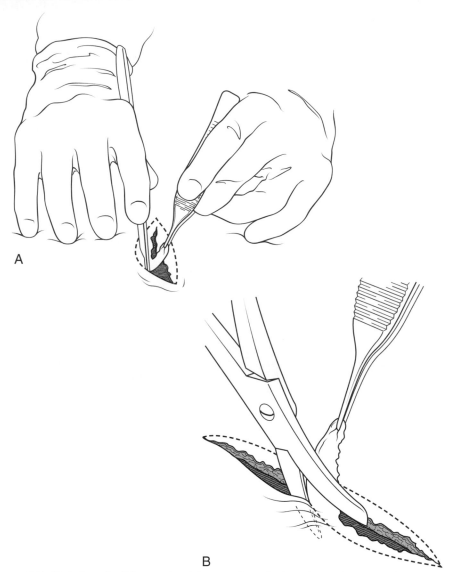

Figure 9-7. Technique for full wound excision. **A,** The scalpel can be used to excise the wound in its entirety. **B,** Tissue scissors can be used to follow the original wound outline created by the "scoring" of the epidermis and dermis with the scalpel blade.

- Significant lacerations in patients with preexisting valvular heart disease
- Presence of disease or drugs causing immunosuppression or altered host defenses (e.g., diabetes)

The initial intravenous antibiotic of choice is usually a first-generation cephalosporin, such as cefazolin (Kefzol, Ancef). For penicillin-allergic patients, ciprofloxacin and clindamycin are reasonable alternatives. For animal bites, the recommended agents are discussed in Chapter 15. It is recommended that a wound culture be taken, before initiation of antibiotics, to assist in later modification of therapy if necessary.

GUIDELINES FOR CONSULTATION

Inevitably, physicians are faced with wounds, lacerations, and related problems that cause them to consider consulting a specialist. There are no definitive rules governing consultations. Because there are many different circumstances under which a consultation might be considered, it is impossible to make comprehensive recommendations. In addition, each emergency physician has his or her own level of expertise, experience, and comfort. The following guidelines are based on practice realities governing emergency care.

Standard of Care

Driven largely by the legal system, medical care often is defined in terms of some standard. In the case of wound care, emergency physicians often are held to the same standard of care as might be practiced by a surgical specialist. In reality, there is no fixed standard for any specialty or type of care. Through board certification, emergency physicians are qualified to provide emergency wound care. The "practice" line between an emergency physician and a surgical specialist is blurred, however. Each practitioner of wound care has to understand his or her strengths and limitations and has to act accordingly. It also is important to have knowledge of community-defined patterns of care. In some locales, only specialists perform tendon repairs, whereas in others, emergency physicians comfortably treat extensor tendon lacerations.

Logistics of Care

Certain wounds technically can be managed by emergency physicians, but the time necessary to close the wound would significantly impede the operation of the emergency department. If direct physician involvement time exceeds 30 minutes, consultation might be considered.

Cosmetics and Patient Expectation

Patients or family members often have expectations that "specialists" need to be involved in the care and repair of wounds. Parents frequently request a "plastic" surgeon for their child's facial laceration. If the emergency caregiver can repair the laceration confidently, most parents can be made comfortable with a clear explanation of the actual repair needed and the skills of the caregiver. Some patients or relatives are fixed on the need for a specialist, however. Usually, it is best to accede to those wishes.

Continuity of Care

Certain wounds, particularly wounds of the hand, require close follow-up and rehabilitation. It may be best to involve a specialist in the initial care to ensure continuity. It is a common arrangement between emergency physicians and hand specialists to have the emergency physician do the primary closure with follow-up care going to the specialist. Specific circumstances include uncomplicated injuries to tendon or digital nerves. The emergency physician does the initial injury assessment and skin closure. The specialist can follow the patient and can schedule a delayed repair of the tendon or nerve. This collaboration can be extremely successful and is built on trust between the different caregivers.

References

1. Robson M, Duke W, Krizek T: Rapid bacterial screening in treatment of civilian wounds, *J Surg Res* 14:426–430, 1973.
2. Losken HW, Auchinloss JA: Human bites of the lip, *Clin Plast Surg* 11:159–161, 1984.
3. Dimick AR: Delayed wound closure: indications and techniques, *Ann Emerg Med* 17:1303–1304, 1988.

 4. Stierman KL, Lloyd KM, De Luca-Pytell DM, et al: Treatment and outcome of human bites in the head and neck, *Otolaryngol Head Neck Surg* 128:795–801, 2003.
 5. Bender JS: Factors influencing outcome in delayed primary closure of contaminated abdominal wounds: a prospective analysis of 181 consecutive patients, *Am Surg* 69:252–255, 2003.
 6. Smilanich RP, Bonnet I, Kirkpatrick JR: Contaminated wounds: the effect of initial management on outcome, *Am Surg* 61:427–430, 1995.
 7. Altemeier W: Principles in the management of traumatic wounds and infection control, *Bull N Y Acad Med* 55:123–138, 1979.
 8. Palm MD, Altman JS: Topical hemostatic agents: a review, *Dermatol Surg* 34:431–445, 2008.
 9. Lammers RL: Principles of wound management. In Roberts JR, Hedges JR, editors: *Clinical procedures in emergency medicine*, Philadelphia, 1985, WB Saunders.
10. Edlich RF, Rodeheaver GT, Thacker JG, et al: Revolutionary advances in the management of traumatic wounds in the emergency department during the last 40 years: part 1, *J Emerg Med* 20:1–11, 2008.
11. Roberts JR: Intravenous regional anesthesia, *JACEP* 6:261–265, 1977.
12. Haury B, Rodeheaver GT, Vensko J, et al: Debridement: an essential component of wound care, *Am J Surg* 135:238–242, 1978.
13. Edlich RF, Rodeheaver GT, Morgan RF, et al: Principles of emergency wound management, *Ann Emerg Med* 17:1284–1302, 1988.
14. Haughey R, Lammers R, Wagner D: Use of antibiotics in the initial management of soft tissue hand wounds, *Ann Emerg Med* 10:187–192, 1981.
15. Magee C, Rodeheaver GT, Golden GT, et al: Potentiation of wound infection by surgical drains, *Am J Surg* 131:547–549, 1976.
16. Gravante G, Caruso R, Araco A, et al: Infections after plastic procedures: incidences, etiologies, risk factors and antibiotics, *Aesthet Plast Surg* 32:243–251, 2008.
17. Landes G, Harris PG, Lemaine V, et al: Prevention of surgical site infection and appropriateness of antibiotic habits in plastic surgery, *J Plast Reconstr Aesthet Surg* 61:1347–1356, 2008.
18. Zehtabchi S: Evidence-based emergency/critically appraised topic: the role of antibiotic prophylaxis for prevention of infection in patients with simple hand lacerations, *Ann Emerg Med* 49:682–689, 2007.

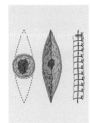

CHAPTER 10
Basic Laceration Repair: Principles and Techniques

Key Practice Points

- Applying the principles of wound closure is key to acceptable wound and scar appearance.
- Matching the layers of the wound surfaces with sutures is critical to scar appearance.
- Because scar tissue contracts over time, wound edge eversion prevents "pitting" of the scar and eliminates a poor result.
- Excessive wound tension, caused by sutures placed too tightly, can cause ischemia of the edges and an increased amount of scar tissue.
- Deep sutures become foreign material when buried in a wound. Placing as few deep sutures as possible is recommended to reduce the risk of infection and the risk of an increase in the amount of scar tissue.
- "Dead" space is created when the skin of deep wounds is closed without deep or subcutaneous sutures to eliminate the dead space.
- The final sutured wound should have all of the knots aligned to one side of the wound. This appearance inspires confidence in the patient and, more important, prevents the knots from interfering with laceration healing.

Each wound and laceration has technical requirements that have to be met to repair a wound effectively. By understanding the basic principles that underlie the technical requisites of wound care, lacerations and wounds can be closed with the best chance for an optimal result. During actual closure, every attempt is made to match each layer evenly and to produce a wound edge that is properly everted. Proper knot-tying technique is paramount to facilitate eversion and to prevent excessive tension on the wound edge. When necessary, dead space is closed, and finally, sutures are spaced and sequenced to provide the best and most gentle mechanical support.

DEFINITION OF TERMS

Several techniques and maneuvers used in wound care are referred to by terms that can be confusing. These terms are defined so that the reader thoroughly understands the material contained in this chapter.

- *Bite:* A bite is the amount of tissue taken when placing the suture needle in the skin or fascia. The farther away from the wound edge that the needle is introduced into the epidermis, the bigger the bite.
- *Throw:* Each suture knot consists of a series of throws. A square knot is fashioned with two throws. Because of nylon's tendency to unravel, several additional throws are necessary to secure the final knot when this material is used.

- *Percutaneous closure (skin closure):* Sutures, usually of a nonabsorbable material, which are placed in skin with the knot tied on the surface, are called percutaneous closures. They also are referred to as skin closures. Recent clinical studies have shown that, in certain circumstances such as lacerations of the face and fingertip, absorbable sutures can be used to close skin.[1,2]
- *Dermal closure (deep closure):* Sutures, usually of an absorbable material, which are placed in the superficial (subcutaneous) fascia and dermis with the knot buried in the wound, are called deep closures.
- *Interrupted closure:* Single sutures, tied separately, whether deep or percutaneous, are called interrupted sutures.
- *Continuous closure (running suture):* A wound closure accomplished by taking several bites that are the full length of the wound, without tying individual knots, is a continuous or running suture. Knots are tied only at the beginning and at the end of the closure to secure the suture material. Continuous closures can be percutaneous or deep.

BASIC KNOT-TYING TECHNIQUES

Several knots can be used to tie sutures during wound closure. The most common is the surgeon's knot (Fig. 10-1). The advantage of this knot is that the double first throw offers better knot security, and there is less slipping of the suture material as the wound is gently pulled together during tying. The wound edges remain apposed while the second and subsequent single throws are accomplished. The knot-tying sequence shown in Figure 10-1 illustrates the proper instrument technique required to obtain a surgeon's knot. The instrument tie can be used for almost all knots, whether for deep or superficial closures.

PRINCIPLES OF WOUND CLOSURE

Layer Matching

When closing a laceration, it is important to match each layer of a wound edge to its counterpart. Superficial fascia has to meet superficial fascia. Dermis to dermis necessarily brings epidermis to epidermis. Failure to appose layers meticulously can cause improper healing with an unnecessarily large scar (Fig. 10-2).

Wound Edge Eversion

Just as important as layer matching is proper wound edge eversion during the initial repair. Because of the normal tendency of scars to contract with time, a wound edge slightly raised above the plane of the normal skin gradually flattens with healing and has a final appearance that is cosmetically acceptable (Fig. 10-3). Wounds that are not everted contract into linear pits that become noticeable cosmetic defects because of their tendency to cast shadows.

Techniques for Wound Edge Eversion

The key to achieving proper wound edge eversion is to use the correct technique for introducing the needle into the skin and for producing the proper suture configuration. As illustrated in Figure 10-4, the point of the needle should pierce the epidermis and dermis at a 90-degree angle before it is curved around through the tissues. To ensure a 90-degree angle, the needle holder has to be held in the manner described in Chapter 8. It is mechanically difficult to maneuver the needle correctly if the operator's fingers remain in the finger rings of the needle holder. Figure 10-4 illustrates the correct and incorrect final configuration of an interrupted suture to achieve wound edge eversion.

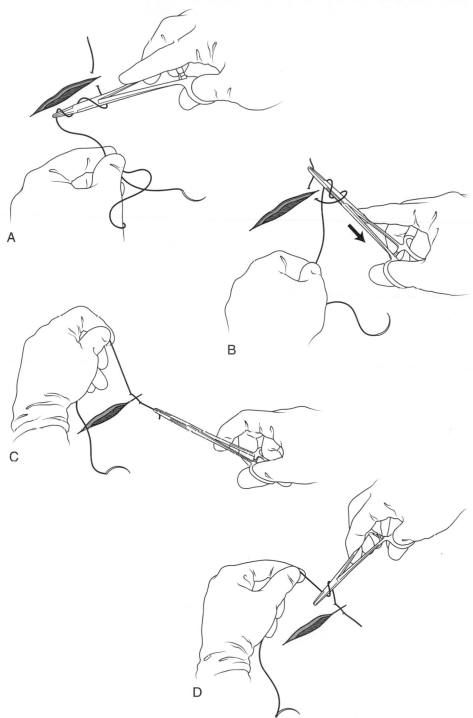

Figure 10-1. **A-G,** Sequence for instrument tie of a standard percutaneous suture closure. Note the surgeon's knot and final square knot configuration in the inset illustration in **G.**

Continued

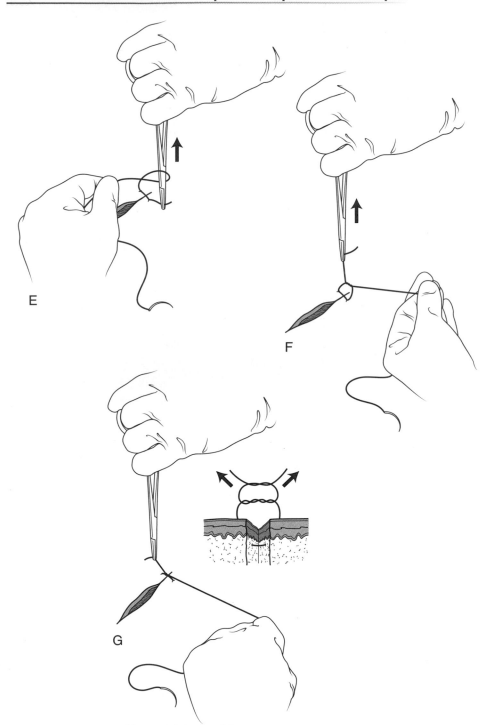

Figure 10-1, cont'd. For legend, see previous page.

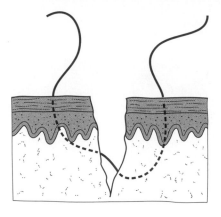

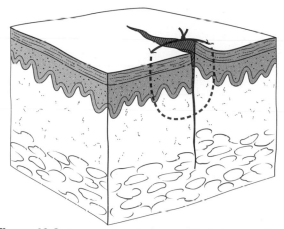

Figure 10-2. Incorrect technique to provide for layer matching.

Vertical Mattress Suture

Another useful method for wound edge eversion is the vertical mattress suture. This suture is placed by first taking a large bite of tissue approximately 1 to 1.5 cm away from the wound edge and crossing through the tissue to an equal distance on the opposite side of the wound. The needle is reversed and returned for a small bite (1 or 2 mm) at the epidermal/dermal edge to approximate closely the epidermal layer (Fig. 10-5). The vertical mattress suture is helpful in areas of lax skin (e.g., elbow, dorsum of hand), where the wound edges tend to fall or fold into the wound. Another advantage of the vertical mattress suture is that it can act as a deep and a superficial closure all in one suture. Some wounds are not deep enough to accommodate a separate, absorbable suture but still need some deep support to close dead space. This technique can meet that need.

A modification of the vertical mattress suture, the shorthand technique, allows the suture to be placed more rapidly.[3] Instead of taking the large bite first, as described earlier, the small bite is taken, then the large one. By placing simultaneous traction on

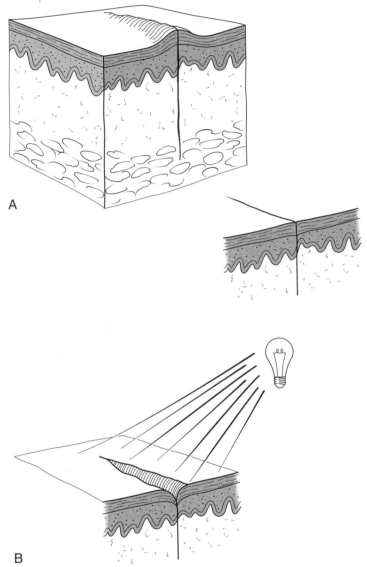

Figure 10-3. Wound edge eversion. **A,** Correct technique allows for a slight rise of the wound edges above the skin plane. These edges eventually contract to flatten out at the skin plane. **B,** Wound edges that are not properly everted contract below the skin plane and allow incident light to cause unsightly shadows.

the trailing and leading portions of the suture after the small bite, the wound edges are elevated so that the needle easily takes the large bite.

Horizontal Mattress Suture

Another technique, the horizontal mattress suture, can be used to achieve wound edge eversion (Fig. 10-6). The needle is introduced into the skin in the usual manner and is brought out at the opposite side of the wound. A second bite is taken approximately 0.5 cm adjacent to the first exit and is brought back to the original starting

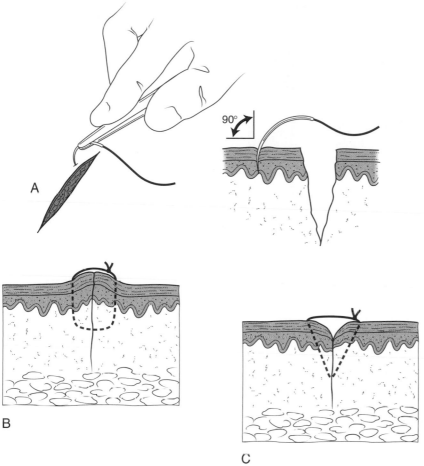

Figure 10-4. Technique for proper wound edge eversion. **A,** The suture needle is introduced at a 90-degree angle to the epidermis. **B,** The proper configuration of the suture should be square or bottle shaped. This configuration is difficult to achieve in practice; however, this figure illustrates the correct principle. **C,** The incorrect technique of needle placement and suture configuration leads to wound edge inversion, which leads to "pitting" of the eventual scar.

edge, also 0.5 cm from the initial entry point. The knot is tied, leaving an everted edge. This is a suture technique often used in closing hand (palm and dorsum) lacerations.

Wound Tension

Whenever wound edges are brought together by suturing, there is inevitable tension and pressure created in the tissue within the suture loop. It is important to minimize tension to preserve capillary blood flow to the wound edge. Excessive force exerted on the tissue leads to ischemia and can cause some degree of cellular necrosis.[4] Necrosis provokes a more intense inflammatory response with the eventual formation of an irregular, cosmetically unacceptable scar. When tying knots, the first throw is crucial. As the wound edges are brought together, they are allowed just barely to touch. Bringing the edges together more forcibly by making the first throw too tight promotes

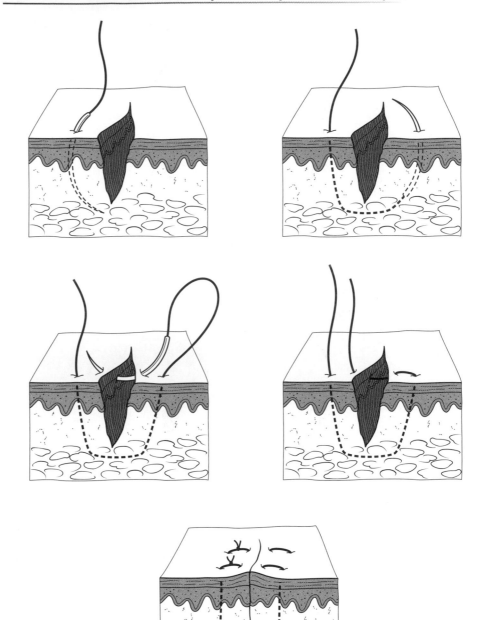

Figure 10-5. Technique for a vertical mattress suture. The second bite barely passes through the dermis to provide meticulous apposition of the epidermal edges.

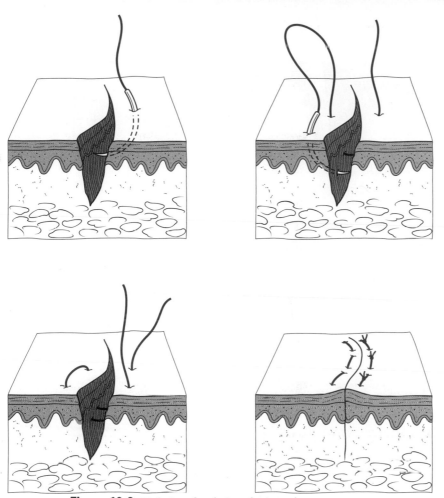

Figure 10-6. Technique for placing a horizontal mattress suture.

ischemia. Wound edges tend to become slightly edematous after repair; a small amount of slack between them disappears. The addition of edema to a suture line that already is too tight can be disastrous.

Techniques for Reducing Wound Tension
Deep Closures
Proper placement of deep closures to bring the dermis close together before suture closure reduces final wound edge tension. Figure 10-7 illustrates the method for placing and tying deep closures. To start this suture, the needle is introduced into the superficial fascia, close to the underside of the dermis. Then the needle is brought up through the dermis. At this point, the needle has to be rearmed with the needle holder. The needle is introduced into the dermis of the matching opposite wound edge and is carried down into the superficial fascia to complete the second bite.

Crucial to this technique is that the trailing and leading portions of the suture remain on the same side of the portion of the suture that crosses from dermis to dermis.

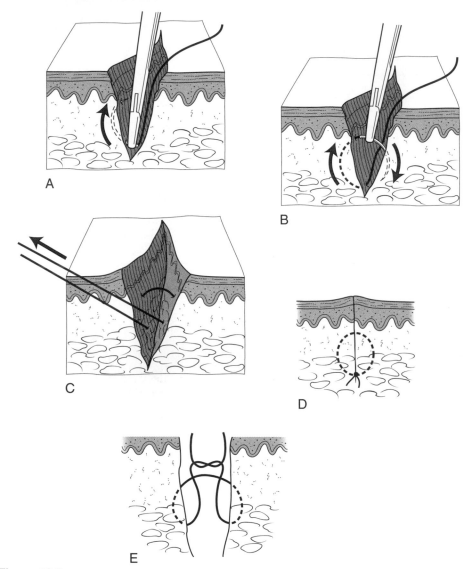

Figure 10-7. Technique for placing a deep suture. **A,** Suture placement is initiated by driving the needle from deep in the wound to superficial. **B,** The needle is driven superficial to deep on the opposite side of the wound. **C,** The leading and trailing sutures come out on the same side of the cross suture. **D,** This same-side technique allows for the knot to be tied deep and away from the wound surface. **E,** If the same-side technique is not followed, the knot is forced to the wound surface by the cross suture and may protrude out of the wound.

In this manner, when the knot is tied, it is buried. If the trailing edges are on opposite sides of the dermal crossing, the knot is pushed superficially and interferes with epidermal healing. Three or four throws are adequate to secure the knot, and the suture ends are cut close to the knot itself, leaving no more than 2-mm "tails." The temptation to place numerous deep closures must be resisted. These sutures act as foreign bodies and become a nidus for wound infection.[5] They also provoke a greater healing response and

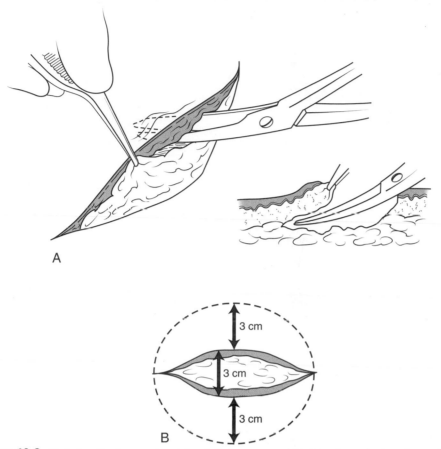

Figure 10-8. Technique for tissue undermining. **A,** Scissors are used for dissection at the dermal-superficial fascia level. Tissue spreading is preferred to cutting the sharp edges. **B,** The zone of undermining

can increase the total bulk of a scar. Only as many sutures as are necessary to accomplish the task of reducing wound tension should be placed.

Wound Undermining
Another technique for reducing tension is wound undermining. Undermining releases the dermis and superficial fascia from their deeper attachments, allowing the wound edge to be brought together with less force. Anatomic areas where undermining is useful include the scalp, forehead, and lower legs, particularly over the tibia, where the skin is under a great deal of natural tension. Caution has to be exercised in deciding to undermine, because this procedure can spread bacteria into deeper tissues and can create a deeper, larger dead space.

The technique for undermining is illustrated in Figure 10-8A. For most minor wound care problems, the proper tissue plane for wound undermining is between the superficial fascia (subcutaneous tissue) and deep fascia overlying the muscle. Staying in this plane maintains the integrity of the blood and nerve supply to the skin (dermis and epidermis). Scissors can be inserted parallel to the deep fascia where it joins the superficial fascia. The instrument is spread gently to create a plane of dissection. Undermining also can be performed with a no. 15 blade on a standard knife handle. The blade is

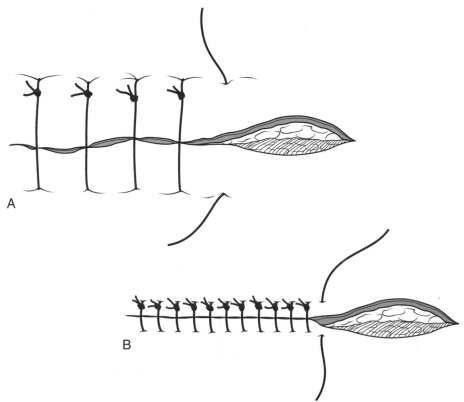

Figure 10-9. A technique for reducing wound tension. **A,** A few sutures, placed far apart and far from the wound edges, will increase wound tension. **B,** More sutures, placed closer together and closer to the wound edges, will reduce tension.

rotated away from the deep fascia and is used as a combination cutting instrument and probe. Actual cutting is kept to a minimum to prevent excessive bleeding.

Wounds are undermined from end to end, to a distance from the wound edge that approximates the extent of "gapping" of the wound edges. In other words, if a wound gaps open 3 cm from edge to edge, undermining is carried out to 3 cm under the dermis, perpendicularly away from the wound edge. A common mistake in using this technique is to fail to include the wound ends. Figure 10-8B illustrates the proper zone of undermining during dissection.

Additional Suture Placement
Placing more sutures closer together also reduces wound tension (Fig. 10-9). Mechanically, a greater number of sutures lessens the total force exerted on each suture, reducing potential tissue compression. The caregiver has to keep in mind, however, that sutures act as foreign bodies and can potentiate infection. When closing a wound, a balance has to be struck between the number of sutures used and the desired tension reduction.

Dead Space
In the past, it was axiomatic that no open or dead spaces should be left behind during wound closure. These spaces tend to fill with hematoma and can act as potential sites for wound infection (Fig. 10-10). Hematoma formation in these areas also can delay

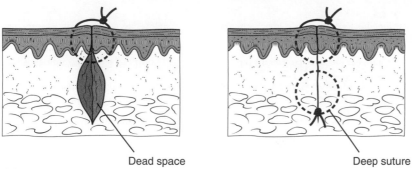

Figure 10-10. Example of dead space and a two-layered closure to obliterate that space.

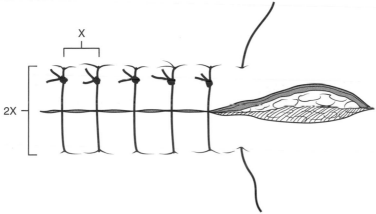

Figure 10-11. Example of closure style and sequence. The knots should be placed evenly on one side of the wound. Knots directly over the wound increase inflammation and scar tissue formation.

wound healing. There is experimental evidence, however, that suture closure of these spaces, when they are contaminated with bacteria, increases the chance of wound infection.[4] It is recommended that deep closures be used only to close dead space in clean, minimally contaminated wounds. Even in these cases, as few sutures as possible should be used.

Closure Sequence and Style

Students learning to care for wounds often ask how close together sutures should be placed. As a general rule, sutures should be placed just far enough from each other so that no gap appears between the wound edges. As a general guideline, the distance between sutures is equal to the bite distance from the wound edge (Fig. 10-11); however, the great variability of lacerations dictates that experience rapidly teaches the practitioner the proper distances at which sutures should be placed to close the wound.

The final appearance of a suture line should be neat and organized. The knots are aligned to one side of the laceration. In addition to appearing orderly, knots are placed away from the wound edge to prevent a further inflammatory response that can be provoked by an increased amount of foreign material directly over the healing surface. Aligning the knots to one side or the other contributes to wound edge eversion.

References

1. Luck RP, Flood R, Eyal D, et al: Cosmetic outcomes of absorbable versus nonabsorbable sutures in pediatric facial lacerations, *Pediatr Emerg Care* 24:137–142, 2008.
2. Karounis H, Gouin S, Eisman H, et al: A randomized controlled trial comparing long-term cosmetic outcomes of traumatic pediatric lacerations repaired with absorbable plain gut versus non-absorbable nylon sutures, *Acad Emerg Med* 11:730–735, 2004.
3. Jones SJ, Gartner M, Drew G, et al: The shorthand vertical mattress stitch: evaluation of a new suture technique, *Am J Emerg Med* 11:483–485, 1993.
4. Crikelair G: Skin suture marks, *Am J Surg* 96:631–639, 1958.
5. Edlich RF, Panek PH, Rodeheaver GT, et al: Physical and chemical configuration of sutures in the development of surgical infection, *Ann Surg* 177:679–687, 1973.

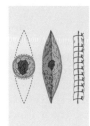

CHAPTER 11
Complex Skin Wounds: Advanced Repair Techniques

Key Practice Points

- Most lacerations can be closed with one or two simple techniques. However, some wounds and lacerations are more complicated and require advanced repair techniques to close.
- Long, straight lacerations can take a long time to close. Techniques to save time include running sutures, staples, and wound adhesives.
- The corner, or flap stitch, is an important suture technique for the surgeon to master to preserve the blood supply of the tip of the flaps or corners in an irregular wound.
- Injured fat in a laceration or in the underside of a flap has no value and can act as substrate for bacterial growth. Injured fat should be débrided before closing the wound with sutures.
- When closing a curving laceration, a "dog-ear" defect can be created. The "dog-ear" technique can repair that defect and can improve the cosmesis of the wound.

Most lacerations and wounds are straightforward and can be closed with the basic techniques described in Chapter 10. Some wounds are more complicated, however, and present with a variety of technical challenges. This chapter describes some of the more complicated wound problems that can be encountered in a wound care setting. Techniques for "solving" these "puzzles" are suggested.

RUNNING SUTURE CLOSURE
Description
Lacerations, usually caused by simple shearing forces, can be quite long and time consuming to close. Lacerations often are caused by slash wounds from a knife or a piece of glass. The continuous "over-and-over" (running) suture technique can be used when a shortage of time is a factor.[1] Wounds longer than 5 cm can be considered for this technique. The time saved is beneficial to the person repairing the wound, because he or she can return quickly to other emergency-department duties. There are drawbacks to this technique. If one loop of the suture breaks or is imperfectly positioned, the whole process has to be repeated. Wound edge eversion can be difficult to control with this technique. Continuous sutures are reserved for straight lacerations in healthy, viable skin that would not collapse in with suturing. If this technique is applied to curved lacerations, it can create a "purse-string" effect that bunches up the wound. Another technique that can be used for long, straight lacerations is wound stapling (see Chapter 14).

Technique for Continuous Over-and-Over (Running) Suture

The technique for continuous over-and-over suturing is shown in Figure 11-1A. The closure is started with the standard technique of a percutaneous interrupted suture, but the suture is not cut after the initial knot is tied (see Fig. 11-1A). The needle is used to make repeated bites, starting at the original knot and making each new bite through the skin at a 45-degree angle to the wound direction (Fig. 11-1B through 11-1F). The cross stays of suture, on the surface of the skin, are at a 90-degree angle to the wound direction. The final bite is made at a 90-degree angle to the wound direction to bring the suture out next to the previous bite exit (Fig. 11-1G). The final bite is left in a loose loop. The loop acts as a free end of suture for knot tying. The first throw of the final knot is made by looping the suture end held in the hand around the needle holder, then by grasping the free loop (Fig. 11-1H). The first throw is snugged down to skin level (Fig. 11-1I). The knot is completed in the standard instrument-tie manner with several more throws at skin level (Fig. 11-1J and 11-1K).

BEVELED (SKIVED) WOUNDS

Description

A common problem in layer matching is the beveled-edge, or "skived," laceration. Beveled edges are created when the striking angle of the wounding object is not perpendicular, but the angle and force are not acute enough to create a true flap deformity.

Technique for Closure of a Beveled Edge

A common misconception about the repair of a beveled-edge wound is that a larger bite is taken from the thin edge of the laceration rather than from the bigger edge. The opposite technique is the solution to proper layer matching. The technique for closing a beveled laceration is shown in Figure 11-2. By taking unequal bites as shown, the edge is brought into correct apposition with the opposite edge. If sufficient tissue redundancy exists in the wound area, excision of the edges can equalize the wound so that simple sutures can close the wound.

PULL-OUT SUBCUTICULAR CLOSURE

Description

A favorite technique of plastic surgeons is the pull-out subcuticular stitch using a nonabsorbable suture material, such as polypropylene (Prolene). This suture material is stiffer and stronger than nylon and allows for easier removal.[2] A newer, nonabsorbable suture material, polybutester (Novafil), is also useful for this technique.[3] The pull-out closure is limited to straight lacerations less than 4 cm long, because the suture would be too difficult to extract at removal time. Children have naturally higher skin tension, so this technique is thought by some clinicians to be superior for children because it prevents suture marks. Despite this fact, the pull-out subcuticular closure has no distinct advantage over percutaneous closure when final wound and scar appearance is compared.[4] Another use for this technique is for closure of lacerations over which splinting materials or plaster will be placed. It also can be used in patients who are at risk for keloid formation to prevent keloid formation at the needle puncture sites.

Technique for Pull-Out Subcuticular Closure

Before placement of a pull-out subcuticular closure, the superficial fascia (subcutaneous tissue) has to be apposed adequately with absorbable suture to bring the dermis

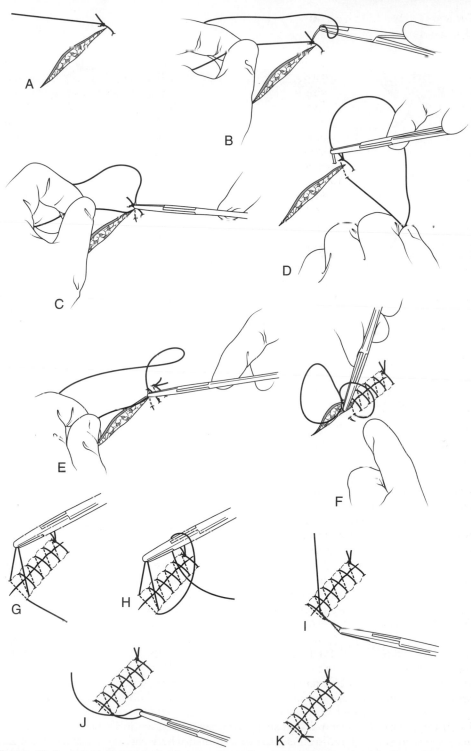

Figure 11-1. **A-K,** Technique for continuous over-and-over suture (running suture). The needle bites are made at a 45-degree angle to the axis of the wound. By taking bites at this angle, the cross stay of the suture at the skin surface is at a 90-degree angle to the wound axis. See text for complete description of technique.

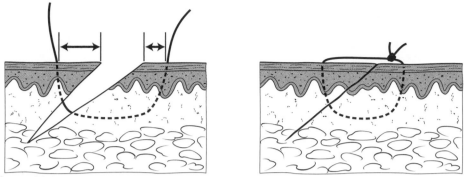

Figure 11-2. Technique for closing a beveled edge. There is a larger bite taken on the larger wound edge; there is a smaller bite taken on the flap portion of the wound edge.

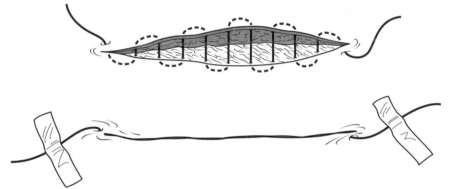

Figure 11-3. Technique for pull-out dermal closure. See text for complete description of technique.

close to approximation. The actual closure is begun by passing the needle of 4-0 or 5-0 nylon or polypropylene 1 to 1.5 cm from the wound end through the dermis layer and bringing it out of the wound parallel to and through the plane of the dermis. Subsequent bites are made (Fig. 11-3) parallel to the dermis at a depth of 2 to 3 mm into the dermis. Each bite should "mimic" the other with regard to bite size and dermal depth on each side of the wound until the "tail" is brought out at the opposite end of the wound. The beginning and final tail can be secured by wound tape. In the face, this suture can remain in place for 7 days. This technique often is used in conjunction with wound taping to match dermal and epidermal layers accurately. The suture is removed merely by pulling on one end with forceps or a needle holder and sliding the suture out of the dermal layer.

SUBCUTICULAR RUNNING CLOSURE

Description

Surgeons often use a subcuticular running closure to close straight incisions. The subcuticular running closure can suffice to close the wound alone, or it can be supplemented with interrupted skin sutures. In wound care, this closure should be reserved for straight, clean lacerations with sharp, nondevitalized wound edges. It can be used to close wounds that have been excised or trimmed where the edges are left fresh and straight.

Technique for Subcuticular Running Suture

An absorbable suture material (e.g., Dexon, Vicryl, PDS, Maxon, or Monocryl) can be used. One strand is used, without interruption, for the entire laceration. As shown in Figure 11-4, the suture is anchored at one end of the laceration. The plane chosen is either the dermis or just deep to the dermis in the superficial subcutaneous fascia. While maintaining this plane, "mirror image" bites are taken horizontally the full length of the wound. The final bite leaves a trailing loop of suture (see Fig. 11-4) so that the knot can be fashioned for final closure. This technique commonly is supplemented with wound tapes, particularly if some degree of gapping of the edges remains.

CORNER STITCH

Description

Many wounds are irregular and jagged, with corners that need to be secured during closure. Corners and flaps are particularly vulnerable because they receive their blood supply only from an intact base. Improper suturing of the tip of a corner can compromise an already tenuous vascularity.

Technique for Closing a Corner

A simple technique to secure a corner without interrupting the small capillaries at the tip is shown in Figure 11-5. The technique used is the half-buried horizontal mattress suture. A nonabsorbable (nylon, Prolene) suture is introduced percutaneously through the skin in the noncorner portion of the wound. The needle is brought through the dermis, is then passed horizontally through the corner dermis, and is brought back to the same plane of dermis on the opposite side of the noncorner portion. Finally, it is led out through the epidermis.

The key to this suture is that the flap portion of the suture passes horizontally through the dermis and not vertically through the epidermis and the dermis. When the tip is in place with the corner stitch, the remainder of the flap can be closed with interrupted percutaneous or half-buried horizontal mattress sutures, which should be placed far enough from the tip to allow for unrestricted dermal circulation.

A single corner stitch can encompass several corners of stellate lacerations by capturing all of the corners of flaps (Fig. 11-6) until the final percutaneous reexposure is completed to tie the knot. The corner suture is one of the most useful suture techniques in emergency wound and laceration care for complex wound closure.

PARTIAL AVULSION, FLAP WOUNDS

Description

Flap lacerations are the result of forces that tear up, or avulse, a flap of skin from the subcutaneous tissue. The vascular supply of a complicated flap is even more tenuous because it derives blood from only its intact dermal attachment. A general rule for viability is that the flap base should exceed flap length by a ratio of 3:1.[5] Flaps with lower ratios are less likely to survive. The rule varies according to anatomic site and other considerations. A long, narrow-based flap is in greater jeopardy than a short, broad-based flap.

Flaps that are distally based have the tip pointing opposite to the natural cutaneous arterial flow. These flaps rely solely on venous backflow for oxygen and nutrients. The repair technique has to be meticulous and gentle, and has to be dictated by the condition of the flap, the width of the total wound, and the anatomic location. Flaps that are proximally based usually have adequate perfusions, but the repair has to be handled no less carefully.

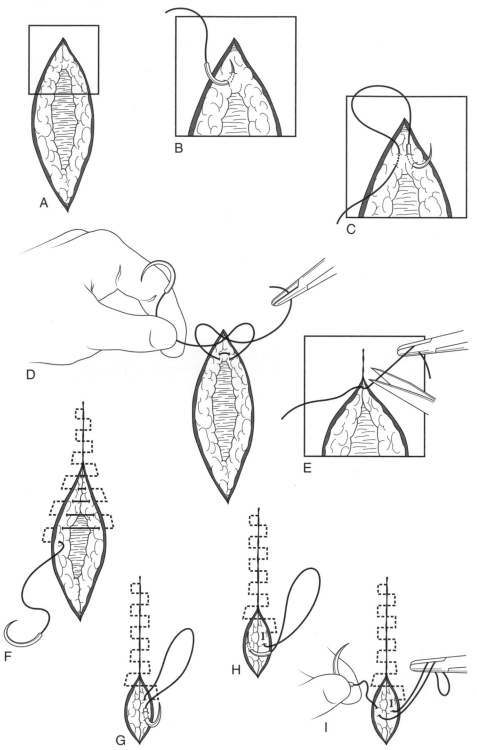

Figure 11-4. **A-I,** Technique for subcuticular running suture. See text for complete description of technique.

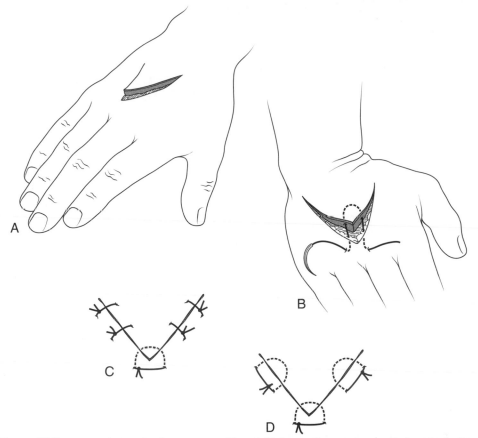

Figure 11-5. A-D, Technique for closing a corner (flap stitch). See text for complete description of technique.

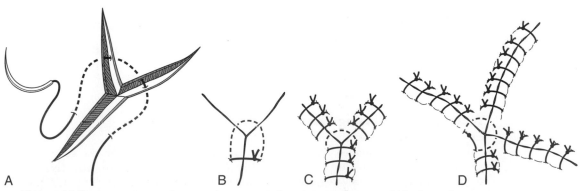

Figure 11-6. A-D, Technique for using the corner stitch to close a stellate or multiflap laceration.

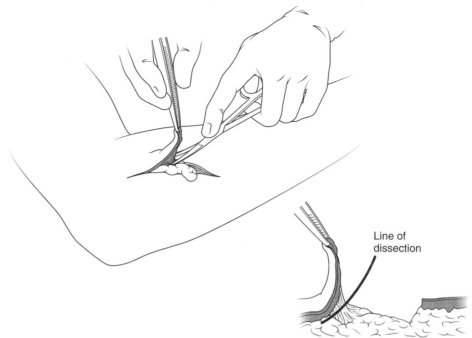

Line of
dissection

Figure 11-7. Technique for defatting the base of a flap for better union and vascularization to occur after suture anchoring. Fat is removed at the dermal–superficial fascia plane.

Technique for Preparing and Repairing a Complicated Flap

Excessive fatty superficial fascia (subcutaneous tissue) on the underside or dermal part of the flap can impair healing when it is secured with sutures. A raw dermal surface is preferable to damaged fat when the flap is replaced in the laceration defect. In this sense, flaps are similar to grafts. To improve the chance of flap survival during early healing, it is best to remove the excessive fat from the flap before suturing (Fig. 11-7). Iris scissors can be used to trim the fat until only a fresh tissue surface remains.

If the flap is otherwise in good condition with viable edges, the initial suture is the half-buried mattress suture described earlier for corner closure. The remainder of the flap can be closed with the same suture technique for the corner closure with simple interrupted percutaneous sutures.

Technique for Closing Flaps with Nonviable Edges: V-Y Closure

Often flaps have damaged edges that are not viable, in which case the edges can be excised to create a smaller but more viable flap. Figure 11-8 shows how this flap is secured by converting a V closure to a Y closure to accommodate the smaller amount of tissue available. With iris scissors, the edges of the flaps are trimmed back to viable tissue. The remaining flap is not large enough, however, to accommodate the resultant defect. By using a modified corner stitch technique, the flap tip can be brought together with the wound edges in a Y configuration. The remainder of the wound is closed with small-bite percutaneous interrupted sutures. Similar to the previously mentioned complicated flap, defatting also is recommended if appropriate.

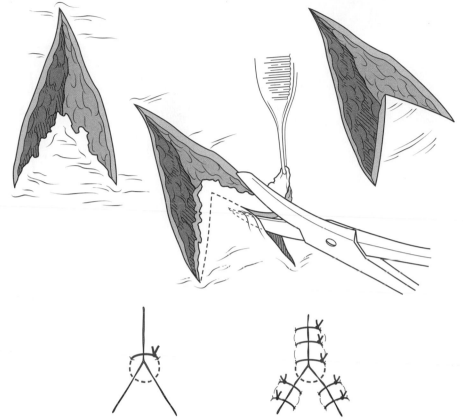

Figure 11-8. Technique for closure of flaps with nonviable edges: the V-Y closure. The edges of the flap are excised. The remaining flap is not large enough to fill the defect; a corner stitch is placed to close the wound as a Y instead of its original V configuration.

Technique for Closing a Wound with a Completely Nonviable Flap

Some flaps are beyond revision or repair. In this case, closure can be achieved by "ellipsing" the flap (Fig. 11-9) and completely closing the wound by following the 3:1 length-to-width ratio rule for ellipse closure (see Chapter 9). In some cases, there is insufficient tissue redundancy so that ellipsing is not feasible, and the wound has to be considered for open healing (secondary intention) or grafting.

GEOGRAPHIC LACERATIONS

Description

One of the most challenging wounds is the geographic laceration, a wound that can be irregular in configuration and depth. These lacerations are caused by differential forces occurring at the same time to create a complex wound. Closure requires some creativity.

Technique for Closure of Geographic Wounds

The first principle in closure of geographic wounds is to appose the natural geographic points (Fig. 11-10). After that, simple percutaneous interrupted sutures might suffice, but a creative mix of different techniques and suture sizes ultimately might be required.

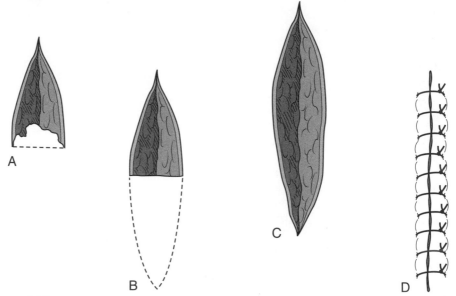

Figure 11-9. **A-D,** Technique for closure of a wound with a completely nonviable flap. In this case, a complete ellipse can be fashioned and closed primarily.

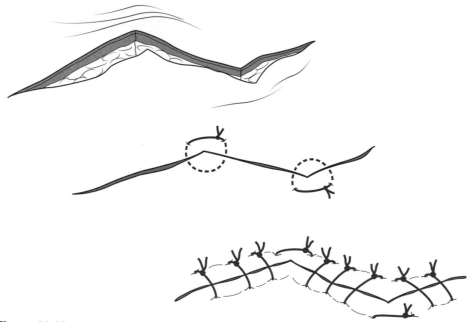

Figure 11-10. Technique for closure of geographic wounds. Obvious geographic points are apposed first with either simple percutaneous sutures or with corner sutures.

Closure techniques may appear unorthodox, but for traumatic wounds, the maxim "whatever works" should be followed to obey basic closure principles and to achieve the best possible result.

COMPLETE AVULSIONS

Description

When tissue is lost or avulsed through the primary wounding event, several considerations have to be addressed. Full-thickness losses are identified by the complete loss of dermis. Superficial fascia (subcutaneous fat) "shows" through the wound. Partial-thickness losses are identified by the raw appearance of underlying dermis without its covering epidermis. Partial-thickness losses, especially when intact dermal elements are visible, heal well without aggressive intervention. Generally, any full-thickness defects, less than or equal to 1 to 2 cm^2 in area, can be left to heal by open healing (secondary intention). This rule also applies to wounds on fingertips.

Full-thickness gaps or defects that are greater in area than 2 cm^2 need to be considered for grafting. Whenever questions arise about the possibility of grafting, consultation with a specialist is recommended. Some defects can be closed primarily, without grafting, and suggested techniques are described subsequently.

Technique for Converting a Triangle to an Ellipse

If the avulsion defect is configured as a triangle, conversion of that defect to an ellipse can be made by extending with excision the "defect" (see Fig. 11-9B through 11-9D). If the basic 3:1 length-to-width rule can be maintained during this process, the whole defect can be closed with a few dermal (deep) supporting sutures and a line of percutaneous sutures with the result of a simple, single suture line. Undermining may be required to bring the wound edges together to reduce wound edge tension. There must be sufficient tissue redundancy to perform this closure successfully (see Chapter 10).

Technique for Closing a Circular or Irregular Defect

The simplest way to close a circular or irregular defect is to turn it into an ellipse as shown in Figure 11-11. If the defect is too great, a double V-Y closure technique can be used. In this case, the defect is covered by two sliding pedicle flaps created by a no. 15 blade (Fig. 11-12). It is crucial not to disturb the fascial attachments of the flaps and not to interrupt the blood supply. The dermis is incised without including the subcutaneous tissue to allow the flaps to move forward on their vascular base into the gap.

DOG-EAR DEFORMITIES

Description

Trying to close a laceration evenly, particularly if it has a curving configuration, can lead to bunching of one or both of the wound edges as the suture closure proceeds. One edge of the wound can become redundant and can lead to the creation of a "dog ear."

Technique for Closing a Dog Ear

To correct a dog-ear deformity, an incision is made with a no. 15 blade, beginning at the end of the wound and at a 45-degree angle from the direction of the laceration on the side of the redundancy (Fig. 11-13). The redundant tissue flap is excised along an imaginary line that directly corresponds with the incision. The remaining

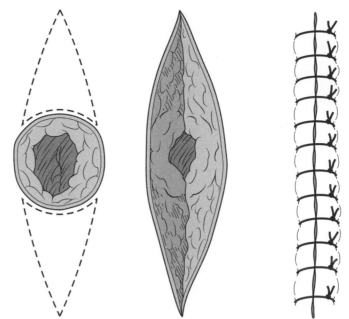

Figure 11-11. Technique for closure of a circular defect by the ellipse method.

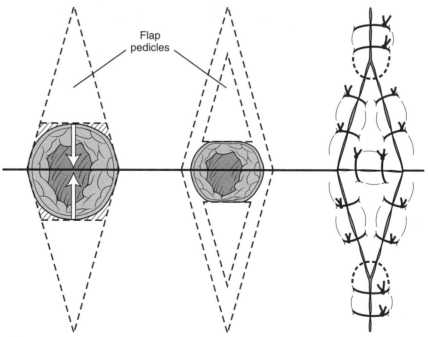

Flap
pedicles

Figure 11-12. Technique for closure of a circular or irregular defect by advancing flap pedicles to effect a double V-Y closure. (Adapted from Zukin D, Simon R: *Emergency wound care: principles and practice*, Rockville, Md, 1987, Aspen Publishers.)

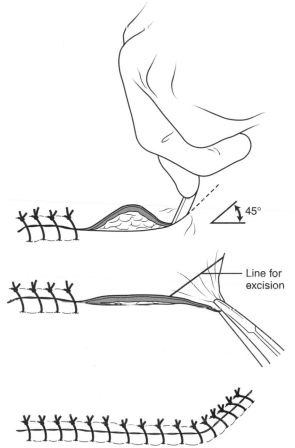

Figure 11-13. Technique for closure of redundant tissue, or a dog ear. The incision is made at an approximately 45-degree angle from the original axis of the wound. See text for complete description of technique.

portion of tissue fits the new configuration of the laceration incision and is appropriately sutured. The final outcome is a slightly angulated wound with a "hockey-stick" appearance.

PARALLEL LACERATIONS

Description

Two or more parallel lacerations that are in close proximity are often the result of self-inflicted wounds on the wrists or forearms. They are usually superficial, but because of the nature of the anatomic site, these wounds can result in significant injuries to the underlying flexor structures of the wrist. Careful functional testing of nerves and tendons with wound exploration often is necessary before closure.

Technique for Closure of Parallel Lacerations

After close inspection and exploration to rule out tendon or nerve damage, the caregiver will choose from several methods for closing parallel lacerations without compromising the blood supply to the tissue "strips" between lacerations. Some wounds can be closed with the horizontal mattress suture, modified to cross all lacerations

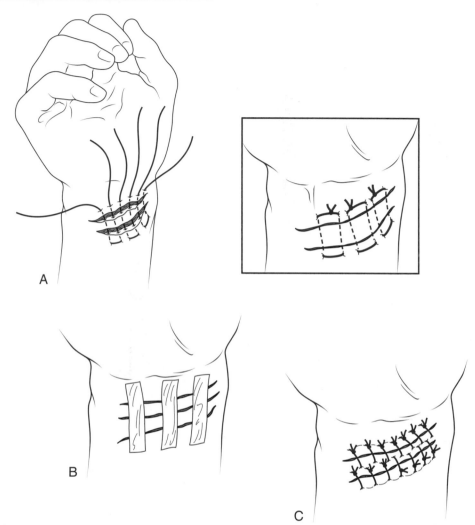

Figure 11-14. Three techniques for closure of parallel lacerations. **A,** The horizontal mattress technique is used to cross all lacerations for closure. **B,** Wound tapes can be used to close these lacerations. **C,** If the island of tissue is wide enough, alternating sutures can be used on each laceration. It is necessary, however, to be careful not to compromise vascular supply when using this technique. (Adapted from Zukin D, Simon R: *Emergency wound care: principles and practice*, Rockville, Md, 1987, Aspen Publishers.)

(Fig. 11-14A). Wound tapes are particularly effective if the lacerations are superficial (Fig. 11-14B). Finally, the alternating percutaneous approach can be used if the vascular supply of the tissue would not be compromised (Fig. 11-14C).

THIN-EDGE, THICK-EDGE WOUNDS

Description

Occasionally a wound can be created in which the thickness of one edge is markedly different from the other wound edge. There is unequal dermal loss during injury. To appose the two edges properly, simple percutaneous interrupted sutures do not suffice. The thin edge has to be elevated to meet the appropriate layers of the full-thickness edge.

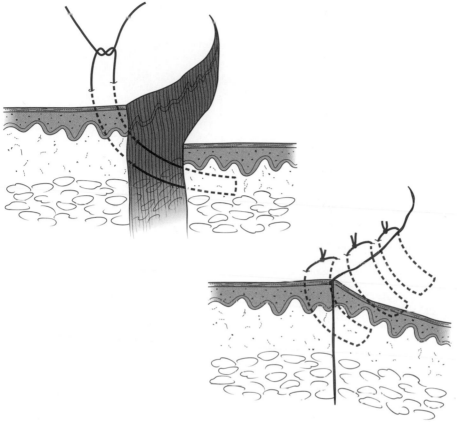

Figure 11-15. Technique for closure of a thin-edge, thick-edge laceration. The horizontal mattress technique is used; however, one portion is buried and is not brought through the opposite side of the wound surface.

Technique for Closing a Thin-Edge, Thick-Edge Wound

A technique for closing a thin-edge, thick-edge wound is to use the half-buried horizontal suture in the manner shown in Figure 11-15. The thin edge (dermis lost) is captured by the suture and is brought up to match the thick edge (dermis preserved).

LACERATION IN AN ABRASION

Description

Another complex wound is the loss of surface skin accompanied by a laceration in the defect.

Technique for Closing a Laceration in an Abrasion

The laceration can be repaired by using the deep (dermal) closure with the knot buried under the wound surface (see Chapter 10). When the laceration is closed (Fig. 11-16), the defect can be managed by allowing it to close by secondary intention or grafting.

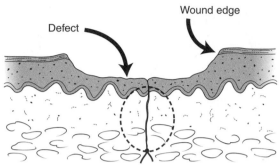

Figure 11-16. Technique for closure of a laceration within a deep abrasion. The deep-suture technique is used, and the abraded surface is avoided.

References

1. Wong NL: Review of continuous sutures in dermatologic surgery, *J Dermatol Surg Oncol* 19:923–931, 1993.
2. Swanson NA, Tromovitch TA: Suture materials, 1980s: properties, uses, and abuses, *Int J Dermatol* 21:373–378, 1982.
3. Bernstein G: Polybutester suture, *J Dermatol Surg* 14:615–616, 1988.
4. Winn HR, Jane JA, Rodeheaver GT: Influence of subcuticular sutures on scar formation, *Am J Surg* 133:257–259, 1977.
5. Grabb WC: Introduction to the clinical aspects of flap repair. In Grabb WC, Myers MB, editors: *Skin flaps*, Boston, 1975, Little, Brown.

CHAPTER 12
Special Anatomic Sites

Key Practice Points

- Although scalp lacerations can appear small and innocuous, they can bleed profusely to the point of hypotension.
- Hair does not increase the risk of wound infection. Shaving hair increases the risk of wound infection. Hair can be clipped or cleaned to prepare the laceration for closure.
- Closing scalp lacerations with absorbable sutures, particularly in children, avoids the need for the patient to return for suture or staple removal.
- The forehead has little redundant tissue. Débride as little as possible to preserve skin for later revision if necessary.
- Face lacerations do not require dressings. Have the patient apply a small amount of antibiotic ointment daily to the sutured laceration to facilitate easy removal of sutures.
- Lacerations near the eye can cause several serious complications, such as hyphemas, tear duct injuries, and other problems. Carefully examine the eye and its structures before closure.
- Never shave an eyebrow. Eyebrow hair does not grow back in some patients, or it grows abnormally.
- Lacerations to the side of the face can injure the parotid gland or the seventh nerve. Examine these structures before repair.
- Injuries to the nose can cause a septal hematoma. Use an otoscope to look in the nares to detect hematoma of the septum or exposed cartilage or bone.
- Lacerations to the ear can involve cartilage. However, it is not necessary to suture cartilage. Closure of skin over the cartilage will bring cartilage into proper position.
- Alignment of lacerations through the vermilion border of the lip is critical to avoid a noticeable cosmetic defect.
- If a tooth is knocked out, the prognosis for salvage worsens by the minute. If not replaced within 30 minutes, it is not likely to remain viable.

Although the wound closure principles and suture techniques discussed in Chapters 10 and 11 can be applied to all lacerations and wounds, several areas of the body have unique anatomic considerations that require special attention. Particular emphasis is placed on facial wounds because of cosmetic concerns. Initial management and wound closure are crucial to the way that scars eventually form and to the final appearance of the injury. Table 8-3 in Chapter 8 presents a reference guide for sutures and closure materials for each anatomic region of the body. Because of the importance and complexity of the hand, this anatomic feature is covered separately in Chapter 13.

SCALP

There are five layers of the scalp: skin (epidermis, dermis), dense superficial fascia, galea aponeurotica, loose areolar connective tissue, and periosteum (Fig. 12-1). The skin is densely covered with hair. Ragged lacerations often are closed without regard to cosmetics because of the assumption that hair will hide the scar. Most men experience some balding in their lifetimes, however, a fact that must be taken into consideration during wound closure.

Underlying the skin is a dense layer of connective tissue that corresponds to the superficial fascia. This layer is richly invested with arteries and veins. Although this profuse vascularity protects against the development of infection, the denseness of the connective tissue tends to hold vessels open when the scalp is lacerated. For this reason, even small lacerations can cause considerable bleeding, leading to hypovolemia, hypotension, and even death.[1] Hemorrhage is worsened if alcohol is present in the blood, which is a finding in 50% of patients with scalp lacerations.[2]

The next layer of skin is the galea aponeurotica (Fig. 12-2). It is a dense, tendon-like structure that covers the skull and inserts into the frontalis muscle of the forehead anteriorly and into the occipitalis muscle posteriorly. Failure to repair large, horizontal lacerations of the aponeurosis can cause the frontalis muscle to contract

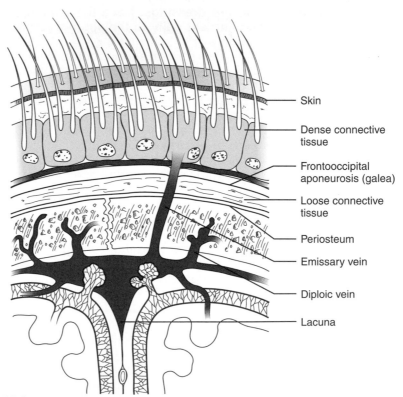

Skin

Dense connective tissue

Frontooccipital aponeurosis (galea)

Loose connective tissue

Periosteum

Emissary vein

Diploic vein

Lacuna

Figure 12-1. Cross-sectional anatomy of the scalp. Note the emissary vein; it can act as a conduit for bacteria to brain tissues if the scalp wound becomes infected.

asymmetrically, which can cause a significant cosmetic deformity of the forehead. Closure of galea lacerations also is important for protection of the loose connective tissue that is vulnerable to infection.

Blood and bacteria can spread easily from a laceration of the skin through the injured galea to the loose connective tissue. Within this layer are emissary veins that drain into the skull and intracranial veins. Infection of this space can lead to osteomyelitis or brain abscess. Beneath the loose connective tissue layer is the periosteum of the skull itself. The periosteum can be mistaken for the galea but is not as dense, and it does not readily accept sutures without the risk of tearing.

Preparation for Closure

Visual inspection and digital palpation of large wounds are recommended to identify galeal or bone injuries. The periosteum frequently is injured during trauma. Injuries to this layer often can be seen or palpated through a laceration. Because of its close adherence to the bone, a laceration of the periosteum can be mistaken for a skull fracture. Computerized tomography is recommended to rule out a true fracture, even if the published criteria for computerized tomography in minor head injury are not met.[2,3]

Hair removal before closure is necessary only if hair interferes with the actual closure and knot tying. Hair is not contaminated with high levels of bacteria and can be cleansed easily with standard wound preparation solutions.[4] In a study of 68 patients with traumatic scalp lacerations, no wound infections were documented in patients whose hair had not been removed before closure.[5] If removal is necessary for mechanical reasons, clipping with scissors or shaving with a recessed blade razor suffices.[6] Shaving at skin level can increase the chance for wound infection.[7,8] Another method to expose the laceration before closure is to apply ointment such as Vaseline or antibiotic ointment to the hair around the wound. The hair is then flattened away from the wound before closure.

Because of the scalp's propensity to bleed profusely, hemorrhage control is necessary before attempting closure. Trying to suture a bleeding scalp wound can be difficult and

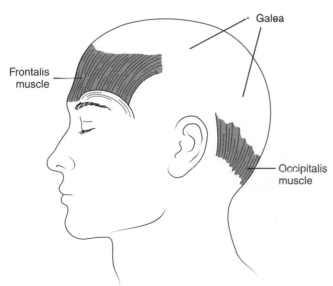

Figure 12-2. Lateral view of galea aponeurotica. Repair of large lacerations of the galea is required to maintain the integrity of facial structures.

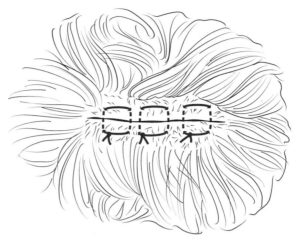

Figure 12-3. Horizontal mattress suture technique for closure of scalp wounds with uneven or macerated edges.

frustrating. The vessels do not lend themselves to easy clamping or ligation because they are encased in the dense connective tissue. Direct pressure, applied in the manner described in the following text, is an effective way to gain hemostasis. First, gross contaminants, if present, are removed immediately with a brief cleansing or irrigation. Then the wound is covered with sterile, saline-moistened sponges and is compressed with an elastic bandage. This bandage can be left in place for 30 to 60 minutes. After compression, significant bleeding is usually under control.

Injection of lidocaine with epinephrine can also control bleeding. It can anesthetize the wound before formal closure or the application of horizontal mattress (Fig. 12-3) or figure-of-eight sutures, which can also aid in controlling bleeding.

Another method to control scalp hemorrhage is the use of hemostatic agents. In a review of the available agents, oxidized cellulose (Surgicel) and gelatin foams (Gelfoam) are effective for use in skin and scalp wounds.[9] Hemostatic agents should be considered as a last resort. These agents can interfere with suturing of a scalp wound and can take 2 to 6 weeks to be absorbed.

Galeal Lacerations
Because the galea is a key anchoring structure for the frontalis muscle, large frontal galeal lacerations need to be repaired separately with 3-0 or 4-0 absorbable sutures to prevent a serious cosmetic deformity from developing. If the frontalis muscle loses its anchoring point at the muscle-galeal junction along the frontal scalp line, facial expressions dependent on that muscle appear distorted and asymmetric. Closure of large galeal lacerations in other areas of the scalp also is recommended to protect the loose connective tissue layer from infection.

Uncomplicated Lacerations
Uncomplicated, shearing lacerations can be closed with nonabsorbable 5-0 or 4-0 monofilament nylon, staples, or fast absorbable gut suture. The fast absorbable gut material often is preferred for children, because suture removal becomes unnecessary. Some practitioners find this strategy equally effective for adults. Absorbable irradiated polyglactin-910 (Vicryl Rapide) also can be used to close scalp wounds, obviating the need for later suture removal.[10,11] Closure outcomes with this material are similar to

outcomes for other methods, in that low rates of dehiscence and infection result.[12] The use of staples is common for scalp wounds. Stapled wounds heal in the same way as wounds treated with standard closure methods.[13,14] In children, the cosmetic outcome of stapled scalp lacerations is no different from the outcome of lacerations closed with standard sutures.[15] In an analysis of stapling versus suturing, stapling was significantly faster and less costly.[16]

A simple, "low-tech" approach to scalp laceration closure is hair braiding. Because hair removal is not necessary for scalp laceration cleansing and repair, the hair itself can become the closure material.[17] This technique works best for straight and superficial lacerations with enough hair to tie in small knots. The wound is cleansed and irrigated (see Chapter 7). About 10 to 20 hairs on each side of the wound are moistened with saline or water and are clumped together to form a "thread." The two threads are tied together in a simple square knot. Forceps can be used to tighten the knot to prevent slippage. A small amount of cyanoacrylate glue (Dermabond) can be applied to the knot to increase security. Sutures and staples provide more overall wound security, but patients must return for removal of these closures.

Compression Lacerations with Irregular Margins

Lacerations of the scalp are often caused by blunt rather than sharp shearing forces. In these cases, the wound and its edges are irregular and macerated. Simple closure with percutaneous, interrupted sutures can be difficult under these conditions. The scalp does not have excessive tissue redundancy, so débridement has to be kept to a minimum, or the wound cannot be approximated without abnormally high tension. The rich vascularity of the scalp allows for eventual successful healing even if less than optimal tissues are brought together. After judicious wound edge trimming, the horizontal mattress suture technique is recommended to approximate the remaining edges (see Fig. 12-3). This technique also is useful for closing an excessively bleeding wound.

Compression injuries can result in complex, stellate lacerations. Judicious débridement is advised. The corner closure (flap) technique, described in Chapter 11, often approximates all of the corners and flaps in one suture. The remainder of the repair is performed with simple percutaneous or half-buried mattress sutures.

Avulsion or Scalping Lacerations

High-speed forces that are delivered in a tangential manner to the scalp can cause large flaps or complete loss of portions of the scalp. Associated intracranial injury also can occur. These wounds are best managed by a consultant. Preserved portions of complete scalp avulsions, similar to other amputated parts, are wrapped in saline-moistened gauze, are placed in plastic bags, and are cooled over ice. It is possible that they might be reimplanted in the defect by grafting or microvascular anastomosis techniques.

Aftercare

After repair, it is sometimes necessary to place a temporary (24-hour), light-pressure compression wrap with an elastic bandage over the scalp dressing of large lacerations to prevent formation of wound hematoma. The patient can be instructed to remove the bandage after the recommended compression period.

Most scalp lacerations do not require dressing, just a thin layer of an antibacterial ointment. Scalp sutures are left in place for 7 to 9 days for adults and for 5 to 7 days for children. Gentle bathing of the scalp can commence 24 hours after closure. Daily application of ointment after cleansing is recommended.

FOREHEAD

The forehead is a common site of injury in children and adults. The forehead is also of paramount cosmetic importance because of its visibility. Three principles govern the initial repair of a forehead injury, as follows:

- Skin tension lines that parallel skin creases play a major role in the outcome of any laceration. A laceration that is perpendicular to dynamic skin tension lines tends to heal with a more visible scar than one that is parallel to these lines (see Chapter 3).
- The forehead has little excess tissue to permit extensive revisions and excisions. The temptation to excise ragged wounds has to be assessed carefully or resisted. A small defect can inadvertently become larger by overaggressive repair efforts.[18] It is often best to preserve as much tissue as possible just by "tacking down" ragged tissue tags so that later cosmetic revisions can be made when conditions are more favorable.
- Whenever possible, avoid the use of dermal (deep) absorbable sutures. Excessive tissue reaction with increased scar size can result from deep sutures.

Preparation for Closure

Anesthesia for small or single lacerations of the forehead can be accomplished by the direct or parallel injection techniques, using an anesthetic with epinephrine to decrease bleeding. Large or multiple lacerations often are managed best by a forehead block (see Chapter 6). This block reduces the number of needle-sticks and prevents distortion of the tissues to allow for more accurate wound edge approximation.

When anesthesia is achieved, the wound can be explored for any bony abnormality or foreign body; radiographs are recommended when the suspicion for either is raised. Large pieces of glass can be discovered under small and innocuous-appearing wounds. After gentle scrubbing with a sponge, after irrigation, and after débridement with the tip of a no. 11 blade, most foreign material should have been removed. Any remaining permanent material can be surgically removed. Every effort is made to remove potential tattooing tar or grit at the time of the first repair. When in doubt, consultation with a specialist should be considered.

Uncomplicated Lacerations

Most lacerations can be closed with the simple percutaneous technique using a 6-0 monofilament nonabsorbable suture. Absorbable sutures, such as Vicryl Rapide, can be used for superficial skin closure as well.[19] Deeper lacerations may require placement of a few supporting dermal (deep) 5-0 absorbable sutures. The percutaneous technique in any laceration should be performed by taking small bites (close to the wound edge) with several sutures rather than large bites with few sutures. This technique reduces wound edge tension and allows for more accurate wound edge apposition.

Complex Lacerations
Multiple Small Flaps, Lacerations,
and Abrasions (Windshield Injury)

One of the most daunting wounds is a "windshield" injury, characterized by multiple lacerations, abrasions, gouges, and small flaps. The anesthetic technique of choice is the forehead block. Flaps that are smaller than 5 mm in width and length are tacked down with single 6-0 percutaneous nonabsorbable sutures (Fig. 12-4). Larger flaps can be closed using the corner technique. Partial-thickness abrasions and shallow gouges (<5 to 10 mm wide and 1 to 2 mm deep) can be left to heal by secondary intention. Other lacerations are closed as necessary with percutaneous sutures. A petroleum-based antibiotic ointment applied three times a day suffices as a dressing. Because of cosmetic concerns, a consultant might be helpful, especially if the wounds are severe.

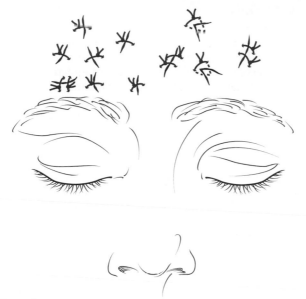

Figure 12-4. Small abrasions/lacerations, caused by a windshield injury, often can be closed by using simple, single, percutaneous sutures or single corner sutures.

Consultation also is appropriate if the estimated time of repair would interfere with an emergency physician's other duties, even if there is little technical challenge.

Ragged-Edge Lacerations, Large Flaps, and Tissue Defects

Lacerations with ragged and macerated edges can be trimmed as described in Chapter 9. If the unevenness or maceration is not extensive, complete excision is an option if the laceration is parallel to the skin tension lines and there is sufficient tissue redundancy. Lacerations perpendicular to skin tension lines have less tissue redundancy and cannot tolerate wide excision. The principle of tissue preservation has to be kept in mind when considering excision. When there is any doubt about tissue availability for excision, the caregiver should try to preserve what is viable or should obtain a consultation.

Large avulsion flaps and near-scalping injuries are prone to what is called the trap-door phenomenon, in which congestion and lymphedema lead to unsightly bulging of the flap after repair. The flaps are U-shaped with the base in a superior position on the forehead. These injuries are best managed by a consultant.

Aftercare

Facial lacerations usually do not require dressings. Daily application of an antibacterial ointment after gentle cleansing is recommended for protection and to allow for easier suture removal (by reducing crusting). Cotton swabs moistened with a mild soap and water solution are useful for cleaning in and around facial lacerations. A small amount of antibiotic ointment applied to the laceration after cleaning makes it much easier to remove the sutures. Facial sutures are removed within 3 to 5 days to prevent suture mark formation. Larger lacerations (>2 cm) are supported by wound tape for 1 week after suture removal.

EYEBROW AND EYELID

The eye and periorbital tissues are susceptible to serious injury by relatively minor trauma. Figure 12-5 illustrates various structures that must be checked for damage before repair proceeds. If any of the important anatomic parts discussed here are involved, immediate referral to a consultant is recommended.

Lacerations of the medial lower lid can injure the tear duct apparatus (lacrimal canaliculus and nasolacrimal duct) or the medial palpebral ligament at the medial canthus. Copious tears running down the cheek of the patient are a sign of possible tear duct injuries. A laceration of the medial palpebral ligament displaces the lid apparatus laterally, giving the appearance that the patient is "cross-eyed."

The levator palpebrae muscle is responsible for maintaining the eyelid in its normal position when open. Interruption of the muscle causes traumatic ptosis. Injury to the muscle is suspected when periorbital fat can be seen to extrude from a laceration of the upper lid. Periorbital fat signifies that the orbital septum has been violated. The levator muscle originates from the septum; any septum injury risks this muscle.

Close inspection of the eye itself is necessary to rule out a hyphema, corneal abrasions, blow-out fracture, and foreign bodies. A complete examination of the eye includes

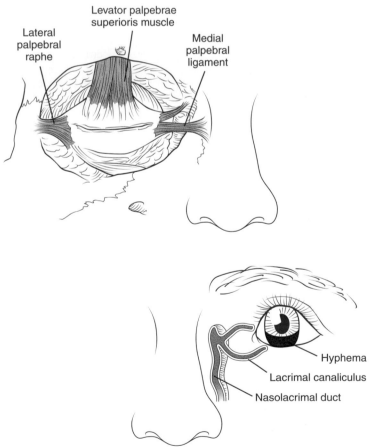

Figure 12-5. Important anatomic structures that can be injured during eye trauma. The integrity of these structures must be confirmed before the closure of any laceration (see text).

extraocular muscle function, pupil reaction, and corneal staining. Of these injuries, hyphema is the most serious. It is caused by a direct blow to the eye and is recognized by a blood layer in the anterior chamber of the eye in patients in the upright position. In patients who are supine, blood distributes evenly in the anterior chamber over the iris and gives the iris a color different from the opposite iris. The patient also complains of decreased vision in the affected eye. Having the patient sit up reveals the hyphema as the blood settles with gravity.

Preparation for Closure

It is best to deliver an anesthetic to the eyelid by direct wound infiltration, using a small 27-G or 30-G needle. Epinephrine-containing anesthetics are not necessary. For the eyebrow, the same technique is used, but epinephrine in the anesthetic can be useful to control minor bleeding. Special care is taken to minimize spillage of cleansing agents into the eye to prevent unnecessary corneal irritation. Povidone-iodine solution (not a detergent-containing solution) diluted 1:10 with saline and nonionic surfactants (Shur-Clens) are the cleansing agents of choice.[20] Inadvertent spilling of these preparations can be prevented by holding a folded 4 × 4 sponge over the closed eyelid margin to absorb free solution. The caregiver should never shave the hair from the lid margin or brow because of the unpredictability of hair regrowth in these locations.

Closure of Extramarginal Lid Lacerations

Extramarginal lacerations are usually horizontal and occur most commonly in the upper lid. If extramarginal lacerations are simple and superficial, they can be repaired with a single layer of 6-0 nonabsorbable suture material (Fig. 12-6). No dressing is applied. These lacerations heal well enough that scars become virtually unnoticeable with time.

Until more recently, nonabsorbable suture was the only material recommended for skin closure of the face. In practice, some physicians have started closing face and eyelid lacerations with rapidly absorbable polyglactin-910 (Vicryl Rapide).[21] The principal advantage of these sutures is that a return visit to the physician for removal is not required. The rapid resorption property of this material causes the sutures to fall away naturally within 7 to 10 days. In a study of periophthalmic skin wounds closed with 7-0 Vicryl Rapide, healing was observed to be equal to healing with nonabsorbable nylon.[22] No suture marks were present at 2 months in the Vicryl Rapide group.

Closure of Intramarginal Lid Lacerations

Intramarginal lacerations involve the lid margin and, similar to lip lacerations, require extremely precise repair to ensure proper alignment. Abnormal eversion (ectropion) or inversion (entropion) is a complication of improper alignment. Intramarginal injuries probably are best left to a consultant for repair (Fig. 12-7).

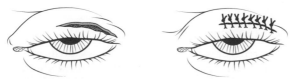

Figure 12-6. Extramarginal lacerations of the upper lid are usually horizontal and can be closed with a simple row of percutaneous closures.

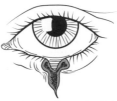

Figure 12-7. A vertical, intramarginal lid laceration is best left to a consultant to repair.

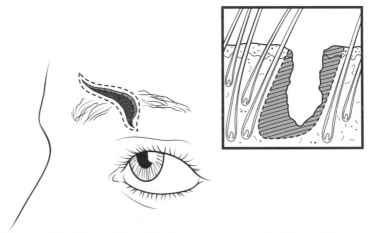

Figure 12-8. Most eyebrow lacerations can be closed without tissue débridement. If macerated or devitalized tissue must be removed, however, it is important to excise this tissue parallel to the hair shaft. This excision technique prevents an unsightly cosmetic defect.

Closure of Eyebrow Lacerations

Simple, uncomplicated eyebrow lacerations can be closed with a 5-0 nonabsorbable monofilament. As previously mentioned, the eyebrow is never shaved or trimmed. Occasionally, one or two dermal (deep) closures are necessary to approximate the superficial fascia. Great care is taken to align the brow margins properly to prevent a cosmetic deformity. Alignment sutures at the superior and inferior margins of the brow hair are placed to initiate closure. Deep sutures, if required, can be placed after the alignment sutures.

If the laceration has particularly ragged or macerated edges, trimming or careful excision can be performed. A basic principle to observe is that any débridement has to be parallel to the brow hair shafts (Fig. 12-8). Failure to observe this principle can lead to an unnecessary defect after the repair.

Aftercare

No dressing is necessary for lid or brow lacerations. Daily cleansing followed by application of an antibacterial ointment is recommended. Sutures are removed in 3 to 5 days in children and adults.

CHEEK OR ZYGOMATIC AREA

There are two major structures underlying the cheek area, just anterior to the ear, that can be injured by penetrating lacerations: the parotid gland and the facial nerve (Fig. 12-9). If the parotid gland is injured, salivary fluid can be seen leaking from the wound. Inspection of the inside of the mouth often reveals bloody fluid coming from the opening of the parotid duct located on the buccal mucosa of the cheek at the level

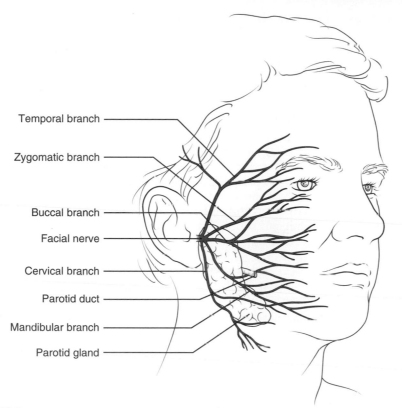

Temporal branch

Zygomatic branch

Buccal branch

Facial nerve

Cervical branch

Parotid duct

Mandibular branch

Parotid gland

Figure 12-9. The parotid gland and facial nerve underlie the zygomatic and cheek areas. Any lacerations anterior to the ear must be assessed carefully for injuries to the various branches of the facial nerve, parotid gland, or parotid duct.

of the upper second molar tooth. The parotid gland is approximately 1.5 cm beneath the skin.

Lacerations of this region also can injure the facial nerve. It is necessary to test all five branches of the nerve to ensure that each one is intact. The temporal branch is tested by asking the patient to contract his or her forehead to elevate the brow. The function of the zygomatic branch is observed by asking the patient to open and shut the eyes. The act of sniffing with flaring of the nasal alae is also evidence for preserved function of that branch. Buccal and mandibular branches innervate the lips during the acts of smiling and frowning. Finally, the cervical branch is tested by requesting that the patient shrug the neck through contraction of the platysma muscle.

Preparation for Closure
The cheek is anesthetized and cleansed in the standard manner described earlier in this chapter and in Chapters 6 and 7. Care is taken to avoid spilling cleansing solutions onto the eye.

Closure of Uncomplicated Cheek Lacerations
The standard percutaneous technique using 6-0 monofilament closes most lacerations. Uncomplicated lacerations can be closed with absorbable gut sutures. These sutures usually dissolve within 7 days. If they do not, the patient is instructed to rub them

off gently to prevent the formation of suture marks. In linear low-tension lacerations, wound adhesives are an option. Many people have natural creases in the skin of the cheek and face. These creases have the same importance cosmetically as the vermilion border of the lip. Proper alignment of the creases requires special attention. Often the initial percutaneous suture is placed in alignment with the crease before proceeding with the remainder of the closure.

Deep or Through-and-Through Lacerations

Complex lacerations that travel deep into the soft tissues of the cheek, or those that penetrate the oral cavity, are at risk for injuring the parotid gland or facial nerve as mentioned earlier. If neither the parotid gland nor the facial nerve is injured, repair can proceed. If there is any doubt, a consultant is required. The oral cavity portion of a penetrating laceration is left open unless it is large (>3 to 5 cm). Large mucosal lacerations are closed with 5-0 chromic gut suture. The external wound is irrigated and is closed with 6-0 monofilament.

Aftercare

Dressings are usually unnecessary for lacerations in the cheek area. Daily cleansing and application of an antibacterial ointment allow for easier suture removal at the 3- to 5-day interval for children and adults.

NASAL STRUCTURES

The nose is composed of a bony and a cartilaginous skeleton. Similar to the ear, direct blows to the nose can cause the formation of a hematoma and a late abscess that compress and injure the nasal infrastructure, including the septum[23] (Fig. 12-10). If not drained, a hematoma can lead to collapse through pressure necrosis of the septum. Lacerations of the nose are common and are often associated with fractures. Radiographs do not always identify fractures, and palpation is a more sensitive indicator of bone injury and displacement.

The skin of the nose is inflexible with little redundancy. It also tears easily with percutaneous suture placement. Consequently, repairs must be performed with great care. Any débridement should be considered only in consultation with a facial specialist.

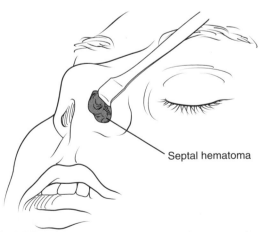

Figure 12-10. Septal hematoma in the area of the anterior nasal septum. Failure to drain this hematoma leads to septal necrosis and collapse.

Preparation for Closure

Before preparation and closure, the nose is inspected for the injuries mentioned in the previous section. Septal hematoma is recognized by its bluish, bulging appearance in the anterior septal area (Kiesselbach's area). The preferred method of examination is with a nasal speculum and an appropriately powerful light source. Penlights and otoscopes may be inadequate.

Anesthesia of the nose is best accomplished by the direct wound infiltration technique with a 27-G or 30-G needle, using an agent without epinephrine. Nasal blocks are difficult to achieve and usually are reserved for major repairs. Cleansing of the nose is done using povidone-iodine solution and saline irrigation.

Skin Lacerations

Most skin lacerations can be repaired with 6-0 nonabsorbable percutaneous monofilament sutures. Sutures are placed with small bites because nasal skin tends to invert. The skin also is torn easily, so great care must be used to avoid creating excessive tension. If tension is present, the placement of one or two deep 6-0 or 5-0 absorbable sutures supports the percutaneous sutures. Complex and irregular skin wounds have to be handled carefully. Because there is little redundancy of nasal skin, débridement must be minimal. The best strategy is to "tack down" small tags or flaps percutaneously or to obtain consultation.

Nostril and Cartilage Wounds

Nostril lacerations involve the rim with skin, cartilage, and mucosal injuries. Alignment of the rim is crucial to prevent "notching." The skin is closed with 6-0 nonabsorbable suture, and the mucosa is sutured with 5-0 or 6-0 absorbable suture. Placement of sutures in the cartilage is not necessary during repair. Closing the skin and mucosa over the cartilage ensures adequate healing. Complete coverage of cartilage is mandatory because of its tendency to develop chronic chondritis if exposed. Avulsion and mutilating injuries of either the skin or the cartilage are best managed by a consultant.

Septal Hematoma

A hematoma over the septal cartilage is drained with a hockey-stick or a crescent-shaped incision (Fig. 12-11). The incision is always made in the dependent portion of the hematoma. To prevent reaccumulation, an anterior nasal pack is placed with gauze that is impregnated with petroleum jelly (Vaseline), and the patient is referred to a consultant within 24 to 48 hours for follow-up. When packing is placed, antibiotics are often recommended to prevent sinus infection. Amoxicillin and trimethoprim-sulfamethoxazole (Bactrim) are reasonable choices.

Lacerations with Bone Involvement

Uncomplicated lacerations of the skin over nondisplaced nasal fractures can be closed using previously described techniques. Complex lacerations with fracture displacement, mucosal injury from bone fragmentation, or extensive cartilage involvement are best managed by a consultant. An uncommon but serious complication of nasal injuries is cerebrospinal fluid leak. It can be detected if clear fluid or diluted blood is seen dripping from the nose. A drop of this fluid placed on filter paper will leave a clear "halo" around a central bloody point.

Aftercare

Dressings are optional for nasal lacerations. Often a simple Band-Aid suffices. Percutaneous sutures are removed in 3 to 5 days in children and adults. The value of antibiotics for nasal lacerations is unclear. The natural vascularity of the face is protective against

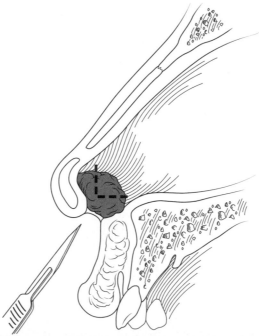

Figure 12-11. Technique to drain a septal hematoma. A no. 11 blade is used to create a hockey-stick incision. After drainage, the nose is packed with gauze impregnated with petroleum jelly (Vaseline). (Adapted from Zukin D, Simon R: *Emergency wound care: principles and practice*, Rockville, Md, 1987, Aspen Publishers.)

infection. Any decision to use antibiotics is based on the circumstances of individual cases. Injuries with fractures should be referred to a specialist. If these injuries are edematous and the anatomy is obscured, referral is planned for 3 to 5 days following the injury.[24] When the underlying deformity and anatomy are revealed after the swelling is reduced, a more accurate repair of the broken nasal bones can be performed with a better cosmetic result.

EAR

The ear consists of a cartilaginous skeleton covered by tightly adherent skin with little intervening superficial fascia (subcutaneous tissue). A direct blow to the ear can cause a hematoma to form, usually in the area of the antihelix, with a resultant breakdown of the cartilage caused by pressure between the skin and cartilage (Fig. 12-12). The eventual result is the well-known "cauliflower" ear. The most important objective for repair of open wounds is the coverage of any exposed cartilage. Failure to do so leads to chondritis and breakdown.

Preparation for Repair

In addition to inspecting the external ear for hematoma formation and cartilage injury, the internal canal and tympanic membrane are visualized to complete the examination. Blunt injuries to the ear can cause perforations of the tympanic membrane. The most significant injury that can accompany lacerations to the ear is a basilar skull fracture, which can be recognized by hemotympanum or Battle's sign (ecchymosis of the mastoid area).

Small, uncomplicated lacerations to the ear can be anesthetized by direct infiltration with a 27-G or 30-G needle using an anesthetic solution without epinephrine.

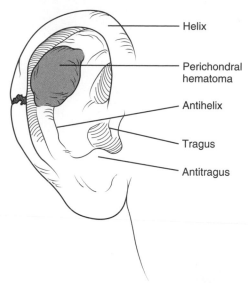

Helix

Perichondral
hematoma

Antihelix

Tragus

Antitragus

Figure 12-12. Anatomy of the external ear. Note the presence of perichondral hematoma; hematoma formation can occur after blunt trauma to the ear and can accompany lacerations.

The needle is introduced carefully between the skin and the cartilage, and only a small amount of anesthetic is deposited to minimize distortion of the wound edges. For large, complex lacerations and wounds, the ear block described in Chapter 6 can be used. Cleansing is done with povidone-iodine solution and irrigation. Because of the complicated topography of the ear, cotton-swab applicators can be particularly useful for cleansing and removing dried blood in crevices.

Uncomplicated Lacerations

Simple lacerations of the helix and lobule that do not involve cartilage can be closed with interrupted 6-0 nonabsorbable monofilament sutures (Fig. 12-13). To prevent wound edge inversion, small 1- to 2-mm bites are taken. If débridement is necessary, it should be kept to a minimum to prevent exposure of the cartilage. Sutures are removed 4 to 5 days after repair.

Lacerations Involving Cartilage

Sharp, shearing lacerations that penetrate cartilage can be managed by carefully apposing the skin overlying the cartilaginous interruption. The skin is sufficiently adherent and supporting so that sutures do not have to be placed through the cartilage itself to bring together the lacerated cartilage edges. In addition, cartilage tears easily and does not hold sutures well. Sharp, through-and-through lacerations can be managed by suturing the anterior and posterior portions of the laceration. The cartilage comes together without sutures. Care is taken to ensure that the skin over the helix rim is everted so that scar contraction does not cause notching.

Irregular wounds that involve cartilage must be managed with two principles in mind: (1) Débridement must be kept to a minimum, and (2) no cartilage must be left exposed. If cartilage is exposed and the skin cannot be brought together over it without undue tension, it can be débrided conservatively to match the skin and cartilage edges. A total of 5 mm of cartilage can be sacrificed without deforming the cartilaginous skeleton. No sutures are placed in the cartilage (Fig. 12-14). Complex cartilage injuries require consultation.

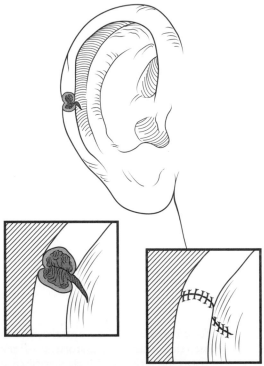

Figure 12-13. Simple noncartilaginous lacerations of the ear are closed with either interrupted or running percutaneous skin sutures.

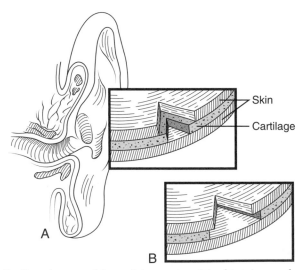

Figure 12-14. **A,** Cartilage that extends beyond the margins of the skin injury can be trimmed back, using tissue scissors, to ensure complete coverage anteriorly and posteriorly by skin. **B,** Skin is closed with simple percutaneous sutures. No sutures are necessary for the cartilage. (Adapted from Zukin D, Simon R: *Emergency wound care: principles and practice*, Rockville, Md, 1987, Aspen Publishers.)

Perichondral Hematoma

When a perichondral hematoma is present, it has to be drained adequately. There is a 72-hour window for hematoma drainage beyond which the risk of cauliflower ear increases.[25] A small incision is made over the hematoma, and the hematoma is evacuated from the space between the perichondrium and the cartilage. Placement of a small rubber drain is optional. After drainage, a mastoid dressing is placed (see Chapter 20). The dressing is removed within 24 hours, and the site is inspected for reaccumulation. More often than not, complex lacerations and hematomas of the ear are best cared for by or under the guidance of a consultant.

Aftercare

Because the ear is difficult to dress, it is often left open. Daily gentle cleansing, followed by application of an antibacterial ointment, is recommended. If there is any question of possible perichondral blood accumulation after the patient is discharged, a mastoid dressing is recommended (see Chapter 20) as discussed above. Sutures are removed after 4 to 5 days for adults and after 3 to 5 days for children. When cartilage is involved or a septal hematoma has been drained, antibiotic prophylaxis is recommended. Choices include dicloxacillin, a first-generation cephalosporin, or amoxicillin with clavulanate. Erythromycin or clindamycin can be used in a penicillin-allergic patient. Uncomplicated, noncartilaginous injuries do not require antibiotics.

LIPS

Lacerations of the lip can cause devastating cosmetic defects if not properly and meticulously repaired. A misalignment by 1 mm of the vermilion border, or "white line," can be noticed by a casual observer. It is a defect that cannot be revised easily after primary healing has taken place. Other important anatomic structures include the mucosal border (the portion of the lip that divides the intraoral and extraoral portion of the lip) and the underlying orbicularis oris muscle. Each of these structures requires careful and exact apposition to achieve the best structural and cosmetic result. Vertical through-and-through lacerations often violate all three of these structures.

Preparation for Closure

Although the mouth is replete with bacteria, and a lip laceration would not remain clean during the repair procedure, cleansing is performed only to remove gross debris and dirt. If any teeth are broken, a careful search is made in the wound for teeth fragments. Retained tooth particles can cause marked inflammation and infection leading to a complete breakdown of any attempted repair. Whenever a portion of a tooth cannot be accounted for, a lateral radiograph of the face using the soft tissue technique can reveal the missing fragment.

Anesthesia for lip repairs is best accomplished by either an infraorbital nerve block for the upper lip or a mental nerve block for the lower lip (see Chapter 6). Direct infiltration of the laceration can cause excessive distortion of the lip and can create difficulties when an attempt is made to align wound edges properly.

Uncomplicated Lacerations

Most lip lacerations do not require extensive revision or débridement. The key to closure is proper alignment of the anatomic structures listed previously. If the vermilion border is violated and the laceration is superficial, the repair begins with placement of the first suture, with careful precision, through that border on each side of the

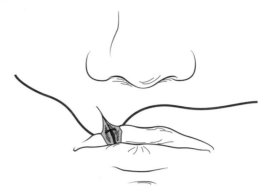

Figure 12-15. The major goal when closing any lip laceration is to align the appropriate borders. Initial suture placement and alignment of the vermilion border are shown. When the vermilion border or white line is aligned, the remainder of the laceration is closed.

wound (Fig. 12-15). When alignment is judged to be appropriate, the remainder of the wound is closed with 6-0 nonabsorbable monofilament sutures. If the mucosal border is violated, it also is aligned meticulously. As a general rule, if the laceration extends beyond the mucosal border into the oral cavity, 5-0 absorbable suture, such as chromic gut, is used to close that portion. Irradiated polyglactin 910 (Vicryl) is also recommended because it does not "stiffen" as much as gut, and it is absorbed rapidly.

Complicated and Through-and-Through Lacerations

In contrast to many other structures of the face, the lip can be revised, and significant portions of devitalized tissue (25% of the upper or lower lip) can be excised in a V shape without causing significant deformity except for the area of the upper lip just below the nose, the philtrum, and the oral commissures. Considerable judgment is required to handle these cosmetic problems in image-conscious patients who have high expectations for excellent results. Consultation is advised for lacerations and injuries that would affect the patient's appearance.

Repair of a vertical through-and-through laceration is illustrated in Figure 12-16. The repair begins with closure of the vermilion border. Next, the orbicularis oris muscle is reapproximated carefully with deep 5-0 absorbable suture material, such as polyglycolic acid. The deep sutures should include the fibrous covering of the muscle to ensure anchoring. The remainder of the repair proceeds with 6-0 nonabsorbable sutures for the skin and exposed lip. For the oral cavity portion inside the mucosal border, 5-0 absorbable sutures are used.

Aftercare

No dressing is placed on the lips. The patient is reminded not to bring excessive pressure to bear on the suture line while the sutures are in place. Rinsing the mouth after eating is recommended to prevent small particulate matter from penetrating the suture line. Extraoral sutures are removed after 4 to 5 days in adults and after 3 to 5 days in children to prevent the formation of suture marks. A controlled study of intraoral lacerations suggests that there is some benefit to administering oral penicillin V potassium (Penicillin VK) four times daily for 5 days as prophylaxis against infection.[26] Erythromycin or clindamycin may be considered as alternatives for a penicillin-allergic patient.

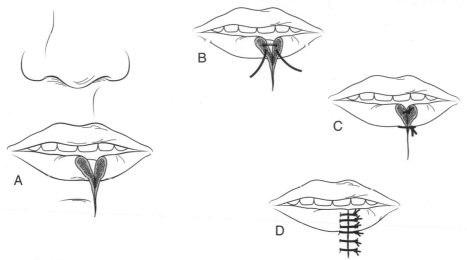

Figure 12-16. **A,** Demonstration of a through-and-through laceration of the lip involving the orbicularis oris muscle. **B,** Closure of the orbicularis oris muscle is performed by the use of absorbable deep sutures, such as polyglycolic acid. **C,** When the orbicularis oris muscle is approximated, the vermilion border or white line is approximated. **D,** The remainder of the laceration is closed with simple percutaneous monofilament nylon sutures.

ORAL CAVITY

The oral cavity consists of several structures, each of which requires separate considerations during management and repair. These are the buccal mucosa, gingiva, teeth, salivary glands and ducts, tongue, mandible, and alveolar ridge of the maxillary bone. Injuries to the oral cavity can be a potential threat to airway patency.

Preparation for Repair

Other than airway considerations, the most important part of the evaluation of the oral cavity is the determination of the integrity of salivary structures, bone, and teeth. Visual inspection and palpation are necessary to complete the examination. Particularly troublesome are teeth, fragments of which must be accounted for if possible. They can lodge easily in the mucosa and the deep tissue of the lip, where they can cause severe inflammation and infection if not removed before closure. If there is any question about the location of a tooth or fragment, radiographs of the soft tissues should be obtained.

Buccal Mucosal and Gingival Lacerations

As a general rule, lacerations of either the buccal mucosa or the gingiva heal without repair if the wound edges are not widely separated or if flaps are not present. Wounds that gape open (usually ≥2 to 3 cm) need only one to three sutures for closure. Flaps that interpose between teeth can be excised or closed; 5-0 chromic gut or another absorbable material can be used. The oral cavity tissues heal remarkably quickly, and most lacerations, even large ones, close without sutures. After repair, the patient is instructed to eat soft food and to rinse the mouth gently after each meal.

Occasionally a flap of tissue overlying the mandibular or maxillary ridge is created during injury to the gingiva. Because of the lack of support provided by thin supporting tissues, the gingival flap cannot be sutured easily. A technique illustrated in Figure 12-17 shows how sutures are brought circumferentially around teeth to

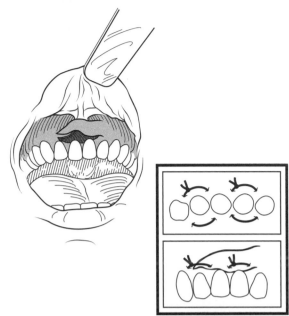

Figure 12-17. Avulsion of gingival/mucosal tissue. The technique to close this injury is shown. The sutures are brought around the teeth and through the avulsed tissue flap. (Adapted from Zukin D, Simon R: *Emergency wound care: principles and practice*, Rockville, Md, 1987, Aspen Publishers.)

provide the necessary anchor for the repair; 4-0 or 5-0 chromic gut or other absorbable material is used.

Tongue Lacerations

Repairing a lacerated tongue can be challenging. Small lacerations ≤1.5 cm, which do not gape widely when the tongue is extended, heal without intervention. Lacerations that gape widely, actively bleed, are flap shaped, or involve muscle probably need closure. The key to repairing these lacerations is to gain the confidence of the patient. With frightened children, gaining confidence is often difficult, and the patient may be best served in a surgical setting where sedation and anesthesia can be delivered. An assistant is required to control the tongue with dry gauze sponges, or a towel clip is placed in the previously anesthetized tip. A bite-block can be fashioned to prevent injury to the assistant or to the operator. The wound area is anesthetized by direct infiltration without epinephrine. The tongue heals rapidly and can be closed with an absorbable suture (e.g., 4-0 chromic, polyglycolic acid, or Vicryl). The sutures are placed in large bites to include the mucosa and muscle.

Aftercare

For the first 2 or 3 days after repair of an intraoral laceration, soft foods and liquids are recommended. Rinsing the oral cavity after eating also is helpful.

Dental Trauma

Teeth often are loosened by trauma to the oral cavity. Minimal loosening (<2 mm), as determined by gentle "rocking" of the tooth between the examining fingers, usually reverses without intervention. Marked loosening or subluxation with an accompanying fracture of the alveolar ridge needs to be repaired with dental stabilization.

Intact teeth also can become avulsed. These teeth can be replaced in an anatomically intact socket, but the prognosis for salvage decreases with each minute that passes. On arrival in the emergency department, an attempt should be made to insert the avulsed tooth in the socket if possible.[27] If the socket contains debris, gentle removal is tried. Vigorous intervention should be avoided. The tooth can be handled by the crown but not by the root. To avoid damage to the periodontal ligament, cleaning of the tooth is not recommended. Even saline may be harmful to ligament cells.

If the tooth cannot be reinserted easily, it can be "stored" in one of three ways until a dentist or an oral surgeon can be consulted. The three storage methods are (1) between the buccal mucosa and gum of the patient's mouth, (2) in Hank's solution, or (3) in milk.[28] Saline is avoided. After 30 minutes outside of the socket, the prognosis for salvage worsens rapidly. Even if the periodontal ligament survives and the tooth reattaches, later root canal intervention is necessary to deal with the sequelae of the loss of neurovascular supply.

PERINEUM

Injuries to the perineum (i.e., penis, scrotum, and female introitus) can involve important structures that need special attention. During the examination of wounds of the perineum, the urethra, corpora, testicles, and rectum must be assessed. Blood coming from the urethral meatus, or difficulty urinating, suggests urethral injury. The shaft of the penis is covered by thin skin; violation of the corpora cavernosa or spongiosum often accompanies lacerations of the penis. The testicle is covered with a capsule-like fibrous covering called the tunica albuginea. Interruption of the corpora or tunica requires repair by a specialist. Most labial lacerations are uncomplicated, but occasionally the female urethra or rectum is involved.

Preparation for Closure

Wounds to the perineum are prepared with a cleansing agent and are irrigated with saline as previously described. Uncomplicated lacerations can be anesthetized directly with lidocaine or bupivacaine. Care is taken not to use epinephrine-containing solutions for anesthetizing the penis because of potential ischemia and constriction of end arteries.

Lacerations of the Penis and Scrotum

Because the skin of the penis is so thin, lacerations are closed with a single layer of nonabsorbable suture (e.g., 5-0 nylon). Closure of the scrotal skin is carried out with chromic gut sutures that fall out within 10 days. If chromic material is unavailable, another absorbable suture material can be substituted, but it may not fall out as soon. Healing occurs rapidly, and removal of sutures from the rugated skin, which can be difficult, is unnecessary.

Lacerations of the Introitus

Lacerations of the labia can involve the deeper supporting muscles. In this case, closure must occur in two layers to ensure reapproximation of the muscles. The skin over the labia majora can be closed with a nonabsorbable material, such as nylon or polypropylene. The labia minora is covered with mucosa and can be closed with absorbable material. Uncomplicated lacerations of the vagina, unless they are extensive, heal without sutures. Extensive or complex wounds are best referred to consultants.

Aftercare

Dressings for the genital area are hard to fashion. Gauze sponges supported by an athletic supporter are an option for men. Perineal pads are suggested for women. Hygiene of the genital area is important; daily gentle cleansing with soap and water is acceptable.

Topical antibiotic ointment (Neosporin) applied after bathing and before application of the dressing is recommended. Sutures of the penis are removed in 7 to 10 days for adults and 6 to 8 days for children.

KNEE

Careful examination of knee lacerations is important because of the structures that can be damaged. The peroneal nerve, patellar tendon, medial and lateral collateral ligaments, and patella all have to be tested for function and integrity before repair. Of particular importance is the joint space itself. If penetration is suspected, 50 mL of normal saline with a few drops of methylene blue is injected into the joint, in a sterile fashion, at a site distant from the laceration. Arthrocentesis technique is used. If the capsule is violated, the dye leaks out of the laceration. For more subtle injuries, fluorescein dye can be used with an ultraviolet light detection lamp.

Knee lacerations can be contaminated with grit and ground-in dirt. Although time consuming, meticulous cleansing, irrigation, and débridement are often necessary to render the wound ready to close. Uncomplicated, nonpenetrating lacerations are closed with monofilament nylon after local anesthetic infiltration. Occasionally, deep (dermal) sutures using an absorbable material are required.

Aftercare

The key to good healing of knee lacerations is proper immobilization and elevation for several days. Crutches can be used for at least 48 to 72 hours if the extensor surface of the knee is involved or if the wound is extensive. Knee flexion can be reduced by the application of a bulky dressing. Sutures are removed in 10 to 14 days for adults and 8 to 10 days for children.

LOWER LEG

The most vexing consideration related to lower leg (shin) lacerations is the significant tension that occurs at the wound edge. Skin overlying the tibia is under higher natural tension than most other regions of the body. Figure 12-18 illustrates a technique for approximating the wound edges with as little tension as possible; 4-0 monofilament nylon is passed through sterile, cotton-retaining pledgets obtained from the operating room. This technique allows for even distribution of tension along the wound edge without tearing. This pledget technique is particularly useful for older and thinner skin. Undermining and deep suture placement can assist in reducing tension.

Another technique for the closure of avulsion/flap wounds of the shin in older patients is the use of wound tapes[29] (see Chapter 11). Tapes avoid the problem of skin tearing that can occur with sutures and staples. Tapes can be left on until they naturally fall off. This technique allows for minimal potential disruption of the healing wound.

Aftercare

Elevation is an important element for lacerations and wounds of the lower leg. Dependent edema should not be allowed to develop. Sutures are removed after 8 to 12 days for adults and 6 to 10 days for children.

FOOT

The foot is anatomically complex and in that way is similar to the hand. Complete lacerations to the flexor tendons need to be repaired, as they also need to be repaired in hands (see Chapter 13). Extensor tendons can be treated with primary skin closure and splinting. Consultation is recommended under these circumstances. Anesthesia for the plantar surface of the foot is best achieved by a posterior tibial nerve or sural nerve

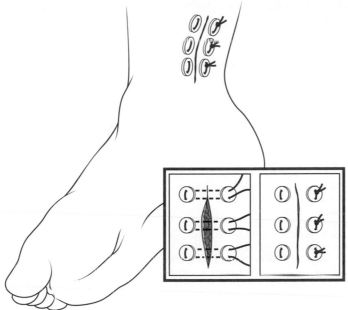

Figure 12-18. Because of the high tension usually associated with lacerations in the lower leg (shin area), sterile cotton pledgets can be used as support for 3-0 or 4-0 monofilament nylon sutures. (Adapted from Zukin D, Simon R: *Emergency wound care: principles and practice*, Rockville, Md, 1987, Aspen Publishers.)

block (see Chapter 6). Occasionally, this method of administering anesthesia needs to be supplemented by local infiltration. Superficial dorsal lacerations are closed with 4-0 or 5-0 monofilament nylon. Lacerations of the plantar surface, or sole, can be closed with 3-0 monofilament. Lacerations of the web spaces between the toes have the same significance as lacerations of web spaces of the hand. There are no crucial structures passing through these areas, and repair of the skin alone should suffice.

Aftercare
Similar to any lower extremity injury, elevation is an important adjunct to care. Crutches are useful, particularly for wounds on the plantar surface. Sutures are removed in 10 to 12 days for adults and 8 to 10 days for children.

References
1. Hamilton JR, Sunter JP, Cooper PN: Fatal hemorrhage for simple lacerations of the scalp, *Forensic Sci Med Pathol* 1:267–270, 2010.
2. Fullarton GM, MacEwen CJ, MacMillan R, et al: An evaluation of open scalp wounds, *Arch Emerg Med* 4:11–16, 1987.
3. Stiell IG, Clement CM, Rowe BH, et al: Comparison of Canadian CT head rule and the New Orleans criteria in patients with minor head injury, *JAMA* 294:1511–1518, 2005.
4. Pecora D, Landis R, Martin E: Location of cutaneous microorganisms, *Surgery* 64:1114–1117, 1968.
5. Howell JM, Morgan JA: Scalp laceration repair without prior hair removal, *Am J Emerg Med* 6:7–10, 1988.
6. Edlich R: Special considerations in wound management, *Am J Emerg Med* 19:1089, 1990.
7. Cruse P, Foord R: A five year prospective of 23,649 surgical wounds, *Arch Surg* 107:206–209, 1973.
8. Seropian R, Reynolds B: Wound infections after preoperative depilatory versus razor preparation, *Am J Surg* 121:251–254, 1971.
9. Achneck HE, Sileshi B, Jamioilski RM, et al: A comprehensive review of hemostatic agents: efficacy and recommendations for use, *Ann Surg* 251:217–228, 2010.

10. Tandon SC, Kelly J, Turtle M: Irradiated polyglactin-910: a new synthetic absorbable suture, *J R Coll Surg Edinb* 40:185–187, 1995.
11. Missori P, Polli FM, Fontana E, et al: Closure of skin or scalp with absorbable sutures, *Plast Recon Surg* 112:924–925, 2003.
12. Aderiotis D, Sandor GK: Outcomes of irradiated polyglactin 910, *J Can Dent Assoc* 65:345–347, 1999.
13. George TK, Simpson DC: Skin wound closure with staples in the accident and emergency department, *J R Coll Surg Edinb* 30:54–56, 1985.
14. Roth JH, Windle BH: Staple versus suture closure of skin incisions in a pig model, *Can J Surg* 31:19–20, 1988.
15. Abu NGA, Dayan PS, Miller S, et al: Cosmetic outcome of scalp wound closure with staples in the pediatric emergency department: a prospective, randomized trial, *Pediatr Emerg Care* 18:171–173, 2002.
16. Orlinsky M, Goldberg RM, Chan L: Cost analysis of stapling v. suture skin closure, *Am J Emerg Med* 13:77–81, 1995.
17. Aoki N, Oikawa A, Sakai T: Hair-braiding closure for superficial wounds, *Surg Neurol* 46:150–151, 1996.
18. Duschoff IM: About face, *Emerg Med* Nov:25–77, 1974.
19. Parell GJ, Becker GD: Comparison of absorbable with nonabsorbable sutures in closure of facial skin wounds, *Arch Facial Plast Surg* 5:488–490, 2003.
20. Edlich RF, Rodeheaver GJ, Morgan RF, et al: Principles of wound management, *Ann Emerg Med* 17:1284–1302, 1988.
21. Luck RP, Flood R, Eyal D, et al: Cosmetic outcomes of absorbable versus nonabsorbable sutures in pediatric facial lacerations, *Pediatr Emerg Care* 24:137–142, 2008.
22. Talbot AW, Meadows AE, Tyers AG, et al: Use of 7/0 Vicryl (coated polyglactin 910) and 7/0 Vicryl-Rapide (irradiated polyglactin 910) in skin closure in ophthalmic plastic surgery, *Orbit* 21:1–8, 2002.
23. Dubach P, Aebi C: Cavesaccio: Late onset of posttraumatic septal hematoma and abscess formation in a six-year-old Tamil girl—case report and literature review, *Rhinology* 46:342–344, 2008.
24. Rohrich RJ, Adams WP: Nasal fracture management: minimizing nasal deformities, *Plast Reconstr Surg* 106:266–273, 2000.
25. Burr WE: Auricular hematoma: treatment options, *Aust N Z J Surg* 57:391–392, 1987.
26. Steele MT, Sainsbury CR, Robinson WA, et al: Prophylactic penicillin for intraoral wounds, *Ann Emerg Med* 18:847–852, 1989.
27. Bringhurst L, Herr RD, Aldous JA: Oral trauma in the emergency department, *Am J Emerg Med* 11:486–490, 1993.
28. Trope M: Clinical management of the avulsed tooth, *Dent Clin North Am* 39:92–112, 1995.
29. King MT: Flap wounds of the skin, *Injury* 12:354–359, 1981.

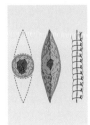

CHAPTER 13
The Hand

Key Practice Points

- Patients with hand injuries are treated in the supine position to prevent syncopal falls induced by pain.
- Remove all jewelry from the injured hand to prevent constriction and ischemia secondary to swelling.
- The "golden period" for repair of hand lacerations and wounds is 6 to 8 hours from the time of injury. Beyond that period, the risk of infection rises.
- Although two-point discrimination is the standard test to measure sensation following possible nerve injuries to the hand, a normal test does not rule out nerve injury if the patient has a subjective feeling of numbness.
- Innocuous-appearing wounds, such as punctures, can cause significant wounds to tendons and nerves. Careful testing is still necessary.
- Tendons can appear to function normally after wounding because of partial injury or cross-linking of extensor tendons. It is prudent to explore wounds over tendons to detect these types of injuries.
- Absorbable sutures are becoming more common in the closure of hand wounds, because they produce the same results as nonabsorbable sutures.
- If the nail is attached firmly to the nail bed, subungual hematomas (even if the subungual hematoma is >50% of the nail surface) can be treated with trephination alone without nail removal or nail bed repair.
- Fingertip avulsions, without nail bed disruption or bone exposure, heal well without surgical intervention or grafting.
- Tendon or nerve injuries can undergo delayed repair. The skin is closed at the time of injury and the patient is referred to a specialist for nerve or tendon repair of the hand.
- Infections and antibiotic prophylaxis of hand wounds have recently become more complicated because of the appearance of community-acquired methicillin-resistant *Staphylococcus aureus* (CA-MRSA).

INITIAL TREATMENT

Before a thorough and careful examination of a patient with an injured hand can take place, certain preparatory steps must be taken. Except for the most trivial injuries, the patient is best managed by placement on a stretcher on arrival at the medical care facility. Hand injuries often are painful and provoke anxiety. Placing the patient in a supine position prevents unexpected vasovagal syncope. The recumbent position allows for easy placement of the hand in an elevated position to decrease the swelling that occurs after injury.

Any rings or constricting jewelry are removed to prevent ischemia of a digit. Most rings can be removed by using a lubricant and applying gentle, persistent traction. Ring removal from swollen fingers can be accomplished by using a specially designed ring cutter and spreading the ring open with two Kelly clamps applied to the edges of the cut portion (see Fig. 2-1). Patients who are concerned about damaged rings can be reassured that jewelers can restore rings to their original condition. Another method for the removal of rings is shown in Figure 13-1. Umbilical tape or O-silk suture can be wrapped firmly around the finger and passed under the ring with a small forceps. The ring is extracted as the tape or suture is unwound proximally to the ring.

Occasionally, a patient arrives with a ring or band made of hardened steel or even titanium. If routine removal procedures, including cutting, do not succeed in removing the ring, the following procedure can be tried[1]:

- Wrap elastic tape, 1 inch in width, tightly around the finger starting from the tip of the finger and moving toward the ring. Extra wraps adjacent to the ring may be needed, because more edema accumulates in that area.
- Elevate the hand above heart level for 15 minutes. Securing the arm gently to an IV pole will help. Apply an ice pack to the finger as well.
- After 15 minutes, apply a blood pressure cuff to the upper arm and inflate it to 250 mm Hg to prevent blood refilling the arm and finger.
- Quickly remove the tape, apply a light coating of lubricant to the finger, and remove the ring.
- If this procedure does not work the first time, there may be residual edema. The procedure can be repeated.

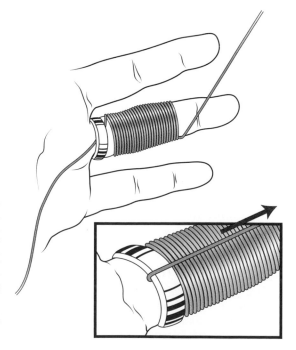

Figure 13-1. The technique to remove a ring by finger wrapping with large silk suture or umbilical tape. The suture is begun distally over the distal interphalangeal joint and is brought back to the ring. The tail end portion of the wrap is brought under the ring, usually with a small hemostat. The removal of the ring is begun by unraveling the wrap and tugging on the string that is proximal to the ring portion. As it unravels, the ring gently travels forward distally over the finger.

Most patients attempt to bandage the injured hand before proceeding to a medical care facility. These hastily fashioned, unsterile dressings should be removed carefully. Until treatment can be administered, sterile sponges moistened with normal saline should be applied, followed by a 2- or 3-inch gauze wrap. Any active bleeding requires manual pressure with gauze sponges. An extremity tourniquet rarely is needed to stop excessive hemorrhage.

If the wound is grossly contaminated with soil or other debris, and if there will be a delay before treatment can be administered, the hand is cleaned gently with a wound-cleansing agent followed by irrigation with normal saline.[2] The chance of infection increases with each passing hour from the time of injury to repair. Early cleansing and irrigation can extend this safe period.

It is a common but unsupported practice to soak hand injuries in a wound-cleansing solution before repair. Soaking is believed to loosen debris and to help kill contaminating bacteria, but there is no scientific evidence to support these beliefs.[3,4] Brief extremity immersion is recommended only to help remove gross soil and debris from the area surrounding the wound before proper skin cleansing and wound irrigation is undertaken.

TERMINOLOGY

Knowledge of conventional terminology is required to properly document and communicate information about injuries to the hand and fingers. All lacerations and wounds can be located accurately by the use of appropriate terms. A ½-inch laceration on the back of the index finger at the first knuckle is described accurately as "a 1-cm superficial laceration of the index finger on the dorsal surface at the proximal interphalangeal joint." Figures 13-2 and 13-3 illustrate the various descriptive landmarks and joints. The back of the hand is the *dorsal* surface, whereas the palm side is the *palmar* or *volar* surface. Common landmarks of the palm are the thenar and hypothenar eminences. The digits are best remembered and recorded, when necessary, as the thumb, index, middle, ring, and little finger. Each segment of the finger is named for the underlying bony phalanx. Although the joints are descriptive of their location, it is the convention to use the abbreviations noted in Figure 13-2.

Instead of using terms such as *inside* and *outside* or *medial* and *lateral,* the sides of the hands and fingers are referred to as *radial* and *ulnar.* This convention eliminates the confusion elicited by the other terms. Any injury to any surface on the side of the hand or finger corresponding to the radius is so described. A laceration of the side of the little finger is either radial or ulnar depending on whether it is on the side of the ulna or on the side of the radius (see Fig. 13-3).

PATIENT HISTORY

Certain key historical facts help determine the timing and choice of repair and other supportive treatment. As previously discussed, the amount of time that has elapsed from the time of injury influences the decision of when to repair the wound. Clean wounds that are caused by shearing forces probably can be safely repaired 6 to 8 hours after the injury. Wounds caused by tension and compression mechanisms are more vulnerable and should be considered for closure sooner. Severely contaminated wounds, or wounds caused by mutilating forces, are best left for consultation and possible delayed closure. This decision is made on a case-by-case basis.

A seemingly innocuous mechanism of injury is the puncture wound of the hand. Although the entry point is quite small and appears innocent, special care has to be taken not to miss a transected nerve or tendon. In addition, the possibility of a foreign body being retained in a puncture wound has to be considered, and a radiographic examination should be performed when the suspicion is raised.

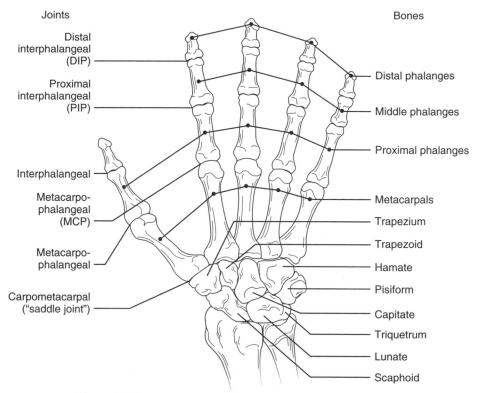

Joints

Distal
interphalangeal
(DIP)

Proximal
interphalangeal
(PIP)

Interphalangeal

Metacarpo-
phalangeal
(MCP)

Metacarpo-
phalangeal

Carpometacarpal
("saddle joint")

Bones

Distal phalanges

Middle phalanges

Proximal phalanges

Metacarpals

Trapezium

Trapezoid

Hamate

Pisiform

Capitate

Triquetrum

Lunate

Scaphoid

Figure 13-2. Descriptive anatomy of the joints and bones of the hand.

Other historical points of importance are the patient's hand dominance, history of previous hand deformities, profession, and hobbies. Although these considerations are seemingly not very important for patients with emergency lacerations and wounds, a simple matter of a mismanaged fingertip injury can significantly affect an activity such as playing the guitar. For a guitar player, every step is taken to preserve the nail matrix. Preservation attempts might not be as crucial for an individual who does not require this anatomic part for either a job function or for a hobby.

Any allergies the patient may have should be verified when taking the history. Many drugs, including tetanus toxoid, local anesthetics, pain medications, and a variety of antibiotics, are administered to patients with hand injuries.

EXAMINATION OF THE HAND

The actual examination of the injured hand consists of careful inspection of the wound and thorough functional testing. Nerve function is evaluated by assessment of motor and sensory components. The integrity of tendons most often can be determined by specific functional maneuvers. Because tendons often are only partially severed, and function is preserved, direct visualization by exploration may be necessary. For wounds in emergency situations, circulation is so profuse that severed, bleeding vessels, which travel in neurovascular bundles, often are better indicators of nerve injury than actual threats to perfusion of the hand or finger. When necessary, radiographs are obtained to assist in the examination to rule out fractures or foreign bodies. Finally, there is no substitute for exploration and direct visualization to discover if there is structural damage of any type.

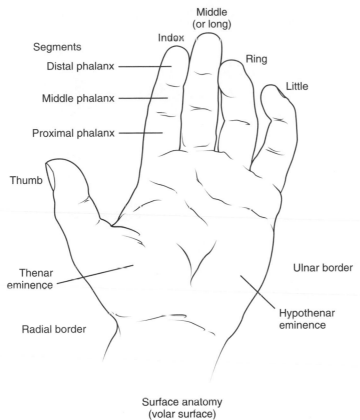

Segments
Distal phalanx
Middle phalanx
Proximal phalanx
Index
Middle
(or long)
Ring
Little
Thumb
Thenar
eminence
Radial border
Ulnar border
Hypothenar
eminence

Surface anatomy
(volar surface)

Figure 13-3. Descriptive anatomy of the surface of the hand. Note the ulnar and radial borders.

Nerve Testing
Motor Function

Three major nerves are responsible for motor and sensory function of the hand. The radial nerve innervates the extrinsic muscles of the forearm that are responsible for extension of the wrist and fingers. This nerve does not innervate any muscle within the confines of the hand itself. The motor function of this nerve is tested by having the patient dorsiflex his or her wrist and fingers against a resisting force, such as the examiner's hand (Fig. 13-4). Intact motor strength, as provided for by an intact radial nerve, should prevent the examiner from overcoming the dorsiflexed wrist when a good deal of counterforce is applied.

In addition to the flexor carpi ulnaris and part of the flexor digitorum profundus, the ulnar nerve innervates most of the intrinsic muscles of the hand itself, including all of the interossei muscles and the little and ring finger lumbricals. The motor portion of this nerve is responsible for the ability of the fingers to spread and close in a fanlike manner. A specific test for ulnar motor function is to have the patient adduct (close) the fingers against an object, such as a pen (Fig. 13-5). With an intact nerve, the examiner cannot easily remove the object. Each finger can be tested in this manner.

The median nerve provides motor innervation to wrist flexors, the flexor digitorum superficialis, part of the flexor digitorum profundus (shared with the ulnar nerve), and the remaining intrinsic muscles of the hand, most notably the muscles of the thumb

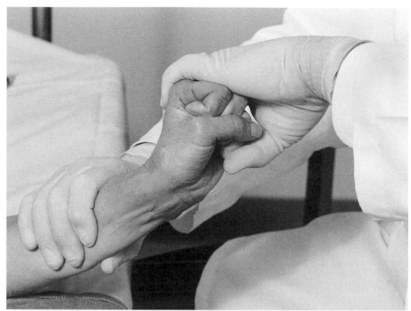

Figure 13-4. Testing for radial nerve function. With the patient's fist dorsiflexed, the examiner tries to "break" the resistance created by the dorsiflexion.

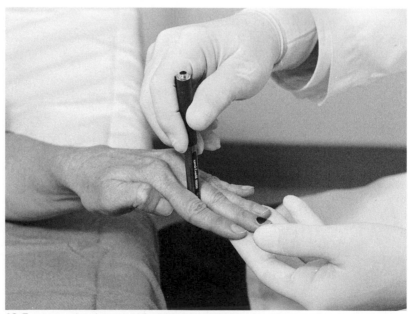

Figure 13-5. Testing for ulnar nerve function. The patient is asked to resist the examiner's attempt to pull an object, such as a pen, from between the adducted fingers.

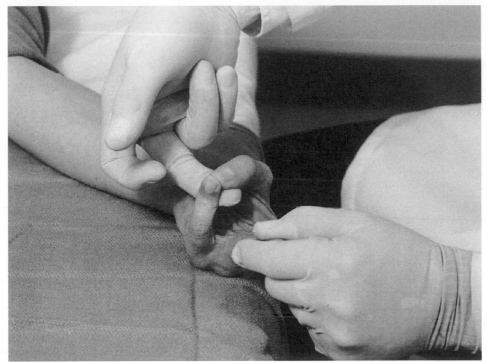

Figure 13-6. Testing for median nerve function. The thumb is apposed to the little finger to form a tight ring. This ring should not be easily broken by the examiner.

that are responsible for opposition. To some degree, opposition also is mediated by the adduction component of the interossei as supplied to the ulnar nerve. The testing maneuver is completed by having the patient oppose his or her thumb with the tip of the little finger. A properly made "ring," consisting of the thumb and little finger, should be difficult to break by the examiner if the median nerve is intact (Fig. 13-6).

Sensory Function

A variety of stimuli can be delivered to the skin of the hand to test sensory function. Gross touch with a blunt object is the easiest but is the least specific. Gross touch can be useful, however, for rapid screening to assess the possibility of nerve damage, especially when comparison testing of the injured and noninjured hands is done. If there is a nerve injury, the patient often is able to report a difference in feeling. Pinprick stimulus is the most commonly used modality for testing. Pinprick is useful when alternated with blunt stimulus. In a complete nerve transection, the patient cannot tell the difference between a blunt and a sharp stimulus. Pinprick testing nevertheless is difficult to assess on the fingertips, especially in a manual laborer whose fingerpads are covered with thick calluses.

A more accurate method of assessing sensory function is two-point discrimination.[5] A paper clip can be fashioned so that two ends can be opened or closed to varying distances from each other (Fig. 13-7). Because the ulnar and radial side of each finger has separate innervation, testing each side of the finger is necessary. A patient with a normally innervated finger should be able to distinguish two simultaneously delivered stimuli that are 6 mm or more distant from each other. Most patients can tell a

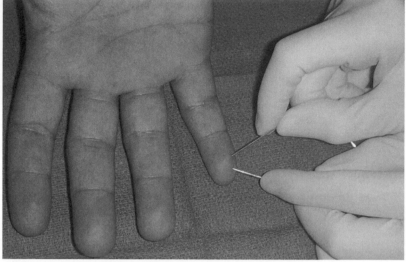

Figure 13-7. Technique for testing sensory nerve function by two-point discrimination. A paper clip is bent in a manner to provide variable distance stimuli. See text for a complete description.

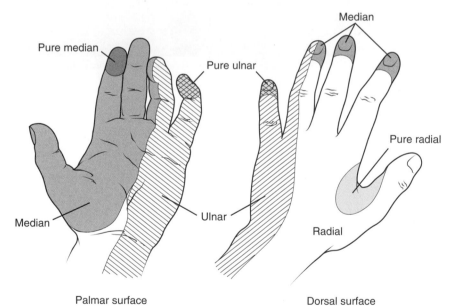

Palmar surface   Dorsal surface

Figure 13-8. The distribution of the three major nerves providing sensory innervation of the hand. Note the areas of pure median, ulnar, and radial sensation.

difference down to 3 mm. When identification of separate stimuli is reported by the patient at 8 mm apart or more, the examination is clearly abnormal.

Of the major nerves, the radial nerve provides the least important sensory innervation to the hand. This nerve supplies sensation to the radial portion of the dorsum of the hand, the dorsum of the thumb, and the proximal portion of the dorsal side of the second and third digits and half of the ring finger (Fig. 13-8). To test gross radial

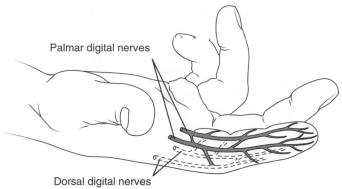

Figure 13-9. Each digit is supplied by four digital nerves. The palmar digital nerves predominate and provide most of the sensation to the volar aspect of the finger and fingertip proximal to the distal interphalangeal joint. The nail bed often is included in the palmar digital nerve distribution.

sensory function rapidly, a stimulus is supplied to the first web space, which is an area of pure radial distribution.

Sensory distribution of the ulnar nerve includes the dorsal and volar surfaces of the ulnar side of the hand, the entire fifth digit, and the ulnar half of the fourth digit. To test an intact sensory component of the ulnar nerve, an appropriate stimulus is delivered to the area of purest ulnar distribution: the tip of the fifth digit.

The remainder of the hand is innervated by the median nerve. The area of sensory distribution comprises the radial side of the palm; volar surfaces of the thumb, index, and middle fingers; and the radial half of the ring finger. As depicted in Figure 13-8, median nerve innervation extends to the fingertips of the thumb, index, and middle fingers, including the dorsal portion of the distal phalanges. Pure median sensation can be found at the tip of the index finger.

More common than injuries to the major nerves are injuries and lacerations to the digital nerves that lie within the hand itself. There are four digital nerves for each digit. The two palmar nerves (Fig. 13-9) are the largest and most important. (The others are the dorsal digital nerves.) Sensation is carried through these two nerves to the palmar surface and the nail bed area of the fingertip. A laceration or puncture wound to the palmar or dorsal surface of the hand or to any individual digit requires careful sensory testing of the digits distal to the injury.

As previously described, a variety of stimuli can be used for sensory testing. The most accurate method of detecting a nerve injury in this setting is the two-point discrimination test. Objective documentation of digital nerve injuries is not always possible at the time of the first examination immediately after injury. Patient pain, anxiety, and factors such as the presence of callused hands can interfere with two-point testing. Even though stimulus testing is inconsistent and does not clearly document nerve injury, any subjective "numbness" reported by the patient has to be taken seriously, and consultation with a hand specialist should be considered. Under these circumstances, it is common to close the skin and to refer the patient for evaluation within a few days after the initial care.

Tendon Function
Extensor Function
Extensor tendon function can be tested simply by having the patient extend his or her fingers against the force of the examiner (Fig. 13-10). Although this maneuver appears to be easy enough, there are complexities of the tendon anatomy that can cause confusion

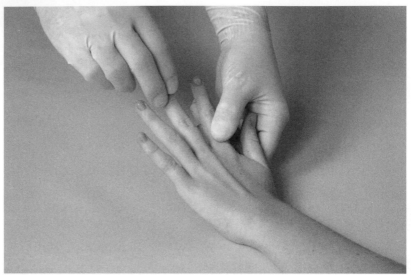

Figure 13-10. Testing the extensor tendon function. Each finger is extended against a resisting force. This force should not be easily overcome.

when results of the examination are interpreted. The wrist itself has three main extensor tendons that are responsible for proper extension at the wrist. If these tendons are cut, the wrist can be extended by the finger extensors but with far less force, and that force can be overcome easily by the examiner. The thumb is served by an abductor and two extensor tendons. If one extensor is cut, the second still can function. Each finger has one main extensor tendon responsible for extension with power. The second and fifth digits, however, have small accessory tendons that can extend these fingers weakly if the main extensors are knocked out of action.

Another anatomic point that can possibly cause misinterpretation in the examination for extension of the digits is the fact that as extensor tendons cross the wrist, they flatten out and interconnect with other extensors over the dorsum of the hand (Fig. 13-11). Weak extension of a severed tendon can occur by the action of the adjacent interconnecting tendon. These interconnections also can prevent severed extensor tendons from slipping back into the forearm after they are cut. This anatomic property of extensors makes anastomosis easier for extensors than for flexor tendons, because the two severed ends can be readily retrieved during repair.

When there is doubt about extensor tendon function, careful exploration has to be performed through the laceration itself. Extensor tendons are superficial and can be identified easily with proper and gentle exposure. A key factor to remember is that the position of the hand at the time of examination and exploration may be different from the position of the hand during injury. If that should be the case, the actual laceration to the tendon may be at a location away from the laceration on the skin (Fig. 13-12). Active flexion/extension of the finger to cause the tendon to slide back and forth is encouraged during the exploration.

Flexor Function

The thumb has only one flexor tendon, but the index, middle, ring, and little fingers have two main flexor tendons. The volar surface of the wrist is a complex and vulnerable area, replete with important structures. As illustrated in Figure 13-13, the median

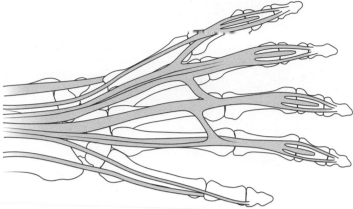

Figure 13-11. Extensor tendon anatomy of the hand. Note in particular the cross-linkages of extensor tendons at the distal metacarpal level. Severance of an extensor tendon proximal to these cross-linkages can give the examiner the false sense that the affected digit can be extended because of the help that cross-linkage provides through the adjacent tendon.

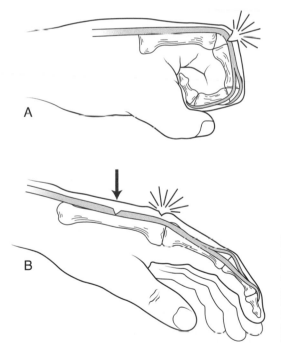

Figure 13-12. Tendon-skin wound mismatch. **A,** A tendon can be partially lacerated in one position, such as a closed fist. **B,** When the wound is explored, however, the tendon injury might be missed because the site of the tendon injury has retracted when the hand is extended for care. The examiner must perform the exploration by trying to re-create the position of the hand during injury.

nerve lies just deep and radial to the palmaris longus, the most superficial tendon. Even lacerations to the wrist that appear trivial can cause serious tendon and nerve damage.

The flexor tendons to each finger are paired. The flexor digitorum profundus tendons are responsible for power and mass action, such as is needed for gripping. These tendons run deep to the flexor digitorum superficialis tendons, but at the level of the middle phalanx, the profundus splits through the superficialis and goes on to attach to the distal phalanx (Fig. 13-14). To test profundus function, the action of the sublimis

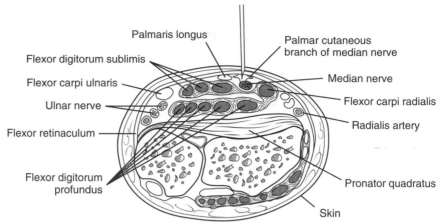

Figure 13-13. Cross-sectional anatomy of the wrist. Note in particular the superficial location of the median nerve. Any visible tendon laceration, such as to the palmaris longus, has to raise the suspicion of an injury to the median nerve.

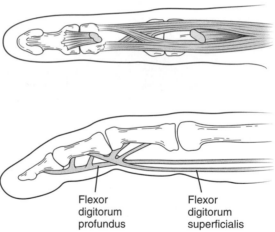

Figure 13-14. Note the relationship of the flexor digitorum profundus to the flexor digitorum superficialis. The profundus splits through the superficialis, which is attached on the middle phalanx. The profundus attaches to the distal phalanx.

tendon has to be blocked by holding each digit, one at a time, in extension at the middle phalanx (Fig. 13-15). The patient is asked to flex the distal phalanx, which now can be accomplished only through the action of the profundus. During this maneuver, 60 degrees of flexion is normal.

The flexor digitorum superficialis tendons are responsible for the positioning of the fingers so that power flexion can occur. These tendons run superficial to the deep tendons until they are split at the distal portion of the middle phalanx by the profundi. The superficialis tendons attach to the proximal portion of the middle phalanx. To test for superficialis action, the profundus group has to be blocked by the examiner. As illustrated in Figure 13-16, the examiner holds all the fingers in extension except the one being tested. The patient is asked to flex the finger fully at the metacarpophalangeal and proximal interphalangeal joint. If the superficialis is lacerated, the patient is unable to flex that finger.

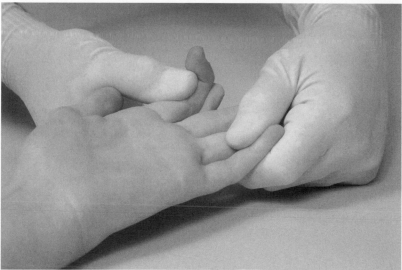

Figure 13-15. Testing for function of the flexor digitorum profundus. The distal phalanx of the finger is forcibly flexed, while the action of the superficialis tendon is blocked. Only the profundus can flex the distal phalanx.

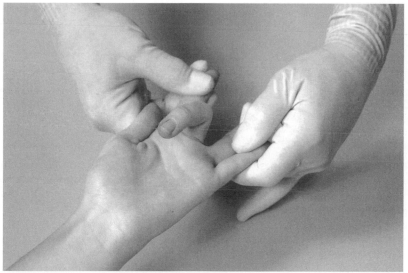

Figure 13-16. Testing for function of the flexor digitorum superficialis. The mass action of the profundus can be blocked by holding the nontested fingers in extension. The tested finger can be flexed only at the proximal interphalangeal joint by the superficialis tendon.

CIRCULATION

The circulation of the hand is extraordinarily rich and redundant (Fig. 13-17). Most people can have complete loss of either the radial or the ulnar arteries and can maintain adequate perfusion. Loss of perfusion because of damage to the vessels is usually the result of an extensive injury not ordinarily repaired by emergency wound care personnel, and consultation is obtained. Although pulses are always documented in any

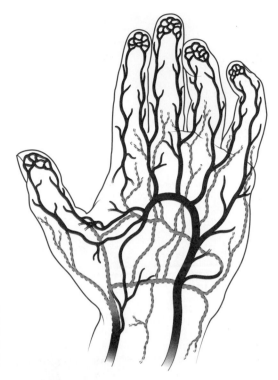

Figure 13-17. The profuse and redundant vascularity of the hand. It is common to be able to sacrifice either the radial artery or the ulnar artery and still have complete perfusion of the hand. Lacerations of the digital arteries arouse suspicion of a lacerated digital nerve.

hand injury, the best indicators of perfusion are color, skin blanching with pressure, temperature, and capillary refill at the nail bed. Because arteries travel with nerves in neurovascular bundles, profuse arterial bleeding of the digit should raise the suspicion of an accompanying digital nerve injury.

RADIOGRAPHY

Radiographs are used liberally to assist in the evaluation of the hand. For any blunt trauma associated with a laceration, underlying fractures must be ruled out. Not only do hand fractures require careful and sometimes specialized management, but also a fracture with a laceration has to be considered an open fracture. Open fractures usually are managed by consultants. Foreign bodies frequently are associated with hand injuries. Radiographic examinations are particularly useful to detect metal and other debris. Contrary to a common misconception among clinicians, almost all types of glass, in 90% of cases, are easily detectable by radiographs (see Chapter 16).[6]

WOUND EXPLORATION

Ultimately, each laceration of the hand should be explored gently and carefully just before repair. Despite normal functional testing, partial tendon lacerations and violation of joint capsules might remain undetected until exploration is performed. This procedure usually is accomplished by retracting the wound with an Adson forceps or a skin hook and using a mosquito clamp to spread open the deeper tissue for a good look, preferably in a bloodless field. Because small wounds can harbor serious injury to underlying structures, extension of the skin laceration sometimes is necessary to gain adequate exposure. Chapter 9 provides further details concerning tourniquet application, wound extension, and exploration. If there is a doubt about an injury to an important structure of the hand, the advice of a specialist should be sought.

SELECTED HAND INJURIES AND PROBLEMS

Although there is a large variety of wounds and lacerations to the hand, the wounds and lacerations described here are those that are commonly managed and repaired by emergency wound care personnel. Serious, complex injuries, especially ones that cause functional deficits, are best cared for by specialists. Animal bites and burns to the hands are discussed in Chapters 15 and 17.

Uncomplicated Lacerations

The principles and techniques of wound repair discussed in Chapter 10 also apply to closing hand lacerations. Most lacerations of the dorsal and volar surfaces of the hand can be anesthetized by direct wound infiltration (see Chapter 6). Large lacerations can be managed by wrist blocks. Wounds beyond the proximal phalanx are best anesthetized with digital blocks.

Débridement of the hand, when indicated, is carried out with great caution. Excessive removal of skin can lead to failure of adequate coverage, eventual wound contraction, and a resulting functional deficit. Fat is a good substrate for bacterial growth, and less care has to be taken when débriding away contaminated and devitalized tissue. Injured fat does not regenerate, however, and the padding role that fat provides the volar surface of the hand can be endangered. In cases in which large amounts of fat must be sacrificed, the opinion of a consultant is recommended.

Because of the number of important structures that lie within the small confines of the hand, deep closures with any suture material are discouraged. Any "foreign" material can provoke inflammation and tissue scarring that might interfere with such important and vulnerable functions as tendon gliding. By closing the skin alone, little dead space is left behind in hand injuries. In addition, natural tension across the wound usually is minimal in hand lacerations, and deep closures are not needed to reduce that tension.

The recommended suture material for skin closure is 5-0 nonabsorbable monofilament nylon. The volar surface of hand lacerations can also be closed with absorbable sutures such as gut and rapidly absorbing Vicryl Rapide.[7] When compared to nonabsorbable sutures, the outcome is no different than closure with absorbable sutures. Nonabsorbable sutures are recommended for the dorsal surface of the hand, because flexion stress requires longer support.

Only as many sutures as are necessary to achieve appropriate wound edge approximation are placed. Hand lacerations heal with little scarring, and no purpose is served by excessive sutures in search of the perfect repair. Simple interrupted technique suffices for most wounds. Skin on the hand tends to invert with closure, however, particularly on the dorsal surface. In this case, the horizontal mattress technique is useful.

Fingertip Injuries

The management of fingertip injuries is controversial. There are few actual controlled studies of fingertip and fingernail problems. The strategies and choices of repair techniques vary considerably among personnel who care for these problems. The issue of whether to remove the nail after an injury evokes widely varying opinions. Certain principles guide the repair process, however. These are preservation of finger length, nail growth capacity, fingertip padding, and sensation.[8]

The fingertip and fingernail apparatus form a complex anatomic and functional unit (Fig. 13-18). The fleshy volar pad is replete with nerve endings and capillaries. There is

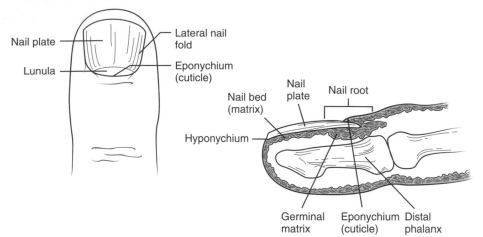

Figure 13-18. Anatomy of the distal finger and nail components.

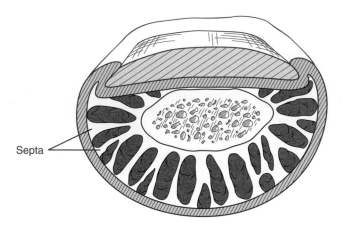

Figure 13-19. The fibrous septa that connect the skin to the underlying phalanges. The septa provide stability to the soft tissue of the finger.

sufficient soft tissue to pad the fingertip and distal phalanx effectively against undue trauma. Preservation of sensation of the fingertip is crucial to all manual activities. Even with full-thickness loss of the fingerpad, healing and regeneration of tissue usually can be relied on to restore a functional pad. Numerous fibrous bands called *septa* anchor the skin to the underlying bone structure (Fig. 13-19). These structures prevent sliding or slipping of the skin during use of the fingers. Septa should be kept anatomically intact whenever possible.

The nail apparatus has several components. The nail itself is divided into the nail root, which is the portion that lies under the eponychium, and the nail plate, which adheres to the sterile matrix. The matrix also has two parts, the germinal matrix, from which new nail is generated, and the sterile matrix, or nail bed, over which the nail passes during normal growth. The eponychium, commonly referred to as the cuticle, is the fold of skin that overlies the nail root. One of the main principles of nail management is to prevent the eponychium from adhering and scarring down onto the germinal matrix. Should this take place, nail regeneration can be impaired significantly. Techniques to prevent this occurrence are discussed in the following sections.

Fingertip injuries can be divided into three groups: (1) blunt injuries (subungual hematoma), (2) nail and nail bed lacerations, and (3) avulsion injuries with tissue loss. Foreign bodies lodged under a fingernail are discussed in Chapter 16.

Blunt Injuries (Subungual Hematoma)

It has been thought and taught that the presence of a large hematoma (>50% of the nail surface) signifies a probable laceration of the nail bed and the need for nail removal and repair.[9] Studies have shown, however, that nail plate removal and bed repair is not necessary when the nail is still intact over a large subungual hematoma. In a study of 45 patients with subungual hematoma who were followed for at least 6 months posttreatment, all patients, including 16 patients with a 50% hematoma and 14 with distal phalanx fracture, had trephination as their only treatment.[10] They were splinted for protection for 1 week. The outcome was uniformly good, with no wound infections, osteomyelitis, or significant later nail deformities. Excluded from the study were patients with nail disruption and previously existing nail deformities.

A more recent comparison of simple trephination versus nail removal and bed repair showed a better outcome in the simple trephination group.[11] There were more complications in the repair group, and the cost was four times that of trephination. Both of these studies are consistent with the author's experience. Regardless of the size of the hematoma or the presence of a tuft fracture, simple trephination is preferable if the nail remains well attached to the bed.

Nail trephination can be carried out by a variety of methods. A heated paper clip creates an appropriate-diameter drainage hole, but this technique requires considerable practice and skill. The clip has to be heated until it is red hot and transferred quickly to the nail. Heat is lost quickly, and the procedure commonly has to be repeated to gain full nail penetration. To create a drainage site, 18-G needles and no. 11 scalpel blades can be used by employing a rotating or drilling motion. The drainage holes are often small and close prematurely with a blood clot. There is considerable pressure brought to bear on the fingertip when applying this technique. More effective and less painful is a battery powered drill.

The most efficacious and least painful device is the disposable electric cautery, which can be handled like a pencil and placed with ease and precision over the hematoma (Fig. 13-20). The drainage hole is adequate, and the patients tolerate the procedure well when they understand that the heat tip will not burn them. With appropriate technique, when the heat tip passes through the nail, heat is rapidly dissipated by the underlying hematoma.

The following guidelines are offered for the evaluation and management of subungual hematomas:

- Trephination alone is appropriate for subungual hematomas of any size in which the nail remains attached and there is no deformity of the fingertip suggesting a displaced fracture. Even if a nail bed laceration or nondisplaced tuft fracture is present, healing proceeds without event, and full function is restored to the finger with splinting.
- Nail removal is reserved for patients in whom the nail is already partially avulsed, torn, or deformed from this injury. Under these circumstances, when the nail is removed, as described in the following section, the bed is inspected, and lacerations are repaired with 6-0 absorbable suture.
- Although subungual hematomas with associated fractures technically can be considered open fractures, in reality they do not need to be treated as such. Antibiotics are not indicated if the nail is left in place.

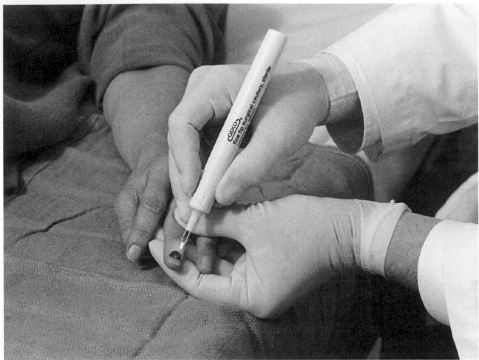

Figure 13-20. Electric cautery to penetrate a nail to drain a subungual hematoma.

Nail Bed Lacerations

Exposed nail bed lacerations of the matrix, caused by blunt trauma, are repaired by careful reapposition of the wound edges and suturing with 5-0 or 6-0 absorbable suture material. If intact, an avulsed or removed nail can be replaced, for temporary splinting purposes, under the eponychium (Fig. 13-21). The main reason for using the nail as a splint is to prevent adhesions and granulation tissue buildup between the eponychium and the germinal matrix of the bed. The nail also serves to splint any accompanying fracture and to mold the healing wound site. To maintain the nail in place, two 5-0 nonabsorbable sutures can be placed through trephined holes (see Fig. 13-21). If the nail cannot be used, a small piece of nonadherent dressing, such as Adaptic or a Penrose drain, can be tucked under the eponychium (Fig. 13-22). The nail or packing is usually left in place for 7 to 10 days.

Crush injuries of the fingertip in children can be complicated, and the extent of the injury may not be evident during the first emergency-department visit.[12] The swelling, pain, and tissue distortion can make treatment decisions difficult. For these complex injuries, cleansing, tissue preservation, antibiotics, dressing, and referral are recommended. Closure can be delayed up to 2 weeks with good long-term results.[12]

In less complicated injuries, it is common for the nail root to avulse partially from the bed under the cuticle (eponychium). The nail root is excised, and the eponychium is packed with a nonadherent dressing material for 7 to 10 days for the same reasons described earlier (Fig. 13-23). A new nail eventually grows out and extrudes the remaining portion of the old nail.

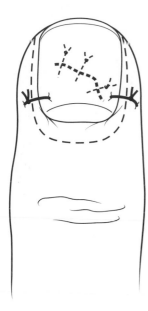

Figure 13-21. Nail bed injury. If the decision has been made to remove the nail, and a laceration of the bed is discovered, this laceration is repaired with 6-0 absorbable suture (e.g., polyglycolic acid). The nail, if removed intact, can be replaced as a splint for 7 to 10 days. The nail prevents adherence of the germinal matrix to the eponychium. The nail is anchored by placing sutures as shown in the lateral aspect of the plate.

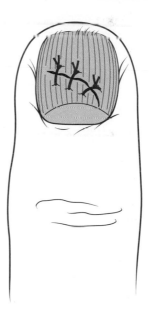

Figure 13-22. Nail bed injury. If the nail is not in a condition to be replaced, a small stent is fashioned to separate the eponychium from the germinal matrix. This stent or packing is removed within 5 to 7 days.

Lacerations of the fingertip and nail apparatus caused by sharp or shearing forces usually can be managed by simple suturing. Transverse lacerations through the nail plate and matrix can be repaired by removing the distal portion of the nail plate to expose the lacerated nail bed. Repair of the matrix is performed with 6-0 absorbable suture (Fig. 13-24). Maintaining the integrity of the nail root prevents nail growth problems with the germinal matrix.

Longitudinal lacerations through the matrix and eponychium require careful repair of both structures. The nail bed is repaired with 6-0 absorbable suture (Fig. 13-25). The eponychium and surrounding skin are closed with either nonabsorbable or absorbable material such as gut or rapidly absorbing Vicryl. If the nail plate is removed in its

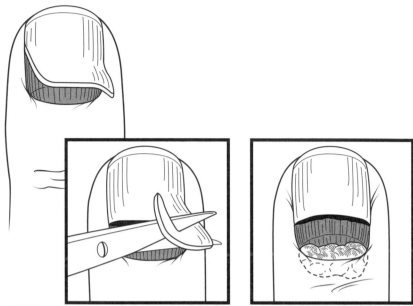

Figure 13-23. Nail root avulsion. If the nail root cannot be replaced, the nail root can be excised, and a small Penrose drain or Adaptic packing is placed under the eponychium for 5 to 7 days. A new nail germinates and extrudes the remainder of the old portion.

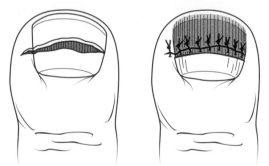

Figure 13-24. Transverse lacerations of the nail bed often can be managed by leaving the nail root intact. The proximal portion of the nail is excised with tissue scissors proximally to the injury. The nail bed is repaired with absorbable suture. The nail continues to grow over the suture line well after the sutures have been absorbed.

entirety, a nail replacement or packing for 10 to 14 days, as previously described, is necessary to prevent eponychial adherence to the germinal matrix. Only the nonabsorbable sutures are removed after 10 to 12 days.

Nail Removal Technique

When the decision is made to remove the nail, the techniques illustrated in Figure 13-26 are suggested. A small hemostat or iris scissors is inserted under the nail plate along the nail bed. The instrument is advanced slowly as it is spread open to lift the nail plate off the matrix. This process is carried back through to the nail root and germinal matrix area. Care is taken to avoid undue injury to the nail bed and germinal matrix. The eponychium also is gently pushed away from the nail plate. When the nail plate

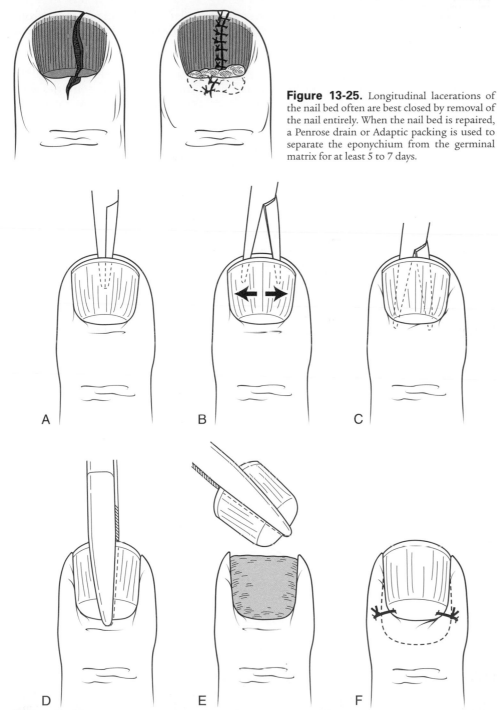

Figure 13-25. Longitudinal lacerations of the nail bed often are best closed by removal of the nail entirely. When the nail bed is repaired, a Penrose drain or Adaptic packing is used to separate the eponychium from the germinal matrix for at least 5 to 7 days.

A   B   C

D   E   F

Figure 13-26. Technique for removal of a nail. **A,** Introduce a small hemostat or iris scissors between the nail and the nail bed. **B,** Gently dissect the nail from the nail bed. **C,** Extend the dissection all the way back to the germinal matrix. **D,** Grasp the nail firmly and remove it from the nail bed **(E). F,** If the nail plate remains intact, it can be replaced as a splint or stent and anchored as shown with two 5-0 nonabsorbable sutures.

has been loosened, a hemostat is used to grasp the nail plate firmly and pull it out from under the eponychium. The nail does not always come off easily, and some measure of force must be applied.

Avulsion Injuries

Another area of controversy in fingertip management surrounds avulsion injuries with loss of tissue (Fig. 13-27). At issue is whether to close these avulsions by grafting or whether to leave them to heal spontaneously. There is consensus that any fingertip avulsion with <1 cm² area of tissue loss and no accompanying bone or nail bed injury can be managed by allowing spontaneous healing to occur.[13] Also at issue are avulsion injuries of larger areas or bone exposure. Losses of 1.8 × 2.6 cm, even with bone exposed, in pediatric and adult age groups, have been treated successfully without grafting.[14-18] When bone was exposed, spontaneous soft tissue covering of the distal phalanx occurred with adequate pad formation.[18,19] When comparing complication rates and time lost from work, conservative management is comparable to grafting.[20] In one study, the infection rate of the conservatively managed group was markedly lower than that of surgically grafted patients.[21] To summarize, nonoperative management of fingertip avulsions heal in 20 to 30 days; the regrown pulp is of high quality with good size, bulk, and function; two-point discrimination returns to an average of 2.5 mm (near normal); and 90% of patients are satisfied with the result.[22] The one area in which conservative management seems less optimal compared with more meticulous surgical repair is when the nail bed is involved and repair is indicated. Unrepaired nail matrices tend to lead more frequently to deformed nails.[21]

Guidelines for the management of avulsion injuries are offered as follows:

- If the defect is <1 cm in diameter and no bone is exposed, spontaneous healing is the treatment of choice.
- For losses >1 cm, but with an intact nail apparatus and no bone exposure, conservative management can be considered as an alternative to grafting. Children do well with conservative treatment. Local practice, which may necessitate consultation, often dictates the management of these injuries.
- For avulsions with nail apparatus involvement, repair or revision of the matrix is necessary. Consultation may be required.

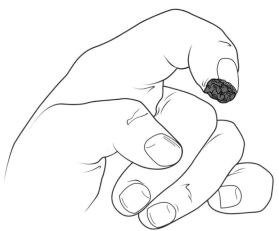

Figure 13-27. Avulsion injury of the fingertip.

- For injuries with exposed bone, consultation is recommended to assist in the decision regarding the treatment choice.
- Proper dressings for fingertip avulsions include a nonadherent base, such as Xeroform or Adaptic, with a sponge covering and gauze wrapping as described in Chapter 20. As discussed later, antibiotics are suggested for injuries with exposed bone.

Tendon Lacerations

All lacerations of flexor tendons (in the upper or lower extremity) are referred to specialists for care. An emergency wound care setting is not the place to repair flexor tendon injuries. Besides requiring a controlled surgical environment, these tendons are managed most effectively by trained surgeons using the proper instruments and magnification. Under the best of circumstances, flexor tendon injuries present considerable technical challenges, and repair can be fraught with complications. Injuries in zone II, known as *no man's land*, present the greatest challenge to the caregiver (Fig. 13-28).

In many cases, flexor tendon lacerations can be repaired primarily 3 weeks postinjury.[23] Anastomoses done within 7 to 10 days may have a better outcome.[24] After 3 weeks, reconstructive procedures must be used. With agreement from the consultant, the skin can be closed and arrangements can be made for follow-up evaluation and a decision regarding formal tendon repair. The skin closure is done after standard skin cleansing and irrigation. A splint is placed. An intravenous dose of a first-generation cephalosporin is administered in the emergency department, followed by oral cephalosporin or dicloxacillin. Clindamycin can be given to the allergic patient. Immediate

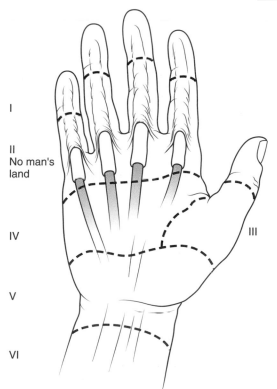

I

II
No man's
land

IV

III

V

VI

Figure 13-28. Zones of tendon repair. The hand can be divided into zones that have different implications when considering tendon repair strategy and technique. Injuries in zone II, also referred to as *no man's land,* are difficult to repair because of the complex and close relationship of the tendons and surrounding structures.

operative intervention may be necessary for injuries with excessive contamination, skin loss, unstable bony skeleton, or missing tissue.

Simple, single lacerations of an extensor tendon on the dorsum of the hand, between the distal wrist and the metacarpophalangeal joints (zone VI), can be repaired in the emergency wound care area by appropriately trained wound care personnel.[25] It is recommended that training for extensor tendon repair include several supervised repairs under the guidance of a specialist. It is important to master appropriate techniques and to understand proper splinting and the necessary follow-up care. The specialist should agree with the plan of care because he or she will take over the aftercare treatment.

Single extensor tendons can be repaired in the emergency department under the following circumstances: (1) if the injury is between the distal wrist and the metacarpophalangeal joints (zone VI), (2) if the skin and tendon wounds are sharp and not heavily macerated or contaminated, (3) if the injury is <8 hours old, (4) if the two ends of the tendon are easily visualized, (5) if appropriate instruments are available to minimize trauma to the tissues, and (6) if the patient is cooperative and will comply with follow-up care. The technique for repairing an extensor tendon is shown in Figure 13-29. A 4-0 nonabsorbable suture, such as nylon or polypropylene, on a straight needle is passed through the tendon in the figure-eight pattern until it is secure. The skin is closed with 5-0 nonabsorbable suture material. A plaster splint is placed on the palmar surfaces of the forearm-wrist-hand-digit, over the appropriate nonadherent base and the gauze sponge/wrap surface dressing. The wrist is placed at a 30-degree angle of extension, and the metacarpophalangeal joints are placed at a 20-degree angle of flexion. The fingers are only slightly flexed. The splint remains in place for 3 weeks; however, the patient is referred much sooner to the consultant for follow-up care.

On careful exploration of a laceration of the hand, it is common to discover partially lacerated extensor or flexor tendons. The management of these injuries is controversial. Unrepaired, these injuries have been reported to rupture, cause "triggering," or become entrapped.[26] Successful treatment of these injuries has been reported with skin closure alone followed by splinting.[26,27] Treatment can be guided by cross-sectional size of the laceration. As a general rule, if the tendon is more than 50% transected, it should be repaired as if fully severed. Lesser injuries can be trimmed to prevent triggering or entrapment. Appropriate splinting, rehabilitation, and follow-up care are carried out under the direction of the specialist.

Nerve Injuries

Lacerations associated with sensory or motor deficits of one of the major nerves of the upper extremity require immediate referral to a consultant. Injuries to the digital nerves can be handled differently, however. Surgical repair is indicated if two-point discrimination exceeds 10 mm.[28] For uncomplicated severed nerves, delayed repair can have significant advantages over early repair.[29,30] The repair setting and time are better controlled, the cut nerve ends and epineurium are better delineated, and early skin closure is an effective barrier against infection. The delayed repair is done through a sterile field and incision. In the emergency department, with consultative support, simple skin suturing is done, a dressing is placed, and the patient is referred to the specialist within 1 to 2 days. Nerve repair can be performed on an elective basis 10 days after the injury. When the injury is complicated by contamination, tissue devitalization, or associated injuries, early consultation is recommended. A recent study of volar digital nerve injuries by using ultrasound can accurately predict transection of the nerve.[31] A 12- to 14-MHz linear array hockey-stick transducer is used. Sonographic exam is performed several days after injury to lessen the effect of distortion from edema.

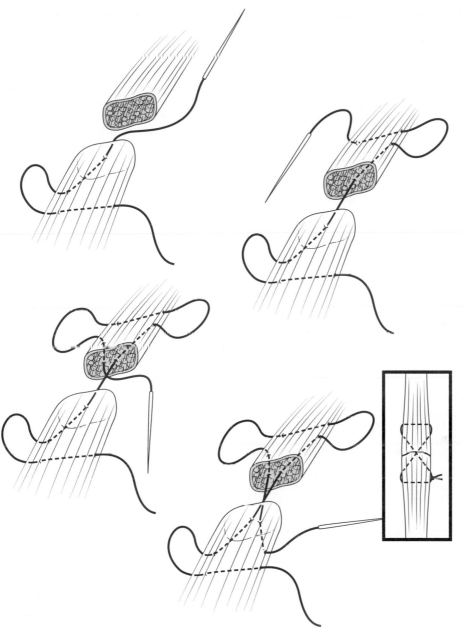

Figure 13-29. The figure-eight technique to reappose sharply divided lacerated extensor tendons. See text for further explanation.

Amputated Parts

Emergency physicians often are involved in the early management of patients with amputated parts. Although the injury is not within the realm of emergency wound care personnel to manage, proper handling of the injured extremity and severed part is important, especially if there is a chance of reimplantation by a specialist.

The injured extremity is gently cleansed and wrapped in lightly saline-moistened gauze sponges followed by gauze wrapping. A tourniquet rarely is needed to stop hemorrhage because natural vasospasm and platelet plugging of the severed vessels occur rapidly after injury. It is common to administer a dose of intravenous first-generation cephalosporins to the patient as prophylaxis.

The severed part is placed in a dry, sterile sponge wrapping. Saline soaking causes unnecessary and unwanted edema and makes reimplantation much more difficult. The wrapped severed part is placed in a small plastic covered cup or bag. The cup and its contents can be put in a container with ice to cool the tissue. Great care has to be taken to ensure that ice does not come into direct contact with the severed part so as not to cause necrosis from freezing. When these steps have been taken, the patient can wait for the specialist or can be transported to an appropriate care facility.

Paronychia

The most common hand infection is a paronychia.[32] A paronychia is an infection of the eponychium, and it usually is associated with a collection of pus between the eponychium and the nail root. The infection is localized most often to one side of the eponychium, in the lateral nail fold. It can include the eponychium in the midline, however, or can proceed in "horseshoe" fashion to involve the entire eponychium. Pus also can invade the space under the nail plate. The most common bacteria found in a paronychia are gram-positive cocci, either *Streptococcus pyogenes* or penicillin-resistant *Staphylococcus aureus*.[32,33]

One of the most serious events in soft tissue infections is the appearance of community-acquired methicillin-resistant *Staphylococcus aureus* (CA-MRSA).[34] This organism has been cultured from hand infections including paronychia.

The simplest and most effective manner to drain a paronychia is to insert a no. 11 blade between the eponychium and the nail plate and gently to sweep the blade to elevate the eponychium (Fig. 13-30). With deft technique in a calm patient, this procedure can be done without anesthesia. Otherwise, a digital block is performed before drainage. After drainage, a simple adhesive bandage (Band-Aid) dressing is applied. The patient is instructed to remove the Band-Aid and to soak the finger in warm, soapy water twice a day. Band-Aids can be reapplied between soakings. Some authorities recommend placing drains under the eponychium. Uncomplicated paronychia in patients, who do not have risk factors such as diabetes, does not necessitate these measures. Antibiotics often are prescribed but are unnecessary if the pus is completely drained and there is no surrounding digital cellulitis. If there is cellulitis, a first-generation cephalosporin or clindamycin (for allergic patients) can be prescribed for 7 days. If CA-MSRA is suspected, recommended antibiotics are trimethoprim-sulfamethosoxazole, clindamycin, or doxycycline.

Occasionally a paronychia extends below the nail plate between the nail and matrix. Pus can be seen through the semitranslucent nail. If pus is suspected to be in this space, partial or complete nail removal is recommended. Merely sweeping a no. 11 blade under

Figure 13-30. Technique for draining a simple paronychia. The no. 11 blade is brought between the nail and the eponychium parallel to the nail plate. This simple maneuver drains most paronychias.

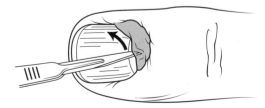

the eponychium does not suffice. Figure 13-31 shows a method of partial nail removal to accomplish the drainage of the paronychia and the pus under the nail plate. A paronychia that involves the entire eponychium and nail root area can be managed as illustrated in Figure 13-32. An incision of the eponychium is made to free the nail root for removal. Occasionally the entire nail must be removed to effect complete drainage.

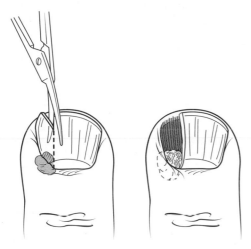

Figure 13-31. When a paronychia extends below the nail and insinuates between the nail bed and the nail plate, partial nail removal must take place. When nail removal is accomplished, a small packing or drain is left in place for 5 to 7 days.

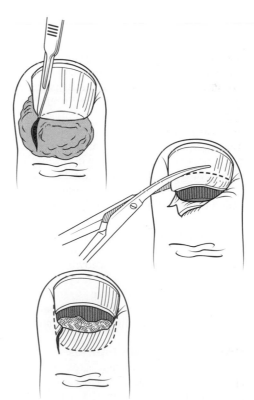

Figure 13-32. A complex "horseshoe" paronychia usually needs to be drained by incising the paronychia directly and removing either a portion or all of the nail. Packing is left in place for 5 to 7 days to prevent adherence of the eponychium to the germinal matrix.

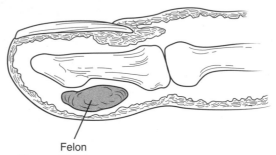

Felon

Figure 13-33. Felon in the pulp of the finger space.

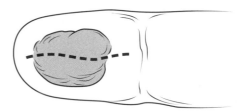

Figure 13-34. Technique for draining a felon. The incision is made directly over the area of maximal tenderness and fluctuance.

Antibiotics often are recommended for complex paronychia. Antibiotics for hand wounds are discussed in the text that follows.

Felon

A felon is an infection with a collection of pus in the pulp space of the fingertip (Fig. 13-33). The finger pad is quite swollen and is exceedingly tender. The most common bacteria found in these infections are *S. pyogenes* and penicillin-resistant *S. aureus*.[32,33] The previous discussion regarding CA-MRSA applies to felons as well. Whenever paronychia and felons are present, the patient needs to be assessed for extension of the infection to the tendon. Suspicion for tenosynovitis is raised if the patient has the four signs of Kanavel[35]:

- Uniform symmetric swelling of the digit
- At rest, digit is held in partial flexion
- Excessive tenderness the whole length of the flexor tendon sheath
- Pain of the tendon sheath and finger with passive extension

Several methods to drain felons have been recommended through the years. The so-called fish-mouth and lateral incisions that cut through the supporting fibrous septa of the finger pad are thought to increase the occurrence of unnecessary sequelae.[36]

The simplest technique to drain a felon is to make a longitudinal incision directly through the finger pad on the volar surface of the digit into the pulp space and pus collection (Fig. 13-34).[36] The incision is kept open with a small, loose-fitting wick made of a nonadherent dressing material or by a small sliver of rubber, such as part of a Penrose drain or a rubber band. The drain is removed at follow-up at 48 hours, after which a soaking routine similar to the one used for paronychia is encouraged. Patients are then started on antibiotics. The treatment protocol should include the possibility of CA-MRSA infection.

Pressure Injection Injuries

An injury to the hand that is caused by a high-pressure injection device, such as a paint sprayer or grease gun, initially seems benign. Through a pinhole, such a device can create a needle-thin stream that can have a pressure of 15,000 psi. A variety of paints, petroleums, and other chemicals can easily pierce the skin and, under the pressure created, spread throughout the hand along natural tissue planes and tendon sheaths. Grease and paint are the two most commonly injected substances.[31]

The entry wound is often no more than a small puncture. The most common site of entry is the tip of the index finger, which happens as a result of "testing" to see if the device works. Some of the injectable chemicals, such as the petroleums, do not cause an immediate reaction or pain. The patient often has minimal complaints. The combination of the small wound and relative lack of symptoms is deceptive. These injuries can progress over hours to marked pain, swelling, and inflammation of the entire hand. They require immediate consultation. Some authorities recommend fasciotomies of the hand, before significant swelling develops, to forestall ischemia created by an increase in tissue pressure from the intense reaction, to remove the chemical, and to débride necrotic tissue. The overall incidence of amputation has been reported to be 48%.[37]

ANTIBIOTICS FOR HAND WOUNDS

The use of antibiotics in patients with hand injuries is largely empirical, because there are few definitive, well-designed studies examining their use. Several studies have shown that prophylactic antibiotics are of no value in uncomplicated lacerations of the hand.[4,12,38] In more complicated injuries, such as avulsions of the fingertip, antibiotics often are prescribed, but there are no definitive studies to support this practice. Some studies have shown that antibiotics are of no value.[15,17]

It is common to treat fingertip injuries with prophylactic antibiotics. In a large study of 299 patients treated without antibiotics for injuries ranging from simple lacerations to avulsions, only two infections developed.[39] One group found a decrease in the infection rate with the use of antibiotics when bone was exposed under severe crushing forces.[40] It has not even been shown in the face of a paronychia that antibiotics improve outcome. Despite this controversy, some recommendations that rely more on traditional practice and clinical judgment can be made. Antibiotics should be used in the following situations:

- Wounds >8 hours old
- Wounds caused by a crushing mechanism in which some tissue compromise is suspected
- Contaminated or soiled wounds in which extensive cleansing and débridement have been necessary
- Fingertip avulsions with exposed bone
- Open fractures
- Tendon or joint involvement
- Mammalian bites (see Chapter 15 for further discussion and special circumstances)
- Complex paronychia with pus under the nail
- Felons
- Immunocompromised patients or patients who have diabetes

The choice of antibiotics for hand injuries also generates debate. First-generation cephalosporins, which are effective against most of the common gram-positive and gram-negative organisms that are implicated in wound care, are a good first choice[41]; these include cephalexin (Keflex) or amoxicillin/clavulanate. For penicillin-allergic patients, the azithromycin (Zithromax) and clindamycin (Cleocin) are appropriate. For antibiotics to have any value, they must be administered as soon as possible in the emergency department, preferably within 3 to 4 hours after the time of injury.[42] For maximal effectiveness, the initial dose should be administered intravenously. A recommended intravenous first-generation cephalosporin preparation is cefazolin (Ancef);

clindamycin (Cleocin) can be used for penicillin-allergic patients. For prophylaxis, the duration of administration is 4 to 5 days. As discussed previously, if CA-MRSA is a possible contaminant, antibiotics that cover CA-MRSA need to be considered. Risk factors for CA-MRSA include children, parenteral drug abusers, men who have sex with men, prisoners, military personnel, and members of athletic teams.[40] Antibiotic choices include clindamycin, TMP/SMX, or doxycycline. It is important to consult local sensitivity patterns for CA-MRSA.

DRESSINGS AND AFTERCARE

The basic finger dressing is described in Chapter 20. Xeroform is a popular nonadherent base, as is Adaptic. As a nonadherent dressing, Adaptic is followed by the application of a gauze pad and a wrap overlay. [43] Adaptic has been shown superior to other dressing for avulsion and fingertip repairs. The latter is probably less adherent in wounds in which there is more exudate and crusting. All fingertips are well padded with gauze sponges. A metal protective splint is recommended for patients who are going to return to work or resume manual activities.

Most hand wounds are best followed up within 48 hours with dressing removal for inspection. If a suture line becomes infected, suture removal and wound cleansing with thorough irrigation are performed as soon as possible. Infections of the hand can be disastrous and can often spread rapidly to important structures from a small nidus. Most sutures of the hand are removed in 8 to 10 days.

References

1. Cresap RC: Removal of a hardened steel ring from an extremely swollen finger, *Am J Emerg Med* 13:218–320, 1995.
2. Custer J, Edlich RF, Prusak M, et al: Studies in the management of the contaminated wound, *Am J Surg* 121:572–575, 1971.
3. Lammers RL, Fourre M, Callahan ML, et al: Effect of povidone-iodine and saline soaking on bacterial counts in acute, traumatic, contaminated wounds, *Ann Emerg Med* 19:709–714, 1990.
4. Roberts AHN, Teddy PJ: A prospective trial of prophylactic antibiotics in hand lacerations, *Br J Surg* 64:394–396, 1977.
5. Gellis M, Pool R: Two-point discrimination distances in the normal hand and forearm, *Plast Reconstr Surg* 59:57–63, 1977.
6. Tanberg D: Glass in the hand and foot, *JAMA* 248:1872–1874, 1982.
7. Shetty PC, Dicksheet S, Scalea TM: Emergency department repair of hand lacerations using absorbable vicryl sutures, *J Emerg Med* 15:673–674, 1997.
8. Margles S: Principles of management of acute hand injuries, *Surg Clin North Am* 60:665–685, 1980.
9. Simon RR, Wolgin M: Subungual hematoma: association with occult laceration repair, *Am J Emerg Med* 5:302–304, 1987.
10. Seaberg DC, Angelos WJ, Paris PM: Treatment of subungual hematomas with nail trephination, *Am J Emerg Med* 9:209–210, 1991.
11. Roser SE, Gellman H: Comparison of nail bed repair versus nail trephination for subungual hematomas in children, *J Hand Surg Am* 24:1166–1170, 1999.
12. Giddins GE, Hill RA: Late diagnosis and treatment of crush injuries of the fingertip in children, *Injury* 29:447–450, 1998.
13. Louis D, Palmer A, Burney R: Open treatment of digital tip injuries, *JAMA* 244:697–698, 1980.
14. Douglas BS: Conservative management of guillotine amputation of the finger in children, *Aust Pediatr J* 8:86–89, 1972.
15. Fox JW, Golden GT, Rodeheaver G, et al: Nonoperative management of pulp amputation by occlusive dressings, *Am J Surg* 133:255–256, 1977.
16. Ipsen T, Frandsen PA, Barfred T: Conservative treatment of fingertip injuries, *Injury* 18:203–205, 1987.
17. Lamon RP, Cicero JJ, Frascone RJ, et al: Open treatment of fingertip amputations, *Ann Emerg Med* 12:358–360, 1983.
18. Young WA, Andrassy RJ: Conservative management of fingertip amputations in children, *Texas Med* 79:58–60, 1983.
19. Farrell RG, Disher WA, Nesland RS, et al: Conservative management of fingertip amputations, *JACEP* 6:243–246, 1977.

20. Holm A, Zachariae L: Fingertip lesions: an evaluation of conservative treatment versus free skin grafting, *Acta Orthop Scand* 45:382–392, 1974.
21. Chow S, Ho E: Open treatment of fingertip injuries in adults, *J Hand Surg Am* 7:470–476, 1982.
22. Martin C: González del Pino J: Controversies in the treatment of fingertip amputations. Conservative versus surgical reconstruction, *Clin Orthop Relat Res* 353:63–73, 1998.
23. Steinberg DR: Acute flexor tendon injuries, *Orthop Clin North Am* 23:125–141, 1992.
24. Tottenham VM: Effects of delayed therapeutic intervention following zone II flexor tendon repair, *J Hand Ther* 8:23–26, 1995.
25. Blair WF, Steyers CM: Extensor tendon injuries, *Orthop Clin North Am* 23:141–149, 1992.
26. McGeorge DD, Stillwell JH: Partial flexor tendon injuries: to repair or not, *J Hand Surg Br* 17:176–177, 1992.
27. Wray R, Weeks P: Treatment of partial tendon lacerations, *Hand* 12:163–166, 1980.
28. Siddiqui A, Benjamin CI, Schubert W: Incidence of neurapraxia in digital nerves, *J Reconstr Microsurg* 16:95–98, 2000.
29. Millesi H: Reappraisal of nerve repair, *Surg Clin North Am* 61:321–340, 1981.
30. Wyrick JD, Stern PJ: Secondary nerve reconstruction, *Hand Clin* 8:587–597, 1992.
31. Umans H, Kessler J, de le Lama M, et al: Sonographic assessment of volar digital nerve in the context of penetrating trauma, *Am J Roentgenol* 194:1310–1313, 2010.
32. Bell M: The changing pattern of pyogenic infections of the hand, *Hand* 8:298–302, 1976.
33. Eaton R, Butsch D: Antibiotic guidelines for hand infections, *Surg Gynecol Obstet* 130:119–121, 1970.
34. Cohen RC: Community acquired methicillin-resistant *Staphylococcus aureus* skin infections: a review of epidemiology, clinical features, management, and prevention, *Int J Dermatol* 46:1–11, 2007.
35. Clark DC: Common acute hand infections, *Am Fam Phys* 68:2167–2176, 2003.
36. Kilgore ES, Brown LG, Newmeyer WL, et al: Treatment of felons, *Am J Surg* 130:194–197, 1975.
37. Vasilevski D, Noorbergen M, Depierreux M: High-pressure injection injuries to the hand, *Am J Emerg Med* 18:820–824, 2000.
38. Worlock P, Boland P, Darrell J, et al: The role of prophylactic antibiotics following hand injuries, *Br J Clin Pract* 34:290–292, 1980.
39. Zook EG, Guy R, Russell RC: A study of nail bed injuries, *J Hand Surg Am* 9:247–252, 1984.
40. Sloan JP, Dove AF, Maheson AN, et al: Antibiotics in open fractures of the distal phalanx, *J Hand Surg Br* 12:123–124, 1987.
41. Levine BJ, editor: *2011 EMRA antibiotic guide*, ed 14, Irving, Tex, 2010, Emergency Medicine Residents Association.
42. Edlich RF, Smith OT, Edgerton MT: Resistance of the surgical wound to antimicrobial prophylaxis and its mechanism of development, *Am J Surg* 126:583–586, 1973.
43. De Alwis W: Fingertip injuries, *Emerg Med Australa* 18:229–237, 2006.

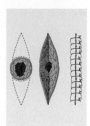

CHAPTER 14

Tissue Adhesives and Alternative Wound Closure

Key Practice Points

- Alternatives to sutures for wound closure include wound adhesives, tapes, and staples. For the most part, all wound closure materials ultimately have the same cosmetic outcome.
- Of the available wound adhesives, octyl cyanoacrylate (Dermabond) has the best wound closure characteristics.
- The proper technique for applying adhesives restricts their use to the skin surface. Adhesives are toxic to subcutaneous tissue.
- Adhesives are in liquid form as they exit the applicator; therefore care is taken to prevent "runoff" of the adhesive into the eyes and the mouth.
- Wound tapes are appropriate for narrow, straight lacerations (commonly on the face), for flaps, and for the fragile skin of the elderly.
- Staples are less reactive than sutures, and staples potentially cause less scarring and infection.
- During the stapling of wounds, it is important to apply the stapler gently to the skin before activating the trigger to prevent driving the staple too deeply.

Through the years, sutures and their alternatives—wound adhesives, tapes, and staples—have become established and are routinely used in wound care. Emergency physicians value staples, because they are easy to apply, they save time, and the outcome of their use is good. Staples are particularly useful for scalp and truncal lacerations. After they were introduced in the 1980s, wound tapes commonly were used for straight lacerations that were under little tension, for surgical incisions, and for supporting lacerations with recently removed sutures. With the advent of adhesives, a new alternative has become available.

TISSUE ADHESIVES

Tissue adhesives are relatively new to wound and laceration closure in the United States; they were approved by the Food and Drug Administration in 1998. Since the 1980s, tissue adhesives have been successfully used in Europe, Canada, the Middle East, and Asia. These compounds derive from the cyanoacrylate adhesives used in common household super glues. Formulated for medical purposes, they are well tolerated, effective, and nontoxic.[1]

Until 1998, n-butyl cyanoacrylate (Histo-Acryl Blue, Indermil) was the most commonly used tissue adhesive worldwide.[2] In 1998, a new compound, octyl cyanoacrylate

(Dermabond), was released for general use.[3] Dermabond has many advantages over Histo-Acryl Blue.[4] Dermabond contains a plasticizer that makes it flexible and useful for irregular or moving surfaces. Dermabond has a bacterial protection effect and a higher breaking strength.[5] Finally, in contrast to Histo-Acryl Blue, Dermabond is packaged sterilely and can be stored at room temperature. In the United States, Dermabond is currently the tissue adhesive with the most desirable characteristics for wound care.

Dermabond can be used in many wounds and lacerations ordinarily closed with sutures, tapes, or staples. It is particularly effective for lacerations on the face. There are no limits to laceration length, and it can be used over joints if properly splinted.[6] Dermabond is an improvement over sutures for the closure of wounds of thin, aged, or corticosteroid-affected skin. If easy approximation can be achieved, Dermabond closes wounds with flaps and corners. Tissue adhesives are not used on mucous membranes or hair-bearing or weight-bearing areas. The following criteria can guide the decision to use tissue adhesives:

- Fresh lacerations that are within the "golden period"
- Laceration under low tension that are easy to approximate
- Lacerations with clean and even edges that can be closed with no gaps
- Lacerations with little or no blood oozing
- Situations in which adhesive runoff can be controlled or avoided

The cosmetic result of wounds closed with adhesives is indistinguishable from that of sutured wounds.[1,7,8] Investigators have followed wounds for 3 months and have used "blinded" observers who could not tell the difference between adhesive-closed wounds and sutured pediatric lacerations.[7] For reasons of convenience and patient comfort, parents prefer closure of their children's lacerations with wound adhesives when asked to compare with previous experiences of standard suturing techniques.[9] It has been reported, however, that children occasionally pick off the glue with their fingers,[10] and in these cases, wounds have been closed successfully with sutures as delayed primary closures. Finally, although not statistically significant, the infection rate for adhesive-closed wounds tends to be lower than that for sutured wounds, and under experimental conditions, adhesive-closed wounds resist contamination more than sutured wounds do.[2]

The most attractive features of wound adhesives are short wound closure time and no requirement for anesthesia. Wound closure time is approximately 20% to 50% of the time necessary for standard suturing.[7,8,10] Adhesives polymerize within seconds after application, and the wound needs manual support for only 30 to 60 seconds after application of the adhesive. Wounds closed with adhesives are at greater risk for breaking open immediately after closure than sutured wounds.[2] After 7 days, there is no difference, however, in tensile or bursting strength between adhesive-closed and sutured lacerations. Breaking strength of adhesives is equivalent to a 4-0 nylon suture.[4] Less technical expertise is required for adhesive closures, and patients do not have to return for suture removal.[1,2] For increased strength in long lacerations, a combination of wound tapes and wound adhesive can be considered.[11]

In emergency wound care, wound adhesives are restricted to skin surfaces, and care must be used to prevent penetration into the wound. Cyanoacrylates applied within tissue can cause acute inflammatory responses, giant cell reactions, inclusion body formation, and seromas.[12] Subcutaneously or within organs, they can remain in tissues for extended periods (1 year).[13] Cyanoacrylates have accumulated an excellent and safe record for use in wound care.[1,14] In large amounts, cyanoacrylates generate exothermic heat that can cause pain. In wound care, small amounts of adhesive are applied externally, and the adhesives peel off after the wound heals.

Adhesive Wound Closure Technique

Dermabond comes in a sterile, plastic-covered glass vial with an applicator tip (Fig. 14-1). Until recently, there was only one choice of adhesive viscosity and applicator tip. Because of concerns about runoff of adhesive from wounds, a new, higher viscosity formulation has been introduced.[1,15] When compared with the low-viscosity formulation, the higher viscosity adhesive had significantly less runoff from the wound area. Otherwise, the outcomes were comparable.[16] The standard applicator tip is rounded and has a tendency to depress or invert the wound edges if excessive pressure is applied during application. A new, chisel tip is more versatile and allows for even application of adhesive without undue pressure on the wound edges to cause inversion. The procedure for application of adhesive is as follows (Fig. 14-2):

- After wound cleansing and any necessary débridement, any significant bleeding should be controlled. The wound does not have to be strictly dry, however, because polymerization occurs in the presence of a liquid, either water or blood.
- The patient is placed in a position so that the wound is facing directly up, and adhesive runoff is prevented. It is advisable to have nearby or to hold a gauze sponge to mop excessive adhesive quickly. A rim of petrolatum ointment placed around the wound helps block runoff.
- The eye is especially vulnerable to "runoff" and inadvertent gluing of the eyelids together. Therefore, if the laceration is above the eye, place the patient in a slight Trendelenburg position.[17] For lacerations below the eye, the patient is placed in the reverse Trendelenburg position.
- When the patient is properly prepared and placed, the plastic Dermabond applicator is crushed and squeezed until adhesive covers the applicator tip.
- The wound is approximated gently with fingers or forceps. In some wounds, a second person can assist with wound edge approximation and excess adhesive removal.
- Adhesive is layered over the wound with a margin of 5 to 10 mm. Finger or forceps approximation is maintained for 30 to 60 seconds to allow for polymerization.

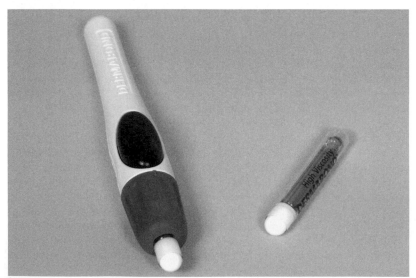

Figure 14-1. Dermabond wound adhesive applicators: *Left,* ProPen. *Right,* Precision tip.

After 15 to 20 seconds, more adhesive can be applied. Three separate layers are recommended to complete the closure. It takes 2.5 minutes for adhesive to reach its full tensile strength.[18]

Histo-Acryl Blue is a combination of adhesive and blue dye. It is not as versatile as Dermabond and is recommended for short, straight lacerations. It comes in a container with an applicator tip but is applied more easily by cutting off the tip and replacing it with a 25-G needle. Because of its consistency, Histo-Acryl Blue requires a different technique for application than does Dermabond. After the wound edges are approximated, small drops, "spot welds," are placed along the wound until it is closed. The wound has to be supported for 30 to 60 seconds to ensure proper polymerization. Histo-Acryl Blue is more brittle than Dermabond and can break more readily.[19]

Adhesive Closure Aftercare

The patient is instructed to keep the wound clean and dry for 24 hours. After this period, gentle cleansing can be done with great care and caution so as not to disrupt the closure. If a wound dehisces, the patient is instructed to return so that delayed primary closure with wound tapes or sutures can be performed. No follow-up is necessary for glue removal because it peels off on its own or comes off with the natural sloughing of keratinized epidermis.

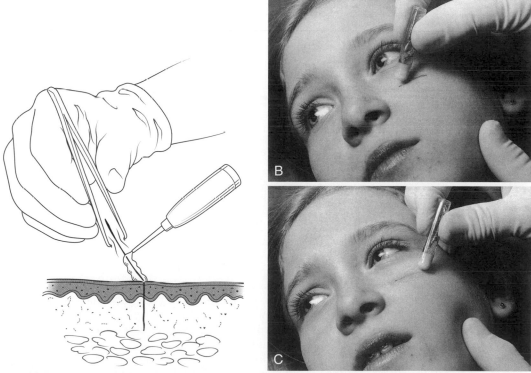

Figure 14-2. Wound adhesive application technique. **A,** Wound edges are apposed with fingertips or forceps followed by application of adhesive. **B,** The applicator tip is drawn gently over the length of the wound. **C,** Three to four layers are applied to complete the closure.

Inadvertent Adhesive Runoff and Removal

Because adhesives are liquid, they can run off the wound area by accident or drip onto unwounded surfaces. Vulnerable areas include the eyes, nose, mouth, ears, and fingers. If possible, the runoff should be wiped up before drying. If polymerization occurs, petroleum ointment can be applied to accelerate breakdown and peeling. Antibiotic ointments can be used for this task. The most effective removal substance is acetone. Because acetone is toxic to delicate tissues, great care must be taken around the eyes. Forceps also can be used when the adhesive is completely dry to flake it away gently.

WOUND TAPING

There are several advantages to wound taping compared with suturing. Advantages include a reduced need for anesthesia, ease and speed of application, even distribution of tension across the wound, no residual suture marks, application by nonphysician personnel, and the elimination of the need for suture removal.[20] Tapes also have advantages in closing flap lacerations and have a greater resistance to wound infection than sutures.[21,22] Tapes do not work well on surfaces that are oily or hair bearing, on joint surfaces, on lax skin, on gaping wounds under tension, or on very young or uncooperative children. The cosmetic outcome is equivalent to adhesive closure.[23]

A bewildering variety of wound tapes are currently on the market. Steri-Strips are the best known; other brands include Shur-Strip, Cover-Strips, Suture-Strip, Clearon, Nichi-Strip, and Curi-Strip. The various brands have differing porosity, adhesion, flexibility, breaking strength, and elongation capability. An early study that compared Clearon and Steri-Strips showed a better overall performance by Steri-Strips.[24] In another comparison study of six tapes (Curi-Strip, Steri-Strips, Nichi-Strip, Cicagraf, Suture-Strip, and Suture-Strip Plus), an overall scoring method was devised to rank their performance under laboratory conditions.[25] The three highest ranking tapes were Nichi-Strip, Curi-Strip, and Steri-Strips. Under experimental conditions, tape closures resisted wound infection better than nylon sutures. Tapes also are well suited for supporting grafts and flaps.

Indications for Taping

Wound taping can be considered under the following conditions:

- Superficial, straight lacerations under little tension. Areas suitable for taping include the forehead, chin, malar eminence, thorax, and nonjoint areas of the extremities.
- Flaps in which sutures might compromise vascular perfusion at the wound edges.
- Lacerations with a greater-than-usual potential for infection.
- Lacerations in an elderly or steroid-dependent patient who has thin, fragile skin.
- Support for lacerations after suture removal.

  Tapes do not work well on irregular wounds, wounds that cannot be made free of blood or secretions, intertriginous areas, scalp, and joint surfaces.

Taping Technique

Most taping of emergency wounds can be done with ¼-inch-wide tape of varying lengths. For wounds that are greater than 4 to 5 cm in length, ½-inch width is preferable. The following steps are performed:

- The wound is cleansed, irrigated, and débrided if necessary. Hemostasis has to be complete and the skin surface completely dried.
- Benzoin is applied to the surrounding skin to increase adhesion. Care is taken not to spill this agent into the wound. Benzoin is left to dry until it becomes tacky.
- Tapes are cut to the length desired while they are still on the backing sheet. Usually 2 to 3 cm of overlap is allowed for each side of the wound.

- One of the perforated end tabs is gently removed to prevent deforming of the tape ends (Fig. 14-3).
- Individual tapes are removed from the backing with forceps by pulling directly away from the backing (Fig. 14-4).
- One half of the tape is securely placed on one side of the midportion of the wound and is held securely. The opposite wound edge is apposed with a finger of the opposite hand (Fig. 14-5). After edge apposition, the tape is completely secured (Fig. 14-6).
- Further tapes are placed evenly adjacent to the original midwound tape. This process is repeated with further tapes until the wound edges are completely apposed (Fig. 14-7). Wound tapes should have a gap between them that is at least 2 to 3 mm wide. Complete occlusion of the wound by tapes can cause normal wound seepage to dissect under the tapes and can lead to premature removal.
- The final step is to place cross stays to prevent elevation of the tape ends and minor skin blistering caused by tension of the tape ends (Fig. 14-8).

Tape Aftercare

Tapes are maintained in place for at least as long as sutures would be for the anatomic area in question. In contrast to a sutured wound, a taped wound cannot be washed or moistened, because premature tape removal can lead to wound dehiscence. Tapes should never be wrapped around a digit in a circumferential manner, because they are not expandable and can act as a constricting band.

WOUND STAPLING

Since the introduction of automatic skin-stapling devices, there has been a reluctance to use them beyond their intended purpose of closing surgically made incisions. Despite the remarkable amount of time saved by placing staples instead of sutures, early

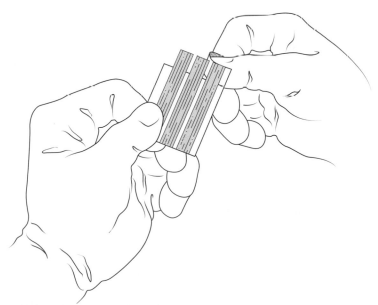

Figure 14-3. The perforated end tab is gently removed to prevent deforming of the tape ends.

animal and clinical investigations included questions about the capacity of staples to appose wound edges as accurately or to promote wound tensile strength as effectively as sutures.[26] Studies in animals have suggested, however, that wound tensile strength is actually greater for staples compared with sutures.[27,28] In addition, less wound inflammatory response has been noted with staples, and they resist infection more effectively than sutures.[29]

Clinical studies of staple use in traumatic lacerations showed that, compared with standard suturing methods, the ultimate cosmetic result as judged by blinded observers is no different.[30,31] In these studies, body regions that were chosen for the comparisons included the scalp, neck, arm/forearm, trunk, buttocks, and legs. Adult and pediatric age groups were studied. The time required for staple closure was approximately four to five times less than that required for suture placement. Cost has been

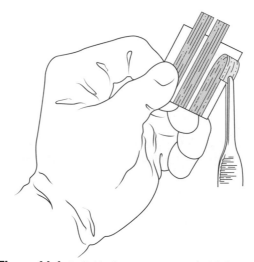

Figure 14-4. Individual tapes are removed with forceps.

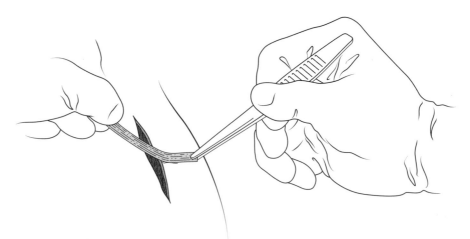

Figure 14-5. The tape is firmly secured on one side of the wound.

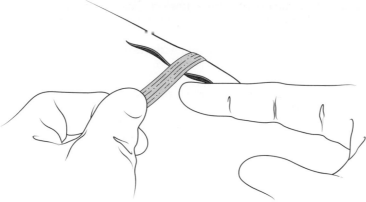

Figure 14-6. The tape is brought over the wound after the wound is apposed with the finger of the opposite hand.

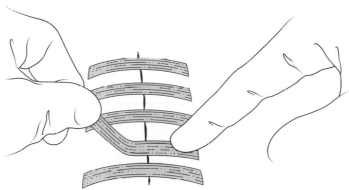

Figure 14-7. Enough tapes are placed so that wound gaping does not occur. Usually there is 2 to 3 mm between tapes.

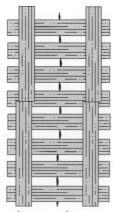

Figure 14-8. Cross stays are placed over the tape ends to prevent skin blistering and premature removal.

cited as a drawback to the use of staples; however, the time saved by a busy physician and the reduced need for wound closure instruments balances that factor.[32] Patients seem to tolerate staples well while they are in place; however, there does seem to be increased discomfort on removal compared with sutures.[27]

Indications for Stapling

Wound stapling can be recommended under the following circumstances:

- Linear, sharp (shearing mechanism) lacerations of the scalp, trunk, and extremities. Although they have been used in hand lacerations, experience is not extensive enough to recommend staples confidently for that area. Stapling similarly is avoided for facial wounds.
- Temporary, rapid closure of extensive superficial lacerations in patients requiring immediate surgery for life-threatening trauma.

Staples are avoided in anatomic areas to be studied by computed tomography or magnetic resonance imaging. Staples can produce streak artifact on a computed tomography scan, but in critical circumstances, clinically useful scans can be obtained despite the presence of staples. Staples can move when magnetic resonance imaging is used, and staples should not be placed if a study is anticipated.

Stapling Technique

Stapling devices have evolved significantly, and many products are available. The Reflex One is representative of a multiple-staple device (35 staples per cartridge) with a wide staple that closes into a rectangular configuration (Fig. 14-9). This stapler commonly is used for surgical incisions or long lacerations of the trunk or extremity. The Precise Ten Shot stapler holds 10 staples that close into a smaller arcuate configuration. This device is useful for shorter, traumatically induced lacerations that might require greater precision and control. In addition to the stapler, the equipment required includes basic wound care instruments and standard anesthetic agents. The following steps are followed to insert staples:

- Forceps are used to evert the wound edges before placement of each staple (Fig. 14-10). When possible, a second operator can help evert the edges while the primary operator uses the stapler.
- Before triggering, the stapler should be placed gently on the skin over the wound without indenting the skin (Fig. 14-11).
- The trigger, or handle, is squeezed gently and evenly to advance the staple into the tissue (Fig. 14-12).
- When the staple is placed, a space should be visible between it and skin. A common mistake in placing staples is to apply excessive downward pressure, causing the staples to seat deep in the wound.
- Because of the configuration of the bending mechanism of the stapler, when the staple is seated, the stapler has to be "backed out" of the staple loop to disengage it.

Staple Aftercare

Staples are kept in place for the same length of time as are sutures in similar anatomic sites. Staple removal requires a special device that is provided by each manufacturer. The lower jaw is placed under the crossbar of the staple, and the upper jaw is closed to open the loop of the staple (Fig. 14-13).

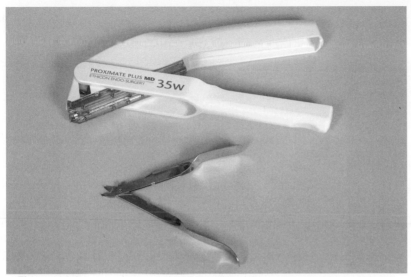

Figure 14-9. Examples of wound stapling device *(top)* and staple remover *(bottom)*.

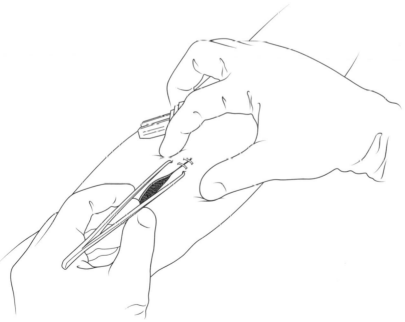

Figure 14-10. Forceps are used to approximate and evert wound edges during stapling.

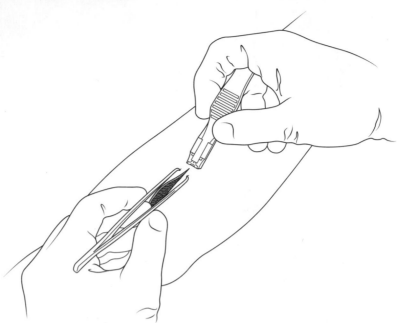

Figure 14-11. During stapling, the stapler is placed gently on the skin before triggering. Indenting the skin with too much pressure causes staples to be placed too deep.

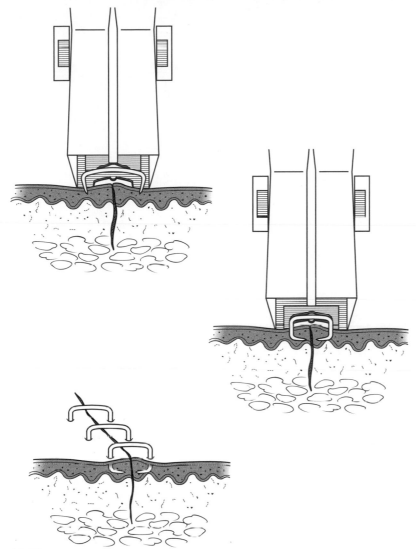

Figure 14-12. During triggering, the staple is reconfigured to approximate wound edges. Do not apply excessive downward pressure on stapler.

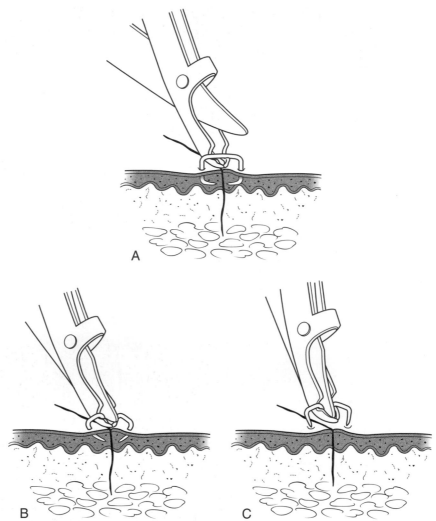

Figure 14-13.   The following procedure is used to remove staples. **A,** The lower jaws of the staple-removing device are positioned under the staple crossbar. **B,** The upper jaw is used to compress the staple gently. **C,** When complete compression has taken place, the staple has been reconfigured for easy, gentle withdrawal.

References

1. Farion KJ, Osmond MH, Harting L, et al: Tissue adhesives for traumatic lacerations: a systematic review of randomized controlled trials, *Acad Emerg Med* 10:110–118, 2003.
2. Noordzij JP, Foresman PA, Rodeheaver GT, et al: Tissue adhesive wound repair revisited, *J Emerg Med* 12:645–649, 1994.
3. Switzer EF, Dinsmore RC, North JH Jr: Subcuticular closure versus Dermabond: a prospective randomized trial, *Am Surg* 69:434–436, 2003.
4. Wackett A, Singer AJ: The role of topical skin adhesives in wound repair, *Emer Med* 41:31–35, 2009.
5. Mertz PM, Davis SC, Cazzaniga AL, et al: Barrier and antibacterial properties of 2-octylcyanoacrylate-derived wound treatment films, *J Cutan Med Surg* 7:1–6, 2003.
6. Saxena AK, Willital GH: Octylcyanoacrylate tissue adhesive in the repair of pediatric extremity lacerations, *Am Surg* 65:470–472, 1999.
7. Quinn JV, Drzewiecki A, Li MM, et al: A randomized, controlled trial comparing a tissue adhesive with suturing in the repair of pediatric facial lacerations, *Ann Emerg Med* 22:1130–1135, 1993.
8. Yaron M, Halperin M, Huffer W, Cairns C: Efficacy of tissue glue for laceration repair in an animal model, *Acad Emerg Med* 2:259–263, 1995.
9. Bruns TB, McLario DJ, Simon HK, et al: Laceration repair using a tissue adhesive in a children's emergency department (abstract), *Acad Emerg Med* 2:427, 1995.
10. Watson DP: Use of cyanoacrylate tissue adhesive for closing facial lacerations in children, *BMJ* 299:1014, 1989.
11. Chigira M, Akimoto M: Use of a skin adhesive (octyl-2-cyanoacrylate) and the optimum reinforcing combination of suturing wounds, *Scand J Plast Reconstr Surg Hand Surg* 39:334–338, 2005.
12. Toriumi DM, Raslan WF, Friedman M, Tardy ME: Histotoxicity of cyanoacrylate tissue adhesives, *Arch Otolaryngol Head Neck Surg* 116:546–550, 1990.
13. Ellis DAF, Shaikh A: The ideal tissue adhesive in facial plastic and reconstructive surgery, *J Otolaryngol* 19:68–72, 1990.
14. Toriumi DM, O'Grady K: Surgical tissue adhesives in otolaryngology—head and neck surgery, *Otolaryngol Clin North Am* 27:203–209, 1994.
15. Singer AJ, Giordano P, Fitch JL, et al: Evaluation of a new high-viscosity octylcyanoacrylate tissue adhesive for laceration repair: a randomized, clinical trial, *Acad Emerg Med* 10:1134–1137, 2003.
16. Blondeel P, Murphy J, Debrosse D, et al: Closure of long surgical incisions with new formulation of 2-octylcyanoacrylate tissue adhesive versus commercially available methods, *Am J Surg* 188:307–313, 2004.
17. Rouvelas H, Saffra N, Rosen M: Inadvertent tarsorrhaphy secondary to Dermabond, *Pediatr Emerg Care* 16:346, 2000.
18. Forsch RT: Essentials of skin laceration repair, *Am Fam Phys* 78:945–951, 2008.
19. Singer AJ, Nable M, Cameau P, et al: Evaluation of a new liquid occlusive dressing for excisional wounds, *Wound Repair Regen* 11:181–187, 2003.
20. Trott AT: Alternative methods of wound closure: wound staples. In Roberts JR, Hedges JR, editors: *Clinical procedures in emergency medicine*, Philadelphia, 1985, WB Saunders.
21. Conolly WB, Hunt TK, Zederfeldt B, et al: Clinical comparison of surgical wounds closed by suture and adhesive tapes, *Am J Surg* 117:318–322, 1969.
22. Efron G, Ger R: Use of surgical adhesive tape (Steri-Strip) to secure skin graft on digits, *Am J Surg* 116:474, 1968.
23. Shamiyeh A, Schrenk P, Steltzer T, et al: Prospective, controlled, blind randomised trial comparing sutures, tape, and octylcyanoacrylate tissue adhesive for skin closure after phlebectomy, *Dermatol Surg* 27:820–877, 2001.
24. Koehn GG: A comparison of the duration of adhesion of Steri-Strips and Clearon, *Cutis* 26:620–621, 1980.
25. Rodeheaver GT, Spengler MD, Edlich RF: Performance of new wound closure tapes, *J Emerg Med* 5:451–462, 1987.
26. Harrison ID, Williams DF, Cuschieri A: The effect of metal clips on the tensile properties of healing skin wounds, *Br J Surg* 62:945–949, 1975.
27. Roth JH, Windle BH: Staple versus suture closure of skin incisions in a pig model, *Can J Surg* 31:19–20, 1988.
28. Windle BH, Roth JH: Comparison of staple-closed and sutured skin incisions in a pig model, *Surg Forum* 35:546–550, 1984.
29. Edlich RF, Rodeheaver RT, Thacker JG, et al: Revolutionary advances in the management of traumatic wounds in the emergency department during the last 40 years: part 2, *J Emerg Med* 38:201–207, 2010.
30. Dunmire SM, Yealy DM, Karasic R: Staples versus sutures for wound closure in the pediatric population (abstract), *Ann Emerg Med* 18:448, 1989.
31. George TK, Simpson DC: Skin wound closure with staples in the accident and emergency department, *J R Coll Surg Edinb* 30:54–56, 1985.
32. Harvey CF, Hume Logan CJ: A prospective trial of skin staples and sutures in skin closure, *Ir J Med Surg* 155:194–196, 1986.

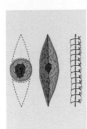

CHAPTER 15
Bite Wounds

Key Practice Points

- All animal bites exhibit similarities, but there are enough differences that each one needs to be evaluated and managed individually.
- The most important steps in bite wound management are cleansing, irrigation, and débridement of devitalized tissue. Dilute povidone-iodine solution (not the scrub preparation) is used for cleansing and irrigation, because it is both bactericidal and virucidal.
- Puncture wounds, especially those caused by cats, have a high risk of seeding deep tissue with bacteria and causing infection with *Pasteurella multocida.* It is important to open those wounds for thorough irrigation.
- Dog bites, which are the most common mammalian bite, have the least virulent bacteria and the lowest infection rate. Cat and human bites have more virulent bacteria with a higher infection rate.
- All of the important bacteria of dog, cat, and human bites are susceptible to ampicillin/clavulanate. For patients allergic to penicillin-based antibiotics, other choices are effective for prophylaxis or for treating established infections, and these antibiotics are listed in the text.
- Because suture material is a foreign body, suturing mammalian bite wounds is not recommended except for cosmetic concerns such as bite wounds on the face. Proper and vigorous local wound care will likely protect a sutured wound from becoming infected.
- Clenched-fist human injuries (striking human teeth) are very likely to penetrate tendon and metacarpophalangeal joints. These wounds often require the advice of a consultant for exploration and irrigation of the wound, tendon, and joint.
- Since 2000, no cases of human rabies have been contracted from domestic animals. The most common cause of human rabies is from bats. No human has contracted rabies from a properly immunized animal.
- Wound care and local injection of rabies immune globulin, as soon as possible after the bite occurs, are the key steps for rabies prevention.
- Optimal timing of postexposure prophylaxis is 48 hours from the bite occurs. However, because the average rabies incubation period is 30 to 90 days, up to 2 years' postexposure prophylaxis should never be denied the patient. Local public health officials and the Centers for Disease Control and Prevention (CDC) can assist in complicated cases.
- Recent recommendations in postexposure rabies prophylaxis from the CDC have reduced the number of postexposure human diploid cell vaccine (HDCV) injections from 5 to 4.

BOX 15-1	Wound Factors That Increase Risk for Infection

Puncture or crush wounds
Bites to hands, face, and feet
Bone, joint, tendon involvement
Delayed presentation, >8 hours from bite incident
Immunocompromised or asplenic host
Wound requiring surgical repair
Presence of prosthetic appliance

Animal and human bites are common wounds managed by emergency caregivers. Bites can be from a multitude of sources, but most are caused by dogs, cats, and humans.[1,2] Despite apparently similar mechanisms of injury, each type of bite has different clinical, microbiologic, and treatment considerations that affect the management of bite wound patients. With animal bites, there is also the possibility of secondary systemic infectious complications, the most important of which is rabies. It is the responsibility of any person caring for an animal bite victim to investigate thoroughly the biting circumstances and to make an appropriate decision about whether or not to administer rabies prophylaxis.

The mechanism of injury from an animal bite or attack plays an important role in predicting the chance of infection and the choice of management technique. All animal bites are to be considered contaminated with potentially pathogenic bacteria. These injuries frequently are associated with crushing, tearing, and avulsion forces and devitalized tissue. The combination of bacterial contamination with accompanying devitalized skin and fascia creates a setting ripe for the establishment of infection. The risk of infection is greater for certain circumstances listed in Box 15-1.

GENERAL BITE WOUND MANAGEMENT

Wound management depends on the type of wound, its severity, and its anatomic location. Simple contusions and superficial bite abrasions, in which no obvious skin puncture, laceration, or avulsion is present, can be treated by thorough cleansing alone. Despite the relatively minor appearance of many of these wounds, the patient still is at risk for developing rabies, and this possibility has to be addressed. For larger wounds that violate the epidermis and dermis, standard wound care techniques are performed as follows:

- Povidone-iodine solution (not the detergent scrub preparation) is the wound cleansing solution recommended for periphery cleansing. [3,4] The standard 10% solution is diluted 10:1 to 20:1 with saline and can serve as the cleansing agent and the irrigant. Povidone-iodine is virucidal and the potential for rabies in animals and human immunodeficiency virus (HIV) in humans make it the preferred bite wound cleansing agent.
- After thorough scrubbing of the wound periphery, copious high-pressure irrigation is the next step, using a 19-G needle, catheter, or splash shield attached to a 20-mL or 35-mL syringe. Delivering diluted povidone-iodine solution directly into the wound enhances its microbicidal action.
- Débridement of all devitalized tissue and wound edges is essential for reducing the possibility of wound infection. Irrigation after débridement is recommended because it provides greater exposure of the wound. Retrospective and prospective studies have shown that wound infection is reduced significantly after débridement.[5-7]
- For fang wounds, particularly slender cat teeth wounds, there is often minimal devitalization of the skin. Edge débridement might not be necessary. The problem of adequate wound cleansing remains, however. To facilitate effective irrigation, after local infiltration of anesthesia, the entry site can be widened with a simple 1- to 1.5-cm incision

across the puncture with a no. 15 knife blade (Fig. 15-1). The new wound is retracted open with a hemostat or forceps to permit irrigation. These incisions are left to close without sutures. If the edges are devitalized, they should be trimmed back to viable skin.

- Purulence or suspected infection is cultured.
- Radiographs are obtained when fracture or joint penetration is suspected.
- Proper tetanus immunization is ensured.
- The wound is covered with a nonadherent base (an antibiotic ointment is optional). The base is covered with gauze pads and tape or a gauze wrap to secure the dressing.
- Assessment and treatment for rabies exposure are performed if necessary.

SPECIFIC INJURIES

The most important steps in the management of animal and human bites are cleansing, irrigation, and débridement. However, the most controversy exists over the choice of antibiotics for prophylaxis and for the treatment of established infections. Antibiotic choices listed here are based on the likely pathogenic organisms in a bite wound and the antimicrobial susceptibility of the available antibiotics. Except for amoxicillin/clavulanate, no single antibiotic covers all of the important organisms. For this reason most of the recommendations include two antibiotics to ensure broad-spectrum

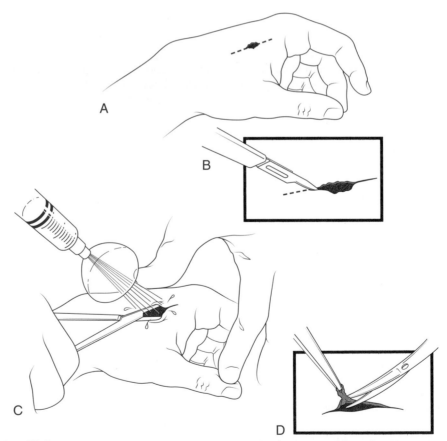

Figure 15-1. Fang wound management. **A,** A fang wound with a suggested line of incision to open the wound for effective irrigation and débridement. **B,** A small 1- to 1.5-cm incision can be made with a scalpel and a no. 15 blade. **C,** When incised, the wound can be exposed with forceps and can be copiously irrigated. **D,** The incision also facilitates wound edge débridement if devitalization or excessive contamination is present.

coverage. Coverage can always be changed based on the clinical course of the patient and available wound cultures.

Dog Bites
Microbiology and Risk for Infection

More than 80% of animal bites are dog bites.[8] The mouths of animals, including dogs, have a bewildering number and variety of bacteria. However, only a few of those bacteria actually cause the majority of established infections.[9] Therefore, prophylaxis should cover at least the likely infecting organisms (Table 15-1). Fifty percent of bacteria recovered from infected wounds are *Pasteurella canis*.[9] Other organisms include *S. aureus,* streptococi, *Moroxella* spp., and anaerobes. An unusual organism, but virulent, is *Capnocytophaga canimorsus.* Multiorgan failure, disseminated intravascular coagulation, and gangrene have been associated with this gram-negative bacillus, but infection most often occurs in immunosuppressed or chronically ill patients. The overall infection rate from dog bites varies from 2% to 20%.[1] Infection is more likely to occur in patients with risk factors, as listed in Box 15-1.

Dog Bite Wound Management

Dog bites are managed according to the general bite wound management guidelines mentioned previously.

Dog Bite Prophylaxis

The most controversial area of dog bite management is the use of prophylactic antibiotics for wounds that appear to be noninfected.[10] The preponderance of evidence is that antibiotics do not reduce the infection rate in low-risk dog bite wounds.[5,11-13] Meta-analyses and systematic reviews of available controlled trials found, however, that prophylactic antibiotics were beneficial in high-risk settings.[14,15] The high-risk setting for which there is the best evidence for the prophylactic effect of antibiotics is for non-infected-appearing hand wounds.[5,14,16] Based on the potentially infecting organisms, ampicillin/clavulanate provides good coverage in this setting (see Table 15-1). Alternatives for penicillin-allergic patients are listed as well.

Suturing

The issue of whether to suture dog bite wounds is controversial. Investigational data and the author's personal experience support the practice of primary suture closure

TABLE 15-1	Outpatient Empirical Antibiotic Treatment (Including Prophylaxis) for Mammalian Bites*
Bite Wound	**Treatment**
Dog, cat, human	**Adults**
	Amoxicillin/clavulanate 875/125 mg PO bid
	Cefuroxime 500 mg PO bid plus clindamycin 300-450 mg PO tid
	†TMP/SMX DS 2 tabs PO bid plus †clindamycin 300-450 mg PO tid
	Children (1-12 yr)
	Amoxicillin/clavulanate 25 mg/kg (amox) PO bid
	Cefuroxime 15 mg/kg PO bid plus †clindamycin 7 mg/kg PO tid
	†TMP/SMX 4-6 mg/kg PO bid plus †clindamycin 7 mg/kg PO tid

*Established infection: treat for 14 days. Prophylaxis: treat for 3-5 days.
†Includes activity against community-acquired community-associated methicillin-resistant *Staphylococcus aureus*.

of low-risk dog bite wounds.[5,6,16-18] In a study by Chen,[19] suture closure of dog bites was 94% successful compared with 97% in nonbite wounds.[4] Caution is recommended for wounds more than 8 to 12 hours old, fang (puncture) wounds, hand lacerations, or wounds that are at high risk.[4] When risk to closure exists, delayed primary closure (tertiary union) or open closure (secondary union) can be considered. Because of the cosmetic concerns associated with facial bites and a low potential for infection, suturing, even after 8 to 12 hours, can be considered.[17] Consultation with a specialist is recommended to assist in the decision. Whenever primary closure of any dog bite is performed, deep closures are avoided to minimize the potential for infection.[4]

Established Dog Bite Infection

For wounds with signs of infection (i.e., purulence, redness, heat, tenderness, and lymphangitis), the initial empirical dose of intravenous antibiotics should be broad spectrum.[20] Ampicillin/sulbactam (Unasyn) provides coverage for the most likely infecting organisms (Table 15-2). If a patient requires admission to the hospital, this agent can be continued until wound culture results are available to determine further therapy. If the patient can be treated as an outpatient, oral ampicillin/clavulanate (Augmentin) can be used after the initial parenteral ampicillin/sulbactam. Culture results can guide outpatient therapy as well. Total treatment time is approximately 14 days; however, the patient is recommended to return in 48 to 72 hours for assessment of treatment effectiveness.

Cat Bites

Microbiology and Risk Factors for Infection

Cat wounds can be inflicted by both teeth and claws. In a study of infected cat bites, *Pasteurella multocida* was found in 75% of cases.[9] It is important to remember that cats lick their paws, which can be covered with *P. multocida*. This organism is particularly virulent. Because cat teeth are long and slender, deep tissue, tendon, or joint seeding can occur. Infection is characterized by rapid onset and spreading (less than 24 hours), pain, and thin grayish discharge. Other organisms that can be cultured are aerobes, including *S. aureus* and streptococci, and anaerobes. Other risk factors for infection are similar to the factors listed for dog bites.

Cat Bite Wound Management

Cat bites are managed according to the general bite wound management guidelines listed previously. Because of the potential for deep penetration, it is important to open fang bites for irrigation to reduce the risk for infection. Injuries to deep structures, such as tendons and joint spaces, can be assessed.

TABLE 15-2	**Initial Empirical Parenteral Antibiotic Choices for Inpatient Treatment of Established Mammalian Bite Infections**
Bite Wound	**Treatment**
Cat, dog, human	**Adults**
	Ampicillin/sulbactam 1.5-3.0 g IV q6h Ceftriaxone 1 g IV q12h plus metronidazole 500 mg q8h TMP/SMX 4-10 mg/kg (TMP) IV q12h plus clindamycin 600 mg IV q8h
	Children (1-12 yr)
	Ampicillin/sulbactam 50 mg/kg IV q12h plus clindamycin 7.5 mg/kg IV q8h TMP/SMX 2-3mg/kg IV q12h plus clindamycin 7.5 mg/kg mg IV q8h

Cat Bite Prophylaxis

Prophylaxis for uninfected-appearing cat bites is less controversial than prophylaxis for dog bites.[10,21,22] Most cat bites, unless they are minor scratches or are limited to the superficial dermis, are candidates for oral prophylactic antibiotics.[23] For prophylaxis to be effective, the first dose should be delivered in the emergency department and, preferably, in intravenous form. Either ampicillin/sulbactam or ceftriaxone plus metronidazole cover the likely pathogens (see Table 15-2). For outpatient management, amoxicillin/clavulanate also can be used. Alternatives and recommendations for children are found in Tables 15-1 and 15-2.

Suturing

Unless tissue coverage and cosmesis are important considerations, cat bite and scratch wounds are probably best left open and unsutured. Cat fangs can penetrate deeply into the soft tissues, and because the infection potential of these wounds is great, the most judicious course of action is to cleanse, irrigate, and débride the wound and to leave it open.[24] Another option is to open the wound with a simple incision as described previously in the section on bite wound management (see Fig. 15-1). Delayed primary closure can be used for wounds that need suturing for cosmetic or functional reasons, but primary closure at the time of wounding is considered too risky for inducing infection. Exceptions to this recommendation include large, easily cleansed lacerations that are not on the hand or the foot. Most lacerations of the face are protected by the good vascular supply of the face, and suturing is recommended for cosmesis. Whenever suturing is chosen, only percutaneous nonabsorbable sutures are used. Deep closures are avoided because of the increased risk of infection.

Established Cat Bite Infections

For initial empirical therapy, as with dog bites, an intravenous dose of ampicillin/sulbactam can be delivered in the emergency department (see Table 15-2). This agent can be continued during inpatient admission until culture results are known. For outpatient treatment, ampicillin/clavulanate can be prescribed for a full course of 14 days. This course can be modified with culture results and can be reviewed at the recommended 48- to 72-hour return visit. Infection with *P. multocida* is often characteristic with onset of symptoms within 24 hours of the bite, with prominent pain and swelling, and with a serosanguinous and grayish exudate.[25] Intravenous antibiotic treatment is administered as soon as possible because of the rapid spread of this organism.

Human Bites
Microbiology

The microbiology of human bites differs from that of cat and dog bites and is more complex. Aerobic organisms recovered from human bite infections include *Streptococcus* (α-,β-hemolytic), *Staphylococcus* (*S. aureus, S. epidermidis*), and *Corynebacterium. Eikenella corrodens* has been recovered from 29% of human bites, including 25% of all clenched-fist injuries.[26-28] *E. corrodens* is a particularly virulent organism that can result in serious, chronic, and indolent infections. Human bite infections in hospitalized or institutionalized patients often are caused by gram-negative organisms, such as *Escherichia coli, Proteus,* and *Pseudomonas.*

Infectious complications of human bites also can derive from viruses and other organisms.[1] Viruses transmitted through human bites include hepatitis B and C and herpes virus types 1 and 2. *Mycobacterium tuberculosis* and *Treponema pallidum* have been reported to be transmitted through human bites. To date, although it is biologically possible, no case of human immunodeficiency virus infection has been reported from transmittal through a human bite.[1]

Bite Wound Management

The basic wound care steps are carried out as previously described. For clenched-fist injuries ("fight bite"), both x-rays and exploration are recommended to rule out fractures and/or penetration of key structures such as joints or tendons. A fist struck against the mouth can drive teeth into the lightly padded knuckles. Suppurative complications are common, and violation to tendon, bone, or joint has been reported in 75% of cases.[29] These injuries require aggressive intervention with exploration, irrigation, débridement, and early parenteral antibiotic administration. Care is best performed in consultation with a specialist.

Prophylaxis

Most authorities and clinicians recommend antibiotic prophylaxis for most human bites with the possible exception of superficial human bite wounds.[30-33] Until reliable clinical studies are performed to clarify the true risk of human bites and the value of prophylaxis, it is best to err on the side of treatment. Uninfected nonhand bite wounds can be treated on an outpatient basis. Simple abrasions or superficial occlusional bites can be cleansed and observed. Antibiotics are given at the discretion of the caregiver (see Table 15-1). Wounds penetrating into the dermis or subcutaneous tissue are best treated with antibiotics. Any bite of the hand needs careful follow-up in addition to antibiotics. Because of the potential seriousness of these bites, consultative support is recommended. To ensure early and appropriate antibiotic levels, an initial parenteral dose of ampicillin/sulbactam should initiate prophylaxis. For children, amoxicillin plus clavulanate or trimethoprim/sulfamethoxazole plus clindamycin can be used.

Suturing

As a general rule, closure of human bite wounds traditionally has been avoided.[1] A study has cast doubt, however, on the practice of not closing human bite wounds.[34] Sutured versus nonsutured hand lacerations from human bites had the same outcome. Further studies are needed to confirm these results. Large, easily cleansed and irrigated proximal extremity or truncal wounds can be closed with a single layer of nonabsorbable material. Facial human bites can be disfiguring. A fresh facial bite (<24 hours old) that does not show signs of infection can be closed safely with sutures.[35] Consultation is recommended when there is doubt about what management steps should be undertaken for human bites. All clenched-fist bite injuries, with penetration of the dermis, should be managed in consultation with a specialist.

Established Hand Infections

For established infections, ampicillin/sulbactam can be initiated intravenously in the emergency department (see Table 15-2). It provides excellent coverage against *S. aureus, E. corrodens,* and the relevant anaerobic species. Most patients with established hand infections are admitted to the hospital for continued intravenous antibiotics, and ampicillin/sulbactam can be continued until culture results are known. An alternative with similar good coverage against the relevant pathogens is ceftriaxone plus metronidazole. Children can be treated with cefuroxime or trimethoprim/sulfamethoxazole plus clindamycin. In human bites inflicted by institutionalized patients, coverage for gram-negative organisms should be considered, and the addition of an aminoglycoside to one of the above mentioned regimens might be indicated.

Rat Bites

Most reported rat bites occur in domestic settings. In a study of 50 cases, *Staphylococcus epidermidis* was the most common organism cultured from the open, fresh wound.[36]

Other organisms included *Bacillus subtilis,* diphtheroids, and α-hemolytic streptococci. Although 30% of wounds had positive cultures, only one case became infected. No patient was treated with prophylactic antibiotics. Antibiotics are recommended only if wound infection is evident. Ampicillin/clavulanate and doxycycline are recommended. Rats do not carry rabies, and patients do not need postexposure prophylaxis.

Fish Bites

People who work with or own fish are susceptible to infection by the small, gram-positive rod *Erysipelothrix*. This organism causes a slowly spreading cellulitis of the affected area, usually the hand. The organism responds to penicillin, ceftriaxone, and ciprofloxacin for patients who are allergic to penicillin.[37]

WOUND AFTERCARE AND FOLLOW-UP

All animal bite victims or members of their families have to be instructed about the signs of infection: pain, redness, swelling, and purulent drainage. Dressings have to be removed approximately 24 hours after the initial visit to the physician so that the wound can be inspected. A wound infection with *P. multocida* usually is apparent by that time.[25] If signs of infection are present, the patient should return to a medical care facility for treatment. A routine follow-up visit for deep, extensive face or hand wounds, 24 (particularly for cat bites) to 72 hours after care, is a prudent recommendation. Tetanus prophylaxis is administered according to the guidelines outlined in Chapter 21.

RABIES EXPOSURE AND PROPHYLAXIS

Since 2000, 31 cases of human rabies have been reported in the United States.[38] Of those cases none were caused by domestic animals. Eight cases were contracted abroad and were diagnosed in the United States. Eighteen of the cases were traced back to bat bites, and 4 other cases were implicated as likely bat exposures. One case was caused by a raccoon, and 4 were transmitted by organ transplantation from a donor before it was determined that the donor was associated with bat rabies.

Because they treat many animal bites, emergency departments (EDs) frequently are the facilities that administer rabies postexposure prophylaxis. The most common exposure treated in EDs is from dog bites.[39] Approximately 6% of dog bites require prophylaxis. Of raccoon and bat bites, 80% receive prophylaxis. Of patients with animal bites that qualify for prophylaxis, 6% of these patients do not receive it. The most common reason for the lack of prophylaxis is the failure to find or account for the status of the biting animal.

Because of the control programs, almost all (85%) of wildlife rabies occurs in skunks, raccoons, and bats.[40] Although canine rabies has been reduced dramatically, it has not been completely eradicated, particularly along the United States–Mexico border. In the rest of the world, including Asia, Africa, and Latin America, dogs remain the most significant threat to humans for rabies transmittal. Eighty-one cases of dog rabies were reported in 2009 in the United States, and 300 cases of cat rabies were reported.[38]

Rabies is a neurotropic virus that, on entering the peripheral nervous system, becomes protected from immune response.[41] For this reason, immediate wound care and postexposure prophylaxis should be initiated to prevent that crucial access. The size of the rabies inoculum, the richness of nerve innervation at the bite site, and the proximity to nerve terminals are crucial risk factors for active disease susceptibility. Animal wounding studies have shown that thorough wound cleansing using soap and water can reduce 90% of the inoculum.[40]

TABLE 15-3	Rabies Postexposure Prophylaxis Guide: United States, 2008	
Animal Type	**Evaluation and Disposition of Animal**	**Postexposure Prophylaxis Recommendations**
Dogs, cats, and ferrets	Healthy and available for 10 days observation	Persons should not begin prophylaxis unless animal develops clinical signs of rabies.*
	Rabid or suspected rabid	Immediately begin prophylaxis.
	Unknown (e.g., escaped)	Consult public health officials.
Skunks, raccoons, foxes, and most other carnivores; bats†	Regarded as rabid unless animal proven negative by laboratory tests‡	Consider immediate prophylaxis.
Livestock, small rodents (rabbits and hares), large rodents (woodchucks and beavers), and other mammals	Consider individually	Consult public health officials. Bites from squirrels, hamsters, guinea pigs, gerbils, chipmunks, rats, mice, other small rodents, rabbits, and hares almost never require antirabies postexposure prophylaxis.

*During the 10-day observation period, begin postexposure prophylaxis at the first sign of rabies in a dog, cat, or ferret that has bitten someone. If the animal exhibits clinical signs of rabies, it should be euthanized immediately and tested.
†Postexposure prophylaxis should be initiated as soon as possible following exposure to such wildlife, unless the animal is available for testing and public health authorities are facilitating expeditious laboratory testing or it is already known that the brain material from the animal has tested negative. Other factors, which might influence the urgency of decision making regarding initiation of postexposure prophylaxis before diagnostic results, are known to include the species of the animal, the general appearance and behavior of the animal, whether the encounter was provoked by the presence of a human, and the severity and location of the bites. Discontinue vaccine if appropriate laboratory diagnostic test (i.e., the direct fluorescent antibody test) is negative.
‡The animal should be euthanized and tested as soon as possible. Holding for observation is not recommended.
From Manning SE, Rupprecht CE, Fishbein D, et al: Human rabies prevention—United States, 2008: recommendations of the Advisory Committee on Immunization Practices, *MMWR Recomm Rep* 57(RR-3):1–28, 2008.

When confronted with a bite victim, the emergency physician has to consider several factors before initiating postexposure prophylaxis, These factors include (1) type of exposure, (2) epidemiology of animal rabies in the area, and (3) circumstances of the exposure incident. Tables 15-3 and 15-4 summarize the current postexposure guidelines and treatment schedule.

Type of Exposure
An exposure to rabies can be considered to have happened if the bite of a potentially rabid animal or exposure of saliva or neural tissue contacts an open wound or mucous membrane. Petting or handling an animal with intact skin exposure to blood, feces, or urine does not constitute an exposure. Any penetration of skin on any body site constitutes a potential risk. A special and potentially dangerous exposure is to bats. Cases have been reported of aerosolized bat rabies in caves and laboratories. Even finding a bat in a room of a person who has slept there can be considered an exposure. Bat contact with humans can be so slight, with transmission of rabies, as to be undetectable by the person exposed. Exposures can occur to unattended children, the mentally challenged, or intoxicated persons. If the bat can be safely caught, it should be transported to public health officials for immediate examination for rabies. The risk of contracting rabies through a bite from a known rabid animal ranges between 5% and 80%.[42] The risk of exposure of rabies to a skin scratch is 0.1% to 1%.

TABLE 15-4	Rabies Postexposure Prophylaxis Schedule: United States, 2010	
Vaccination Status	**Intervention**	**Regimen***
Not previously vaccinated	Wound cleansing	All PEP should begin with immediate thorough cleansing of all wounds with soap and water. If available, a virucidal agent (e.g., povidine-iodine solution) should be used to irrigate the wounds.
	HRIG	Administer 20 IU/kg body weight. If anatomically feasible, the full dose should be infiltrated around and into the wound(s), and any remaining volume should be administered at an anatomic site (IM) distant from vaccine administration. Also, HRIG should not be administered in the same syringe as vaccine. Because RIG might partially suppress active production of rabies virus antibody, no more than the recommended dose should be administered.
	Vaccine	HDCV or PCECV 1.0 mL, IM (deltoid area†), 1 each on days 0,‡ 3, 7, and 14.§
Previously vaccinated¶	Wound cleansing	All PEP should begin with immediate thorough cleansing of all wounds with soap and water. If available, a virucidal agent such as povidine-iodine solution should be used to irrigate the wounds.
	HRIG	HRIG should not be administered.
	Vaccine	HDCV or PCECV 1.0 mL, IM (deltoid area†), 1 each on days 0§ and 3.

HDCV, human diploid cell vaccine; HRIG, human rabies immune globulin; IM, intramuscular; PCECV, purified chick embryo cell vaccine; PEP, postexposure prophylaxis; RIG, rabies immune globulin; RVA, rabies vaccine adsorbed.
*These regimens are applicable for persons in all age groups, including children.
†The deltoid area is the only acceptable site of vaccination for adults and older children. For younger children, the outer aspect of the thigh may be used. Vaccine should never be administered in the gluteal area.
‡Day 0 is the day that dose 1 of the vaccine is administered.
§For persons with immunosuppression, rabies PEP should be administered using all five doses of vaccine on days 0, 3, 7, 14, and 28.
¶Any person with a history of preexposure vaccination with HDCV, PCECV, or RVA; previous PEP with HDCV, PCECV, or RVA; or previous vaccination with any other type of rabies vaccine and a documented history of antibody response to the previous vaccination.
From Rupprecht CE, Briggs D, Brown CM, et al: Use of a reduced (4-dose) vaccine schedule for postexposure prophylaxis to prevent human rabies: recommendations of the Advisory Committee on Immunization Practices, *MMWR Recomm Rep* 59(RR-2):1-9, 2010

Epidemiology of Animal Rabies in a Geographic Area
Wild Carnivores and Bats

Approximately 3% to 20% of all bats submitted for rabies testing are positive for the virus.[40] Bats are responsible for most cases of human rabies in the United States and its territories. Skunks, raccoons, foxes, woodchucks, and wild carnivores should be considered rabid, unless they are in a geographic area known to be free of wildlife rabies. Postexposure prophylaxis should be initiated when patients are exposed to wild carnivores and bats unless (1) the exposure occurred in an area of the continental United States known to be free of terrestrial rabies, and the results of immunofluorescence antibody testing are available within 48 hours, or (2) the animal already has been tested and shown not to be rabid. If the animal cannot be captured or tested, prophylaxis is begun immediately. Because the issue of geographic location and the incidence of wildlife rabies can be complicated, consultation with local public health officials is recommended. If there is any delay in obtaining that consultation, or if the caregiver has any doubt whatsoever about the nature of the biting species, postexposure prophylaxis should be initiated until clinical clarity is obtained. Treatment can be discontinued if it is determined that the risk does not warrant prophylaxis.

Dogs and Cats

The likelihood of a dog carrying rabies varies with geographic area. The area of highest risk in the United States is along the Mexican border; 80% of all dogs submitted for testing in that region have been positive for the rabies virus.[43] Away from the border region, in areas where rabies exists in terrestrial wildlife, only 0.1% to 1% of dogs test positive.

Cats have been reported to have a higher rate of rabies infection than dogs. The region for the greatest rabies risk in cats is the Mid-Atlantic. Transmittal of rabies to cats is probably through raccoons.

No case of animal rabies has been reported from dogs that have been documented to be fully vaccinated (two shots).[40] Only three cases of rabies have been reported in dogs and cats that have been reported vaccinated. In all of these cases, it was discovered that the animals had been incompletely vaccinated and had received only one of the two recommended immunization shots.

Treatment guidelines are as follows: When the animal is known to be rabid or is suspected to be, prophylaxis is initiated without delay. For bites from healthy captured but unvaccinated animals, quarantine for 10 days is recommended. Any illness that develops in that period is followed immediately by initiation of prophylaxis. Treatment is not delayed for animal sacrifice and rabies immunofluorescence testing of the brain. For truly wild, unwanted animals that have been captured, immediate sacrifice and testing can be performed. If the animal cannot be captured and tested, postexposure prophylaxis is guided by the risk of endemic, wildlife rabies in that geographic area. In these circumstances, consultation with public health officials is recommended. In cases in which consultation cannot be obtained within 48 hours of the biting incident, initiation of prophylaxis is recommended if there is any uncertainty regarding the status of the biting animal.

Rodents and Lagomorphs

Rodents include mice, rats, squirrels, hamsters, guinea pigs, gerbils, and chipmunks. Lagomorphs are rabbits and hares. The overall rate of rabies infection in this group is 0.01%. No case of human rabies has ever been documented after a rodent or a lagomorph bite. Woodchucks and groundhogs are an exception because of reported rabies carriage in some regions of the land. In the event of a rodent or groundhog/woodchuck bite, guidance from the local public health officials is recommended.

Exotic Pets

Included among exotic pets are ferrets, exotic wild animals, and domestic animals crossbred with wild ones. The true risk of rabies in these animals is unknown, and it is recommended by authorities that they be sacrificed and tested rather than observed. Rabies prophylaxis can be initiated and terminated if immunofluorescence is negative. Occasionally the animal is of such rarity or value that immunoprophylaxis might be chosen over animal sacrifice. Consultation with public health officials or zoologic experts can assist in these rare cases.

Livestock

Livestock, particularly cattle, are susceptible to rabies infection from skunks. Horses, mules, sheep, goats, and swine also are susceptible but at a lower rate than cattle. Because of the logistical problems created by large animal exposure, consultation in these cases with a veterinarian or public health official is recommended.

Circumstances of Biting Incident

Unprovoked attacks by animals capable of carrying rabies can indicate that the animal might be rabid. Factors to be considered when evaluating a bite incident include local rabies epidemiology, potential exposure of the animals possibly carrying rabies, biting history and behavior of the animal, and vaccination history of the biting animal. Animals should receive their first vaccine at 3 to 4 months of age. The next inoculation is at 1 year and then every 3 years thereafter. It takes 28 days after the initial vaccination to acquire adequate antibody.

Timing of Postexposure Prophylaxis

In optimal circumstances, and because the stakes can be high, every attempt is made to administer postexposure prophylaxis, if indicated, within 48 hours of contact. This timing is based on the fact that the incubation period of rabies can be only 5 days, and a margin of safety is desirable.[43] The incubation period can be 2 years, with an average of 30 to 90 days.[40] For this reason, prophylaxis is administered to any patient found to have a rabies-risk bite or exposure regardless of the interval from contact to treatment. The average interval between exposure and care is 5 days, and that delay has not been found to increase the risk of contracting the disease.[44] Because the risk of canine rabies is low in the United States, other than along the Mexican border, a delay of 10 days is considered acceptable if the animal can be confined for observation. Dogs infected with the rabies virus almost always become clinically rabid well before the 10-day period has elapsed.[43]

Immunosuppression, HIV, and Pregnancy

Corticosteroid administration, immunosuppressive therapy or disease, and antimalarials can impair the protective immune response of rabies prophylaxis vaccination. Rabies postexposure prophylaxis is administered per schedule. Under these circumstances, however, serum testing for rabies antibody response is recommended.[45] HIV patients with a CD4 count <100 are less likely to develop immunity.[45] With counts > 200, adequate antibody formation is likely. In these patients, it is particularly important to cleanse and irrigate the wound thoroughly and to surround the wound locally with rabies immune globulin. Rabies postexposure prophylaxis provides no risk to a fetus; pregnant women are treated in the same manner as other exposed persons. Pregnant women undergo normal delivery of a healthy baby.[46]

POSTEXPOSURE PROPHYLAXIS

The new, currently approved regimen for rabies postexposure prophylaxis includes the administration of human rabies immune globulin and four doses of human diploid cell vaccine.[3] The CDC's Prevention Advisory Committee on Immunization Practices has recommended reducing the number of vaccine doses to four from five[3,47] (see Table 15-4). No additional benefit is conferred with the fifth shot. Virtually all vaccines undergo an appropriate antibody response, and antibody titer testing is not necessary.[48] Alternative vaccine dose schedules, often administered in other countries (e.g., intradermal or intramuscular three doses), are not recommended for use in the United States.[48]

The use of rabies vaccine induces local reactions, such as pain, erythema, swelling, or itching, at the injection site in 30% to 74% of recipients.[40] Approximately 5% to 40% of vaccinees report systemic reactions, such as headache, nausea, abdominal pain, muscle aches, and dizziness. Extremely rare, with only three cases reported in the literature, are neurologic illnesses resembling Guillain-Barré syndrome.[40] All three cases resolved without sequelae within 3 months. Another reaction, occurring in 6% of recipients, is an immune complex–like illness characterized by urticaria, arthralgia, arthritis, angioedema, nausea, vomiting, and fever. Local pain and low-grade fever have been reported with human rabies immune globulin.

Because of the seriousness of rabies, if possible, rabies prophylaxis should not be interrupted or discontinued. Attempts are made to manage local or mild systemic reactions with antiinflammatories and antipyretics. Ultimately, in serious reactions, the risk of acquiring rabies must be weighed against the nature of the reaction. In cases such as these, advice and assistance should be sought from public health officials or from the Centers for Disease Control and Prevention in Atlanta, Georgia.

Postexposure Therapy of Previously Vaccinated Bite Victims

Patients who previously have undergone preexposure or postexposure rabies prophylaxis are treated with two doses of the vaccine alone, one dose immediately and the other 3 days later.[48] Human rabies immune globulin is unnecessary because the vaccination booster provides an effective amnestic antibody response. Cleansing and irrigation of the wound, however, remain just as important for these patients as for those who have not previously undergone preexposure or postexposure rabies prophylaxis.

References

1. Griego RD, Rosen T, Orengo IF, et al: Dog, cat, and human bites: a review, *J Am Acad Dermatol* 33: 1019–1029, 1995.
2. Kizer K: Epidemiologic and clinical aspects of animal bite injuries, *JACEP* 8:134–141, 1979.
3. Rupprecht CE, Briggs D, Brown CM, et al: Use of a reduced (4-dose) vaccine schedule for postexposure prophylaxis to prevent human rabies: recommendations of the Advisory Committee on Immunization Practices, *MMWR Recomm Rep* 59(RR-2):1–9, 2010.
4. Goldstein EJC, Citron D, Finegold SM: Dog bite wounds and infection: a prospective clinical study, *Ann Emerg Med* 9:508–512, 1980.
5. Callaham ML: Prophylactic antibiotics in common dog bite wounds: a controlled study, *Ann Emerg Med* 9:410–414, 1980.
6. Callaham ML: Treatment of common dog bites: infection risk factors, *J Am Coll Emerg Physicians* 7:83–87, 1978.
7. Zook EG, Miller M, Van Beek AL, et al: Successful treatment protocol for canine fang injuries, *J Trauma* 20:243–246, 1980.
8. Strassburg M, Greenland S, Marron JA, Mationey LE: Animal bites: patterns of treatment, *Ann Emerg Med* 10:193–197, 1981.
9. Talan DA, Citron DM, Abrahamian FM: Bacteriologic analysis of infected dog and cat bites. Emergency Medicine Animal Bite Infection Study Group, *N Engl J Med* 340:138–140, 1999.
10. Brandt F: Human bites of the ear, *Plast Reconstr Surg* 43:130–134, 1969.
11. Abrahamian FM: Dog bites: bacteriology, management, and prevention, *Curr Infect Dis Rep* 2:446–453, 2000.
12. Douglas LG: Bite wounds, *Am Fam Physician* 11:93–99, 1990.
13. Rosen RA: The use of antibiotics in the initial management of recent dog-bite wounds, *Am J Emerg Med* 3:19–23, 1985.
14. Medeiros I, Sacanoto H: Antibiotic prophylaxis for mammalian bites, *Cochrane Database Syst Rev* 2:CD001738, 2001.
15. Cummings P: Antibiotics to prevent infection in patients with dog bite wounds: a meta-analysis of randomized trials, *Ann Emerg Med* 23:535–540, 1994.
16. Dire DJ: Emergency management of dog and cat bite wounds, *Emerg Med Clin North Am* 10:719–736, 1992.
17. Guy RJ, Zook EG: Successful treatment of acute head and neck dog bite wounds without antibiotics, *Ann Plast Surg* 17:45–48, 1986.
18. Thomas PR, Buntine JA: Man's best friend? A review of the Austin hospital's experience with dog bites,, *Med J Aust* 147:536–540, 1987.
19. Chen E, Hornig S, Sheperd SM, et al: Primary closure of mammalian bite wounds, *Acad Emerg Med* 7: 157–161, 2000.
20. Goldstein EJC: Bite wounds and infection, *Clin Infect Dis* 14:633–640, 1992.
21. Aghababian R, Conte J: Mammalian bite wounds, *Ann Emerg Med* 9:79–83, 1980.

22. Elenbaas RM, McNabney WK, Robinson WA: Evaluation of prophylactic oxacillin in cat bite wounds, *Ann Emerg Med* 13:155–157, 1984.
23. Dire DJ: Cat bite wounds: risk factors for infection (abstract), *Ann Emerg Med* 18:471, 1989.
24. Veitch J, Omer G: Case reports: treatment of cat bite injuries of the hand, *J Trauma* 19:201–202, 1979.
25. Tindall J, Harrison C: *Pasteurella multocida* infections following animal injuries, especially cat bites, *Arch Dermatol* 105:412–416, 1972.
26. Basadre JO, Parry SW: Indications for surgical debridement in 125 human bites of the hand, *Arch Surg* 126:65–67, 1991.
27. Goldstein EJC, Barones MF, Miller TA: *Eikenella corrodens* in hand infections, *J Hand Surg* 8:563–566, 1983.
28. Patzakis MJ, Wilkins J, Bassett RL: Surgical findings in clenched-fist injuries, *Clin Orthop* 220:237–240, 1987.
29. Malinowski R, Strate RG, Perry JF Jr, Fischer RP: The management of human bite injuries to the hand, *J Trauma* 19:655–658, 1979.
30. Farmer C, Mann R: Human bite infections of the hand, *South Med J* 59:515–518, 1966.
31. Chuinard R, D'Ambrosia R: Human bite infections of the hand, *J Bone Joint Surg Am* 59:416–418, 1977.
32. Guba A, Mulliken J, Hoopes J: The selection of antibiotics for human bites of the hand, *Plast Reconstr Surg* 56:538–541, 1975.
33. Shields C, Patzakis MJ, Meyers MH, Harvey JP Jr: Hand infections secondary to human bites, *J Trauma* 15:235–236, 1975.
34. Bite U: Human bites of the hand, *Can J Surg* 27:616–618, 1984.
35. Thomasetti B, Walker L, Bormby M: Human bites of the face, *J Oral Surg* 37:565–568, 1979.
36. Ordog GJ, Balasubramaniam S, Wasserberger J: Rat bites: fifty cases, *Ann Emerg Med* 14:126–130, 1985.
37. Fidalgo SG, Longbottom CG, Rjley TV: Susceptibility of Erysipelothrix rhusiopathae to antimicrobial agents and home disinfectants, *Pathology* 34:462–465, 2000.
38. Blanton JD, Palmer D, Ruprecht CE: Rabies surveillance in the United States during 2009, *J Am Vet Med Assoc* 237:646–657, 2010.
39. Moran GJ, Talan DA, Mower W: Appropriateness of rabies postexposure prophylaxis treatment for animal exposure, *JAMA* 284:1001–1007, 2000.
40. Human Rabies Prevention—United States, 1999. Recommendations of the Advisory Committee on Immunization Practices (ACIP), *MMWR Recomm Rep* 48(RR 1):1–21, 1999.
41. Mann J: Systemic decision-making in rabies prophylaxis, *Pediatr Infect Dis* 2:162–167, 1983.
42. Hatwick MAW: Human rabies, *Public Health Rev* 3:229–274, 1974.
43. Fishbein DB, Robinson LE: Rabies, *N Engl J Med* 329:1632–1638, 1993.
44. Beck AM, Felser SR, Glickman LT: An epizootic of rabies in Maryland, 1982-84, *Am J Public Health* 77:42–44, 1987.
45. Wilde H: Post-exposure rabies prophylaxis in patients with AIDS, *Vaccine* 27:5726–5727, 2009.
46. Sudarshan MK, Giri MS, Mahendra BJ, et al: Assessing the safety of post-exposure rabies immunization in pregnancy, *Hum Vaccin* 3:87–89, 2007.
47. Mitka M: CDC advisors suggest streamlining postexposure prophylaxis for rabies, *JAMA* 303:1586, 2010.
48. Manning SE, Rupprecht CE, Fishbein D, et al: Human rabies prevention—United States, 2008. Recommendations of the Advisory Committee on Immunization Practices, *MMWR Recomm Rep* 57(RR-3):1–28, 2008.

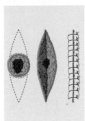

CHAPTER 16
Common Wound Care Problems

───────────────── **Key Practice Points** ─────────────────

■ The most common soft tissue foreign bodies (FBs) are wood, metal, and glass.

■ Foreign bodies, such as wood, should be removed if they are reactive, as wood and other reactive materials can cause infection or granulomas. Nonreactive objects, such as metal, need not be removed if they are in a noncritical area. If these objects can interfere with weight-bearing areas or joints, they should be removed.

■ Lead objects can increase blood lead levels, but if they are in anatomically unimportant areas, they need to be removed only if symptoms of toxicity (fatigue, headache, nausea, or other symptoms) are present, and blood lead levels confirm toxicity.

■ The majority (80%) of foreign bodies, including glass, are visualized directly or indirectly with radiographs. Wood and other organic objects are the least likely to be seen on radiographs. Computerized tomography, MRI, and ultrasound are alternative methods to localize FBs.

■ Exploration and removal of FBs can be difficult and frustrating. As a rule, if exploration exceeds 20 to 30 minutes, assistance from or referral to a consultant is recommended.

■ Clean plantar puncture wounds without visible inflammation or foreign material have a low complication rate, and there is no evidence that prophylactic antibiotics have any value.

■ Plantar puncture wounds with suspected foreign material or contamination should be opened, irrigated and débrided, and treated with antibiotics.

Common nonlaceration problems lend themselves to emergency wound care techniques. These problems include retained foreign bodies and fishhooks, plantar puncture wounds, and abrasions. Although they can appear trivial, each of these problems presents special challenges and occasionally requires sophisticated diagnostic and management procedures. In addition, certain anatomic areas of the body, particularly the structures of the face, hand, and foot, can be fraught with unique difficulties, which are best managed by a thorough understanding of the issues and an application of the proper technique.

FOREIGN BODIES

Any object becomes a foreign body when it penetrates the skin and lodges in the soft tissue. In a study of 490 cases of foreign-body injuries presenting to an emergency department, the majority of the injuries were caused by wood, metal and glass.[1] Other reported foreign bodies were pencil leads, thorns, nails, and plastic objects.[2] Generally, foreign bodies are classified by material—inert (nonreactive) and organic (reactive). The vast majority of patients presented within 48 hours.[1]

Inert (Nonreactive) Objects

Inert objects include bullets, needles, and other metallic items. Although they do not provoke inflammation, these objects can cause chronic pain and discomfort, especially in weight-bearing areas or near joints. Metals that oxidize (i.e., rust) can cause mild to moderate tissue reaction. The clinical decision to remove an inert object has to be weighed against the potential damage that could be created during a search for the object. Inert objects can be left in place if they are inaccessible and will not cause tissue damage or functional deficit. If left alone, noncritical inert foreign bodies encapsulate within soft tissue and cause no further problem.

A question sometimes arises concerning lead foreign bodies, usually bullets, and the risk of lead absorption and toxicity. When compared with controls, patients with extraarticular retained missiles (lead bullets) show a rise in lead levels over time, but the vast majority (96%) of level increases were shown not to be clinically significant.[3] In a study of patients with retained bullets, lead levels averaged 17 μg/dL compared with 7 μg/dL in the control patients ($P < .002$).[4] Levels greater than 10 μg/dL are considered toxic. Clinical signs of toxicity are uncommon, however. Symptoms, such as fatigue, headache, and nausea, can be low grade and vague. If toxicity is suspected, patients are referred for lead level testing and evaluation.

Although glass is considered inert, glass foreign bodies are often symptomatic. If the glass is accessible, removal is recommended except for small, insignificant fragments. Pencil "lead" (i.e., graphite) is inert but can cause tattooing. It also can be accompanied by wood fragments during injury. For these reasons, even though it is inert, graphite should be removed from the injury site.

Organic (Reactive) Objects

Objects that are not inert—wood, bone, soil, stones, rubber, and other organic materials such as thorns—must be removed in their entirety. These materials can cause a variety of bacterial and fungal infections.[5,6] Synovitis from joint penetration, periosteal reactions, foreign-body granulomas, draining fistulas, and pseudotumors of the soft tissue all have been reported with noninert foreign objects.[2,7,8] Retained wood objects have been reported to cause chronic inflammation, drainage, and pain for 7 years after penetration.[7] A missed diagnosis or failure to remove all fragments of a noninert object can lead to prolonged disability and patient discomfort.

Clinical Evaluation

When a foreign object penetrates the skin, patients cannot reliably report its presence. In glass wounds, reliance on the patient's history alone would lead to 50% missed fragments.[9] For cases in which no foreign body is reported, certain clinical settings carry a higher risk for one being present. Any injury with glass should raise the suspicion of a retained fragment. For glass injuries, the head and foot are more likely to have retained fragments.[10] For lip or perioral injuries in which there is traumatic loss of dentition, a tooth fragment might be embedded in the soft tissue. Injuries to the feet or hands with needles, nails, or splinters should be suspected of retention if the patient cannot account for the entirety of the injuring object. If the suspicion is strong, the caregiver is obligated to perform a diagnostic evaluation and local exploration to rule in or rule out the possibility of a retained foreign object.

Before anesthetic is administered, gently running a gloved finger over the suspected foreign-body site can elicit in a patient the characteristic sensation. In the anesthetized wound, gently probing and drawing a closed hemostat in and through the wound can alert the operator to the presence of a wood, glass, or metallic foreign body. The hemostat transmits a distinct "grating" sensation. Probing can reveal the presence of an inert object or a wood splinter before it has been softened by the absorption of tissue fluids.

Imaging
Plain Radiography

For the most part, radiographs are ordered when there is patient belief or clinical suspicion of a foreign object. Most objects (80%) can be visualized directly or indirectly with the use of radiographs.[2] Radiodense objects, even the size of a pinpoint, are easily seen. Metallic objects, with the exception of aluminum, can be visualized in almost all cases. A common misconception is that glass is not visible by radiograph.[11] In experimental conditions, virtually all types of glass (95%) 2 mm in size can be seen by x-ray.[12] Fragments 0.5 mm or larger can be visualized in 50% to 60% of cases. In a clinical study of 98 patients presenting to the emergency department (ED) with foreign-body retention, 24% were radionegative.[1] Other radiodense objects include pencil graphite, some plastics, and gravel.

Nonradiodense objects include wood, thorns, chicken bones, and some plastics. Radiodensity of wood and organic objects depends to some degree on the time in tissue and the absorption of body fluids. Wood has been reported to be visible by radiography in 15% of cases; however, after 48 hours, fluid absorption renders it invisible.[2] Nonradiodense objects (e.g., splinters or plastic fragments) can be revealed as a filling defect or can be outlined by air drawn into the wound during the injury.

Ultrasonography, Computed Tomography, and Magnetic Resonance Imaging

Ultrasonography has become an increasingly important bedside diagnostic aid in emergency departments. Compact portable equipment with versatile transducer probes allows for diagnosis of nonradiodense objects and assisted removal.[13,14] Ultrasonography can detect nonradiodense foreign bodies 1×2 mm or larger.[15] In experimental studies, in which various foreign bodies are introduced to chicken or cadaver flesh, the sensitivity of ultrasound detection varied from 43% to 83%.[16-18] The specificity ranged from 59% to 86%. In a small clinical study of patients with actual nonradiodense foreign bodies, ultrasound detected 21 of 22 foreign bodies found at operation.[19]

Tendons, deep scar tissue, fresh hematoma, and tissue calcifications can produce false-positive ultrasound readings. Similar to any technical procedure, experience increases the accuracy and effectiveness of the operator.

Computed tomography (CT) scans offer an alternative to ultrasound.[20] Not only can a CT scan identify vegetative objects, such as splinters and thorns, but also it can localize objects in relationship to the surrounding anatomic structures. Magnetic resonance imaging has capabilities similar to CT but should never be used to locate objects that contain metal.[21] CT and magnetic resonance imaging are expensive imaging alternatives and require a high degree of patient cooperation, which often is not possible for a pediatric patient.

Radiodense Objects

For objects that are located below the surface and out of direct sight, careful localization is necessary before proceeding with exploration. Radiodense objects can be localized by a variety of techniques using markers and radiographs. A simple technique recommended by the author is to bend a paper clip to form a flat plane with an extended arm. The extended arm is placed directly over the skin entry wound created by the foreign object, and the paper clip is secured with a small piece of tape (Fig. 16-1). Two radiographs are taken exactly at an angle of 90 degrees to each other (anteroposterior and lateral views) using the plane of the clip as a geometric point of reference (Figs. 16-2 and 16-3). In this manner, the location and the depth of the object relative to the extended arm of the paper clip can be determined. Magnification by this technique occurs, and the distance between the object and the clip on the radiograph is greater than the actual distance. After appropriate cleansing and the administering of an anesthetic, a small incision is made, and exploration is performed until the object can be removed. The radiographs are needed for reference in the care area during the removal.

Nonradiodense Objects

If ultrasonography is not available to assist in removal, nonradiodense objects are best approached through a more generous incision and thorough exploration by direct visualization. Incisions permit débridement and removal of tissue that is embedded with foreign material. When the foreign body is located in the hand or the foot, the exsanguination tourniquet technique (see Chapter 9) is recommended. Even a small amount of bleeding can make visualization impossible.

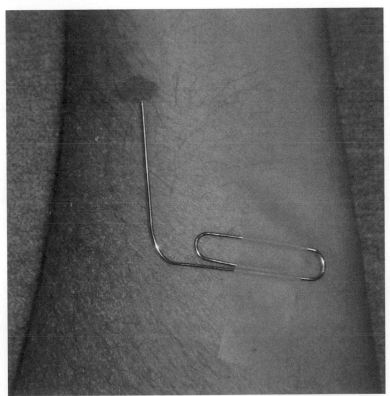

Figure 16-1. Technique for placing a reconfigured paper clip with the extended arm of the clip directly over the entry point of a foreign-body penetration.

Techniques for Removal

When attempts to remove foreign bodies are made by an emergency physician, removal was successful in 89% of cases.[1] Consultation by surgical specialist occurred in 47 cases with a success rate of 65.6% of those cases.[1]

The following steps are recommended for buried foreign bodies:

- The first step is to decide whether a removal attempt should be made in the ED. Removal is likely to be successful if the object has been under the skin for less than 1 week, the object is visible, the entry wound is fresh, the object can be localized with an imaging procedure, the object is radiodense, or the object can be felt during probing. Success is less likely if the object is deep, if it has been present for several weeks or months (as is often the case with needles), if no entry point is present, if the object is nonradiodense, and if the object cannot be localized.
- Ideally, foreign bodies seen in the ED are more easily removed elsewhere in bloodless conditions; however, most FBs are small and superficial enough to be located and removed.
- After the decision is made to remove the FB, the area is cleaned with Betadine or chlorhexidine.
- In order to prevent excessive swelling, anesthesia should be administered by nerve block if possible. Swelling of local anesthesia can make locating the FB more difficult. If no alternative is available, as little local anesthesia as possible should be used.
- A no. 15 scalpel blade is used to make an incision over the entry point, parallel to the axis of the FB if it can be determined.

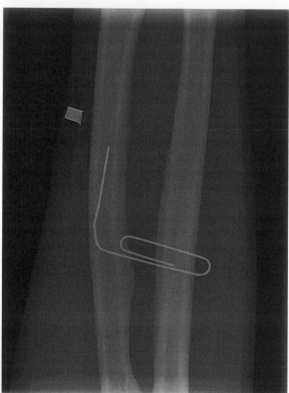

Figure 16-2. Direct anteroposterior view of the paper clip and foreign body.

- A small curved clamp can be used to explore the incision site for the FB. The clamp tip is gently "raked" through the site to feel steel against glass, wood, or metal to assist localization.
- Once localized, the FB is grasped and removed. See the following text for an explanation of the removal of wood or organic objects.
- After removal, the wound is irrigated and a dressing is applied. Incisions, except if they are large and gaping, should not be sutured.

Simple retrieval is not always possible, however. As a rule, if attempts at retrieval exceed 20 to 30 minutes, serious consideration should be given to terminating the procedure and obtaining consultation.

Protruding Objects

For objects that are partially protruding from the skin, the temptation to "grab and yank" must be resisted. If a wood splinter is pulled out injudiciously through a small, tight entry wound, small fragments can be stripped off the splinter and can be left behind to cause future difficulty.[15] The technique illustrated in Figure 16-4 shows how a small incision is made in the finger parallel to the course and angle of the object. By creating an incision, the splinter can be removed without leaving behind smaller splinters. In addition, the wound can be copiously irrigated to decrease the level of bacterial contamination. These small incisions must not be closed with sutures. They should be left open to drain the site, if necessary, and to prevent the accumulation of purulence that might lead to the formation of an abscess.

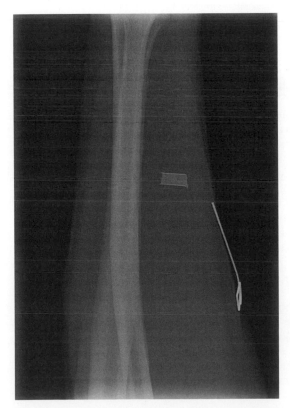

Figure 16-3. Direct lateral view of the paper clip and foreign body. This type of radiograph and that in Figure 16-2 can be used to locate accurately the position of the foreign body relative to the extended arm of the clip by the anteroposterior view and the depth of the foreign body by the lateral view.

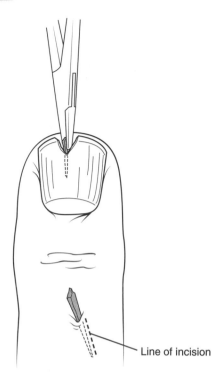

Figure 16-4. *Top,* Technique for removing a small splinter from between the nail plate and the nail bed. A small wedge of nail has been removed to gain exposure to the protruding splinter. A small hemostat is used to extract the splinter gently. *Bottom,* Technique for removing a penetrating foreign body, a splinter, which is protruding from the skin. A small incision is made directly away from the entry point, parallel to the shaft of the foreign body. The splinter can be removed in its entirety without leaving smaller splinters.

Line of incision

Objects under Nail Plates

A common problem is a splinter or other object that is lodged under a nail plate. If the object can be grasped by a hemostat, it can be pulled out carefully from under the nail. Care has to be taken not to strip fragments off a wooden object. For a splinter that cannot be grasped, removal of a small part of the nail plate in a wedge-shaped fashion can be carried out to expose the splinter, as shown in Figure 16-4 (top).

A simple technique for removing small splinters lodged under the nail plate is to bend the tip of a 25-G or 27-G needle so that a small barb equal in size to the diameter of the needle is created.[22] The shaft of the needle is introduced adjacent and parallel to the splinter and is carried back to the most proximal portion of the object. Then the barb is raked along the splinter, and the needle and the foreign object are pulled out from under the nail. Removing objects from under nails is best performed when the patient is anesthetized. The anesthetic usually is delivered via a digital block (see Chapter 6).

Thorns and Cactus Spines

Particularly troublesome are small thorns and cactus spines that can become embedded accidentally in the skin in large numbers, usually in children. In a controlled rabbit experiment, Elmer's Glue-All was applied under a single layer of gauze and was allowed to dry. Gentle peeling successfully removed 95% of all spines.[23] The next most effective method was the manual removal with tweezers, with a 76% rate of spine removal. The combination of tweezer removal of large spines followed by glue application is effective.

When to Consult

Occasionally a foreign body cannot be retrieved successfully by attempts at localization and exploration in an emergency wound care setting. This situation most commonly arises in the case of deep foreign objects in the foot. These foreign bodies are best removed in radiology department suites where ultrasound, image intensifiers, and stereotaxic localization can be applied while a consultant explores the affected area.[24,25]

PLANTAR PUNCTURE WOUNDS

Plantar puncture wounds are a common presenting complaint. Most wounds (≥90%) are caused by stepping on nails.[26] In many cases, the patient seeks only a tetanus shot and does not seek care for the wound itself. Because many patients do not seek care for punctures, the true complication rate is unknown. The complication rate for patients who do seek care, however, ranges from 2% to 8%.[26,27] The time from injury to presentation is significant, because patients who present after 48 hours are more likely to have complications.[28] In actuality, these patients are brought to care because of persistent or worsening symptoms.

In addition to delay of presentation, other circumstances increase the risk for infection and other complications. Punctures suffered outdoors are more likely to be contaminated or caused by rust-covered nails. Remnants of socks or shoes can be carried into wounds, with tennis shoes creating an increased risk for osteomyelitis secondary to *Pseudomonas aeruginosa*.[29,30] The forefoot, including the metatarsal heads and toes, is far more vulnerable to complications, particularly pyarthrosis and osteomyelitis, than are the midfoot and heel. In one study, 34 of 35 serious plantar puncture injuries occurred in the forefoot.[31] Deep punctures can penetrate bone, tendon, or joints. Finally, patients with diabetes, peripheral vascular disease, or immunosuppression carry a greater risk for complications.

Treatment of Puncture Wounds

The management of puncture wounds is controversial and ranges from minimal skin cleansing to surgical management of the puncture wound site.[32] In addition, there are no clinical studies that establish whether antibiotics prevent plantar puncture infection.[33] The following guidelines are based on different clinical presentations.

Simple Punctures

Most patients present with benign-appearing puncture wounds caused by clean objects, such as tacks, needles, or small nails that are exposed and unrusted. These patients often present less than 24 hours after the injury.[34] Realistically, cleaning and irrigating the length and depth of the actual wound might cause more complications than it would prevent. If there are no indications of retained foreign material, if the wound edges are clean and not devitalized, and if the puncture site is not indurated or excessively tender to palpitation, skin cleansing and a small application of antibiotic ointment, followed by an adhesive bandage (Band-Aid), should suffice. The patient is advised to return if signs of infection or foreign-body retention develop.

Puncture with Suspected Retained Material

In puncture wounds with suspected retained material, the puncture is often larger than the small sites noted previously. The wound edges are contaminated, stellate, or appear shredded. Old nails, exposed bolts, and miscellaneous sharp objects are causes of these punctures. By history, the puncturing object is not clean, has broken during the puncture, or possibly has forced sock or shoe fragments into the wound. Patients with these wounds are more likely to complain of significant pain or a foreign-body sensation on palpation of the puncture site. They often present more than 48 hours after the injury after having tried to treat themselves or having ignored the symptoms, without success.[34]

After anesthesia is provided, either through a foot block or by local infiltration, a transverse incision (parallel to the wrinkle line of a curled foot) is made through the puncture site, long enough to provide good exposure of the puncture site and proximal wound track (Fig. 16-5). Any foreign material or devitalized tissue can be débrided. With the wound edges retracted, thorough irrigation is performed. No attempt is made to suture this wound. The wound edges close without difficulty after application of a small amount of an antibiotic ointment and a Band-Aid. For comfort and protection, it is recommended that the patient use crutches to reduce pressure and irritation of the wound. These patients are treated with antibiotics that are effective against gram-positive organisms, and the patients should return for follow-up reexamination within 48 to 72 hours.

Complicated Punctures

In cases in which the puncture site is obviously infected, inflamed, or devitalized, more extensive débridement is performed. Foreign material is suspected until proved otherwise through exploration. In these cases, opening the wound site as shown in Figure 16-5

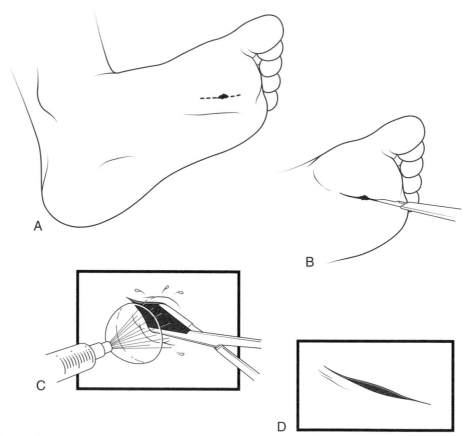

Figure 16-5. Plantar puncture wound management. **A,** A suggested incision line, parallel to the wrinkle lines, through the puncture wound. **B,** The incision can be made with a scalpel and a no. 15 blade through the thick dermis. **C,** A hemostat is used to expose the wound for exploration and irrigation. **D,** The wound edges can be débrided if necessary and can be left unsutured to heal by secondary intention.

can be done to expose the wound track and to provide for the necessary irrigation, exploration, and débridement. Suturing is not recommended, and crutches, as noted earlier, can be used. Antibiotics, as discussed in the following section, might be indicated. Surgical consultation can be considered.

Complicated Puncture with Deep Foot
Symptoms
In cases in which infection has been established, foreign material has had a chance to create significant tissue reaction, or the bone/joint has been violated, the patient complains of deep foot pain. The foot might appear swollen well beyond the puncture site itself, lymphangitic streaks could be evident, or both. In these cases, a radiograph or computerized tomography is recommended to screen for foreign objects, bone injury, or gas pockets. In addition, consultation with a surgical specialist is recommended. Established infection or significant tissue inflammation well beyond the actual puncture site is often a result of a retained foreign body. These patients usually present several days after the original puncture. Every effort has to be made to discover or rule out retained foreign material.

Antibiotics
The use of prophylactic antibiotics in uninfected puncture wounds is not supported by clinical studies.[28,33,35-38] Because *P. aeruginosa* is sensitive to ciprofloxacin in vitro, it has been used as a prophylactic agent. This is not a first-line agent for the treatment of *Pseudomonas*; it is contraindicated in children, which is the group most at risk for this type of infection.[19] Reliance on prophylactic antibiotics is undercut by a study in which cellulitis was shown to occur in nine patients despite receiving appropriate antibiotic coverage.[26] The most important finding of this study was that five of the nine patients had a retained foreign object. In uninfected puncture wounds of the foot, the recommended course of action includes careful instructions to the patient regarding the signs of infection and the arrangement of appropriate follow-up. If an infection occurs, a well-informed patient returns for appropriate treatment. It cannot be overemphasized that, if an infection develops, retained foreign material is the cause until proved otherwise.

In patients with established infection secondary to puncture wounds, the most common organisms involved are *Staphylococcus aureus*, *Staphylococcus epidermitis*, and *Streptococcus* species.[35] *P. aeruginosa* is the most common cause of postpuncture osteomyelitis and is associated with punctures through rubber tennis shoes. In one series of 15 cases of *Pseudomonas* osteochondritis in children, however, half of the children were not wearing shoes at the time of injury.[36] It is common for these patients to have initial improvement after the injury followed by a return of pain and disability. *P. aeruginosa* infection can be suspected if symptoms and signs of infection persist beyond 4 to 5 days despite the use of antistaphylococal and antistreptococal antibiotics.[37] Unless *Pseudomonas* is suspected, established infections should be treated with a broad-spectrum antibiotic with coverage of common gram-positive organisms. The first-generation cephalosporin cefazolin (Ancef), ampicillin/sulbactam (Unasyn), or clindamycin (Cleocin) in allergic patients can be initiated until culture results are known. If *Pseudomonas* is suspected, the addition of an aminoglycoside to any of the previously mentioned antibiotics provides appropriate coverage. In addition, a complete blood count, sedimentation rate studies, and imaging studies should be done to diagnose bone or cartilage involvment.[32]

FISHHOOKS
Many techniques have been described to remove fishhooks. As a rule, hooks with small barbs can be removed with retrograde techniques, and hooks with large barbs often are best managed by the push-through and cut method. In a 1991 study of 97 patients

with fishhook injuries, the most common and successful removal technique was the push-through and cut method.[38] Several methods for fishhook removal are described here, and their success rates accompany the descriptions.

Retrograde Removal

Hooks with small barbs or hooks that are only superficially embedded often can be backed out through the original site of penetration. Gentle pressure is applied to the eye and shank to push the barb away from tissue. Simultaneously a hemostat is applied to the curved portion of the shaft. Traction with the hemostat "backs" the hook out.

Experienced fishermen sometimes make a small incision in the dermis at the entry site and pull the hook out retrograde with needle-nose pliers. Dermis is the most likely layer to resist removal of the hook and barb because of its naturally tough consistency. This extraction procedure can be duplicated easily in an emergency wound care facility. After basic cleansing with an appropriate solution (e.g., povidone-iodine), a small amount of anesthetic is injected adjacent to the penetrating shaft. With a no. 11 or no. 15 blade, a small incision is made in line with the barb, inside the concave portion of the hook (Fig. 16-6). The portion of the shaft at skin level is grasped with a hemostat, and the hook is removed with a sharp, rapid pulling motion. The pulling motion is in direct line with the length of the shaft closest to the barb of the hook.

String Traction

Another method for removing a hook with small barbs requires the use of some string with good tensile strength, such as umbilical tape or 0 silk suture (Fig. 16-7). The string is looped around the curved portion of the shaft of the hook and is gently drawn parallel to and in the opposite direction of the straight portion of the shaft. The straight shaft and eyelet portions are depressed against the skin to rotate the barb slightly from its point of attachment in the skin. The string is given a sharp pull to release the hook. Caution is suggested because bystanders might be in the pathway of the hook's trajectory when it is extracted. This method of hook removal does not require the administration of an anesthetic.

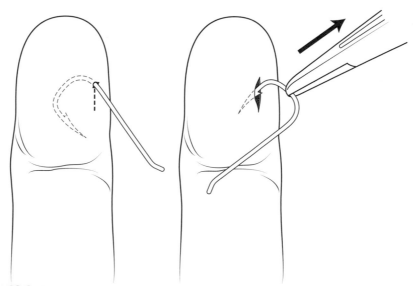

Figure 16-6. Technique for removing a fishhook with a small barb. A small incision is made in line with the concavity of the curve of the hook. The needle is backed out gently through this incision.

Barb Cover Technique

Another removal method uses an 18-G or 16-G needle. As illustrated in Figure 16-8, the needle is introduced into the skin through the original wound entry site. It is passed adjacent to the shaft until the hollow portion of the needle point can be placed over, or "cover," the barb. While both are held firmly together, the needle and hook are brought back out through the wound site. The needle effectively sheaths the barb and prevents it from snagging on tissue during removal.

Hook Push-Through

For deeply embedded hooks or hooks with large barbs, the push-through method is recommended. Trying to back out a deeply penetrated or large barbed hook can cause excessive tissue damage. Basic skin preparation is carried out, and a small amount of local anesthetic is injected at the site through which the hook point is to be extruded. Using a hemostat as a grasping instrument, the hook shaft is manipulated in such a manner so as to push the hook point out through the dermis (Fig. 16-9). The hook is clipped off with wire cutters, and the shaft is backed out of the wound.

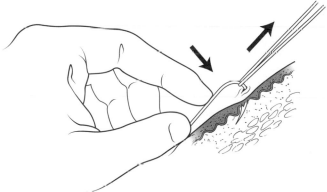

Figure 16-7. Technique for removing a fishhook with a small barb by using traction with 0 silk or umbilical tape. Pressure is applied to the shaft of the hook toward the skin as a swift "yank" of the cord is applied in the direction opposite the barb. Bystanders need to be warned that the fishhook could fly across the room. Placing a small piece of adhesive tape around the hook and string might help avoid this hazard.

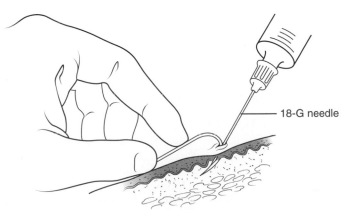

18-G needle

Figure 16-8. Technique for removing a fishhook by placing an 18-G needle on the barb of the hook and backing it out through the puncture wound.

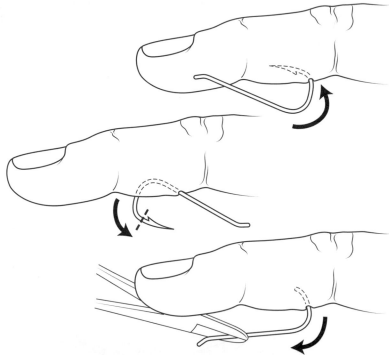

Figure 16-9. The push-through technique for removing hooks with large barbs or removing hooks that are lodged in cartilage or joint spaces. The anesthetic is infiltrated in the area of the hook and the projected exit site. When the exit has been accomplished, the barb is removed, and the shaft is backed out through the original puncture site.

Certain anatomic sites merit separate mention. Hooks embedded in cartilage, most commonly the ear or nose, cannot be backed out successfully. The push-through method is recommended for these sites. Hooks that penetrate into joint capsules also are best removed by the push-through method because barbs can break off in the joint space when backed out. Violation of a joint space can lead to serious complications; consultation is encouraged. Occasionally, fishhooks penetrate the cornea or other part of the globe. This complication constitutes an emergency. No attempt is made to remove the hook in an emergency wound care area. Ophthalmologic consultation is mandatory. If the patient has to be transferred to another facility for hook removal, he or she should be placed in a semirecumbent position to decrease eye pressure. A metal eye shield is taped gently over the eye, avoiding any direct contact or pressure on the eye. Pressure patching with gauze sponges is absolutely contraindicated to avoid extrusion of intraocular contents through the eye wound.

ABRASIONS AND TATTOOING

Abrasions are skin wounds caused by tangential trauma to the epidermis and dermis (i.e., the "skinned knee"). The skin is forced against a resistant surface in a rubbing or scraping fashion. The resultant injury is analogous to a burn. Varying thicknesses of epidermis and dermis can be lost, including tissue as deep as the superficial fascia, and bone can even be lost as well. Abrasions can be small or can cover large body surface areas. Frequently these injuries are impregnated with dirt, debris, and road tar. The principles for management include prevention of infection, promotion of rapid healing, and prevention of "traumatic tattooing" from the retained foreign material. The last-mentioned problem is of special cosmetic importance because when the healing process traps unsightly debris in the epidermis and dermis, it cannot be removed easily by later surgical intervention. At the time of the injury and "tattoo," as much is done as possible to remove the impregnated dirt, because it will become a permanent, unsightly wound. If all of the foreign material cannot be removed, it is best to inform the patient of this reality. Patients can be referred to plastic surgeons or dermatologists who can use instruments such as lasers to remove the particles.[39]

Most abrasions are small and relatively uncomplicated. Similar to burns, however, they are extremely sensitive and painful to the touch. Cleansing has to be gentle, yet thorough. An appropriate wound cleansing solution suffices to remove surface contaminants and to prepare the wound for dressing. Povidone-iodine solution, without detergent, and chlorhexidine (see Chapter 7) are effective in cleaning abrasions. Abrasions, similar to lacerations, are contaminated with bacteria that can lead to infection and cellulitis. Under experimental conditions, cleansing with povidone-iodine within 6 hours of injury can reduce bacterial counts effectively.[40] After 6 hours, the counts remain the same despite cleansing, increasing the risk of local infection.

Cleansing of contaminated and debris-laden abrasions can be tedious and difficult. If the abrasion is small, a local anesthetic can be injected around the area in a "field" or circumferential pattern. When the pain is eliminated, scrubbing can be done with a sponge or a soft surgical brush, using an appropriate cleansing solution. If necessary, meticulous removal of all particulate debris can be aided by using a needle, a no. 11 surgical blade, or a small-jaw tissue forceps.

Large abrasions (i.e., "road rash") that are heavily contaminated are difficult to manage in an emergency wound care area, because the volume of local anesthetic necessary to achieve anesthesia would exceed toxic limits. In these cases, parenteral sedation is recommended, and, in extreme cases, the patient might be better served in the operating room.

One of the most common foreign contaminants of abrasions is road tar or asphalt. If permanently impregnated in skin, tar is a cosmetic disaster because of its dark color. All tar or asphalt particles must be removed during initial wound cleansing and débridement. A cleansing adjunct that is useful for tar removal is polyoxyethylene sorbitan, a nonionic surface-active agent with hydrophilic and lyophilic properties.[41] It is an emulsifying agent that is virtually nontoxic to tissue. This substance is most commonly available as a component of Neosporin antibacterial ointment. Polysporin ointment, with a petrolatum base, is helpful in dissolving tar.[42] The ointment is not as effective, however, and is not water soluble as is the cream. The water solubility of the cream makes it easy to wash off after it has been applied to the tar-laden abrasion. Other effective commercial tar removal agents are citrus-based agents derived from orange peels. They are both effective and nontoxic to skin.

When an abrasion is initially cleansed and débrided, follow-up management is usually the patient's responsibility. The abrasion must be kept clean to prevent secondary infection. Nature's dry "dressing," the scab, ultimately does the job, and most abrasions heal without event (neither infectious nor cosmetic). Wound desiccation has been shown experimentally in humans to slow wound healing, however, and impede epithelial cell covering of the injured surface.[43] Dressings provide a moist environment that promotes rapid and effective healing.

For wounds that can be covered easily with a dressing, any nonadherent dressing can be applied over a thin coating of an ointment, such as Neosporin or Polysporin. A variety of dressing materials are available. Adaptic, Telfa, and Vaseline gauze are the least expensive. Other options include products such as membrane (Tegaderm), foam

(Epilock), and hydrocolloid (Duoderm) dressings.[44] The dressing can be removed every 2 or 3 days for gentle cleansing and redressing.

Experimentally, topical antibiotic ointments alone have been shown to increase the rate of wound reepithelialization as well.[45] It is recommended that wounds that cannot be dressed easily should be kept moist with a thin coating of an antibiotic ointment (e.g., Neosporin or Polysporin).[26] The ointment usually is applied two or three times a day to maintain the moist wound environment.

A new and different approach to managing superficial skin wounds and abrasions is octylcyanoacrylate liquid tissue adhesive (Dermabond). Dermabond currently is used to close lacerations and surgical incisions. This liquid adhesive bandage can be applied directly to fresh abrasions with an applicator brush after cleansing and drying.[46] Compared with standard Band-Aid application, liquid adhesive bandage reduces pain and bleeding. It also stays on the wound for 5 days, which is more than 3 days longer than Band-Aids adhere. The patient is allowed to bathe and can reapply the liquid adhesive bandage as needed. On average, healing is complete in 12 days, which is similar to Band-Aid–treated wounds. Liquid adhesive bandage also has been formulated as a spray that can be applied directly to abrasions.[47]

References

1. Levine MR, Gorman SM, Young CF, et al: Clinical characteristics and management of wound foreign bodies in the ED, *Am J Emerg Med* 26:918–922, 2008.
2. Anderson M, Newmeyer W, Kilgore E: Diagnosis and treatment of retained foreign bodies in the hand, *Am J Surg* 144:563–565, 1982.
3. Nguyen A, Schaider JJ, Mananzares M, et al: Elevation of blood levels in emergency department patients with extra-articular retained missiles, *J Trauma* 58:289–299, 2005.
4. Farrell SE, Vandevander P, Shoffstall JM, et al: Blood lead levels in emergency department patients with retained bullets and shrapnel, *Acad Emerg Med* 6:208–212, 1999.
5. Byron T: Foreign bodies found in the foot, *J Am Podiatr Assoc* 71:30–35, 1981.
6. Rudner E, Mehregan A: Implantation dermatosis, *J Cutan Pathol* 7:330–331, 1980.
7. Cracchiolo A: Wooden foreign bodies in the foot, *Am J Surg* 140:585–587, 1980.
8. Kahn B: Foreign body (palm thorn) in knee joint, *Clin Orthop* 135:104–106, 1978.
9. Steele MT, Tran LV, Watson WA, et al: Retained glass foreign bodies in wounds: predictive value of wound characteristics, patient perception, and wound exploration, *Am J Emerg Med* 16:627–630, 1998.
10. Montano JB, Steele MT, Watson WR: Foreign body retention in glass-caused wounds, *Ann Emerg Med* 21:1365–1368, 1992.
11. Feldman AH, Fisher MS: The radiographic detection of glass in soft tissue, *Radiology* 92:1529–1531, 1969.
12. Tanberg D: Glass in the hand and foot, *JAMA* 248:1872–1874, 1982.
13. Dean AJ, Gronczewski CA, Costantino TG: Technique for emergency medicine bedside ultrasound identification of a radiolucent foreign body, *J Emerg Med* 24:303–308, 2003.
14. Graham DD: Ultrasound in the emergency department: detection of wooden foreign bodies in the soft tissues, *J Emerg Med* 22:75–79, 2002.
15. Lammers RL: Soft tissue foreign bodies, *Ann Emerg Med* 17:1336–1347, 1988.
16. Hill R, Conron R, Greissinger P, et al: Ultrasound for the detection of foreign bodies in human tissue, *Ann Emerg Med* 29:353–356, 1997.
17. Manthey DE, Storrow AB, Milbourn JM, et al: Ultrasound versus radiology in the detection of soft-tissue foreign bodies, *Ann Emerg Med* 28:7–9, 1996.
18. Orlinsky M, Knittel P, Feit P, et al: The comparative accuracy of radiolucent foreign body detection using ultrasonography, *Am J Emerg Med* 18:401–403, 2000.
19. Gilbert FJ, Campbell RS, Bayliss AP: The role of ultrasound in the detection of non-radiopaque foreign bodies, *Clin Radiol* 41:109–112, 1990.
20. Rhoades C, Saye I, Levine E, et al: Detection of a wooden foreign body in the hand using computed tomography: case report, *J Hand Surg* 7:306–307, 1982.
21. Bodne D, Quinn SF, Cochran CF: Imaging foreign glass and wooden bodies of the extremities with CT and MRI, *J Comput Assist Tomogr* 12:608–611, 1988.
22. Davis L: Removal of subungual foreign bodies (letter), *J Fam Pract* 11:714, 1980.
23. Martinez TT, Jerome M, Barry RC, et al: Removal of cactus spines from the skin: a comparative evaluation of several methods, *Am J Dis Child* 141:1291–1292, 1987.

24. McFadden J: Stereotaxic pinpointing of foreign bodies in the limbs, *Ann Surg* 175:81–85, 1972.
25. Wayne R, Carnazzo AJ: Needle in the foot, *Am J Surg* 129:599, 1975.
26. Fitzgerald R, Cowan J: Puncture wounds of the foot, *Orthop Clin North Am* 6:965–972, 1975.
27. Houston A, Roy WA, Faust RA, et al. Tetanus prophylaxis in the treatment of puncture wounds of patients in the deep South, *J Trauma* 2:439–450, 1962.
28. Chisholm CD: Plantar puncture wounds: controversies and treatment recommendations, *Ann Emerg Med* 18:1352–1357, 1989.
29. Fischer MC, Goldsmith JF, Gilligan PH: Sneakers as a source of *Pseudomonas aeruginosa* in children with osteomyelitis following puncture wounds, *J Pediatr* 106:607–614, 1985.
30. Jacobs RF, Adelman L, Sack CM: Management of *Pseudomonas* osteochondritis complicating puncture wounds of the foot, *Pediatrics* 69:432–435, 1982.
31. Patzakis MJ, Wilkins J, Brien WW, et al: Wound site as predictor of complications following deep nail punctures of the foot, *West J Med* 150:545–547, 1989.
32. Chachad S, Kamat D: Management of plantar puncture wounds in children, *Clin Pediatr* 43:213–216, 2004.
33. Harrison M, Thomas M: Antibiotics after puncture wound to the foot, *Emerg Med J* 19:49, 2002.
34. Schwab RA, Powers RD: Conservative therapy of plantar puncture wounds, *J Emerg Med* 13:291–295, 1995.
35. Joseph WF, LeFrock JL: Infections complicating puncture wounds of the foot, *J Foot Surg* 26:S30–S33, 1987.
36. Jarvis JG, Skipper J: *Pseudomonas* osteochondritis complicating puncture wounds in children, *J Pediatr Orthop* 14:755–759, 1994.
37. Baldwin G, Colbourne M: Puncture wounds, *Pediatr Rev* 20:21–23, 1999.
38. Doser C, Cooper WL, Ediger WM, et al: Fishhook injuries: a prospective evaluation, *Am J Emerg Med* 9:413–415, 1991.
39. Kuperman-Beade M, Levine VJ, Ashinoff R: Laser removal of tattoos, *Am J Clin Dermatol* 2:21–25, 2001.
40. Jeray KJ, Banks DM, Phieffer LS, et al: Evaluation of standard surgical preparations performed on superficial dermal abrasions, *J Orthop Trauma* 14:206–211, 2000.
41. Bose B, Tredget T: Treatment of hot tar burns, *Can Med Assoc J* 127:21–22, 1982.
42. Demling R, Buerstatte W, Perea A: Management of hot tar burns, *J Trauma* 20:242, 1980.
43. Hinman C, Maibach H: Effect of air exposure and occlusion on experimental human skin wounds, *Nature* 200:377–378, 1963.
44. Beam JW: Occlusive dressings and healing of standardized abrasions, *J Athlet Training* 43:600–607, 2008.
45. Geronemus R, Mertz P, Eaglstein W: Wound healing: the effects of topical antimicrobial agents, *Arch Dermatol* 115:1311–1314, 1979.
46. Eaglstein WH, Sullivan TP, Giordano PA, et al: A liquid bandage for the treatment of minor cuts and abrasions, *Dermatol Surg* 28:262–267, 2002.
47. Quinn J, Lowe L, Mertz M: The effect of new tissue-adhesive wound dressing on the healing of traumatic abrasions, *Dermatology* 201:343–346, 2000.

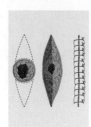

CHAPTER 17
Minor Thermal Burns

Key Practice Points

- The first responsibility of a clinician when evaluating a burn patient is to ensure that there is no airway involvement, inhalation injury, associated trauma, constricting burn, or large burn with potential fluid loss.
- The first treatment step of a minor burn is to cover it with a cool (not cold) wet cloth to stop continued thermal injury and to relieve pain.
- Splash or scalding burns (water or grease) result in superficial injury. Immersion burns (hot liquid or flame) often cause deep tissue injury.
- Signs of inhalation injury include cough, shortness of breath, singed nasal hair, and soot in the mouth or nasal passages.
- The extent of burn is measured by the total area of second-degree and third-degree burns. First-degree burns do not count in that determination.
- Patients with second-degree burns covering <15% of the body surface area can be treated as outpatients.
- Intact blisters act as good burn dressings and do not always need to be removed.
- Burn dressings should be nonadherent so that delicate epidermal and dermal cells will not be torn off during dressing changes.
- Burned patients are at risk for tetanus, and patients' inoculations should be up to date, or patients should receive boosters at the time of treatment.
- There is no evidence that prophylactic oral antibiotics are necessary for minor burns treated on an outpatient basis.

The treatment of burns is a common activity for personnel in facilities that care for emergency wounds and injuries. A thorough understanding of the treatment requirements of burns is necessary for proper selection of patients who can be managed appropriately on an outpatient basis and for selection of patients who need referral for specialized care. The depth, type, and extent of the burn; the anatomic location; and the underlying patient condition all are important factors in making the treatment decision. Although individual treatment aspects of minor burns remain controversial, basic management principles do not vary greatly. The three main principles for treating burn patients are (1) relief of pain, (2) prevention of additional infection and trauma, and (3) minimization of scarring and contracture.[1]

INITIAL MANAGEMENT AND PATIENT ASSESSMENT

No matter how small or how trivial a burn appears, the patient must be assessed for more severe associated problems and injuries. If the patient sustained the burn at the scene of a fire or explosion, immediate evaluation for inhalational injury, carbon monoxide exposure, cyanide exposure, and other trauma is mandatory.[2] Inhalational injury is the most common cause of mortality in fire victims.[3] Clinical signs of inhalational injury include burned nasal hairs, soot on the face, hoarseness, coughing, shortness of breath, and wheezing. Even if these signs are not present at the outset, an inhalational injury must be suspected in patients who were trapped in an enclosed, smoke-filled space. Respiratory tract injury often is delayed, and observation of the patient for 24 hours may be indicated.[4] Carbon monoxide exposure is suspected in any patient who is alert and has a headache or in a patient with confusion or other alteration of mental status.

When the patient has been initially stabilized, when vital signs have been taken, and when unnecessary articles of clothing have been removed from the burned area, attention can be turned to the burn itself. The most salient clinical symptom of minor burns is pain. Epidermal (first-degree) and superficial partial-thickness (superficial second-degree) burns can be extremely painful and require immediate pain relief. The simplest and most rapid manner in which to abolish burn pain is to place moist, cool towels over the burned area.[5] Clinical and experimental evidence shows that the cooling of burned surfaces can decrease the eventual damage to burned tissues.[6-9] The water should not be very cold because excessive cold can compound the burn injury. A water temperature of 8°C (45°F) to 23°C (75°F) seems to be optimal to obtain pain relief and some measure of protection for burned tissue.[7]

Cooling can be effective for 3 hours postburn.[7,10] In a study of children with burns, it was found that only 22% received adequate first aid, including cooling.[11] Immediately on arrival at the care facility, cooling should be initiated to abort the continuing tissue injury. Care must be taken to ensure that large burn areas are not covered with cool, moist towels for excessive periods, because hypothermia can set in. In addition to cool towels and sponges, parenteral pain medicine, such as morphine sulfate or meperidine, can be used, especially for patients who have a significant component of anxiety associated with their burns.

While the patient is being stabilized and pain relief is being administered, a thorough history is taken. Important items in the history include the age of the patient, any associated conditions and illnesses, psychosocial considerations, and drug allergies. Patients younger than 2 years old have thin dermis and immature immune systems.[12,13] These children rarely are treated on an outpatient basis. Likewise, patients older than 65 years tolerate burns poorly and often need inpatient care. Patients with underlying diseases, such as diabetes, pulmonary disease, severe cardiac problems, and disorders requiring long-term immunosuppressive therapy, are at higher risk for additional complications with burns, and these patients require special consideration from hospital management.

Frequently, burn victims have significant psychosocial problems. Similar to automobile trauma victims, burn victims often have alcohol-related or drug-related disorders. Although these impairments may have nothing to do with the treatment of the burn itself, severe alcohol or drug dependency may preclude outpatient management, even for minor burns. The worst psychosocial problem associated with burns is child abuse. Experienced burn care personnel see this catastrophe frequently and tend to think of all children with burns as potential victims of child abuse until proved otherwise. Finally, during the history, a thorough detailing of allergies is necessary, because many drugs may be administered or applied to a burn victim during the course of his or her management.

BURN ASSESSMENT

Cause of the Burn

Knowing the cause of a burn can make a difference in predicting its depth and extent. Brief scalding burns, which occur with the spilling or splashing of hot water, usually result in epidermal or superficial partial-thickness burns. Burns caused by immersion in a hot liquid or contact with a flame more frequently result in deep partial-thickness or full-thickness burns. These burns can be complicated and serious, especially when important anatomic parts, such as the hands or face, are involved. Electrical burns almost always cause full-thickness injuries at the burn site. In addition, electrical injuries can be associated with muscle necrosis, fractures, and cardiac arrhythmias.[14]

Body Location

The anatomic location of a burn is an important factor in determining management. Because of the complexity and crucial function of the hands, extensive partial-thickness or full-thickness burns on the hands are best managed, at least at the outset, in a controlled setting. Not only do hand burns require careful cleansing, débridement, and dressing, but also there is a danger of joint stiffening secondary to the immobility caused by pain and edema. Patients must observe strict elevation of the burned extremity in addition to early motion exercises to prevent "freezing" of the hand. This freezing complication occurs more frequently in patients older than age 50. Partial-thickness burns of the face not only raise the possibility of airway obstruction and inhalational injury, but they also can be difficult to manage surgically.

Burns of the perineum are technically difficult to manage and are extremely uncomfortable for the patient. It is beyond the capabilities of most patients or families to care for these problems at home. Among the most frustrating burns to manage on an outpatient basis are burns of the foot. The dependent nature of this anatomic part and its weight-bearing function cause frequent failure of outpatient management. It is difficult for patients to maintain voluntarily the necessary strict elevation of the legs, and failure to elevate properly can lead to edema, pain, and tissue breakdown at the burn site.

Depth of the Burn

Burns traditionally are divided into four depths of tissue injury: epidermal (first-degree burns), partial-thickness (second-degree burns), full-thickness (third-degree burns), and deep thermal (fourth-degree burns) (Fig. 17-1). Partial-thickness, or second-degree, burns are subdivided further into superficial and deep partial-thickness burns.

- *Epidermal burns (first-degree):* These burns are the most common. Heat induces dermal vasodilation, giving the epidermis its characteristic red color. Blistering does not occur, and these burns heal without treatment. The superficial epidermis sloughs or peels about 5 to 7 days after the burn is sustained, and the vasodilation gradually disappears. Sunburn is the most common example of an epidermal burn. Occasionally, if the heat exposure was especially intense or prolonged, what appears to be an epidermal burn blisters and becomes a superficial partial-thickness burn after 12 to 24 hours.
- *Superficial partial-thickness burns (second-degree):* These burns are so designated because the epidermis and part of the dermis are injured. Superficial partial-thickness burns classically blister and are extremely painful. When the necrotic epidermis is removed,

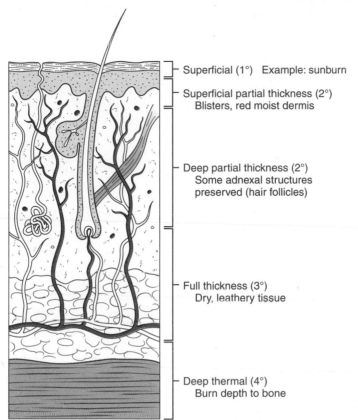

Figure 17-1. Cross section of skin with illustration of different burn depths, including superficial (1°) to deep thermal (4°).

the injured dermis is homogeneously pink and moist in appearance. It is extremely sensitive to touch but heals without scarring over 2 to 3 weeks. The dermis and dermal appendages, such as pilosebaceous units and eccrine sweat glands, survive and give the skin a chance to regenerate epidermis.

- *Deep partial-thickness burns (second-degree):* Clinically, it is important to distinguish between superficial and deep partial-thickness burns. There are important differences in the time they require to heal and in eventual cosmetic appearance. Deep partial-thickness burns are not as painful to touch, and they appear drier and whiter when débrided. Sometimes the surface of these burns is interspersed with reddish spots, indicating underlying dermal appendages such as sweat glands and hair follicles. There still is some awareness of pinprick, however, and some of the dermal appendages are preserved. New skin can grow from these appendages, but some need supplemental grafts. These burns take longer than 3 weeks to heal.
- *Full-thickness burns (third-degree):* With full-thickness, or third-degree, burns, the dermis and the dermal appendages are totally destroyed. A dry, taut, leather-like surface that is insensitive to examination or pinprick characterizes the appearance of these burn injuries. The color of these burned areas can vary from white to brown to black. There is frequent difficulty in distinguishing between deep partial-thickness

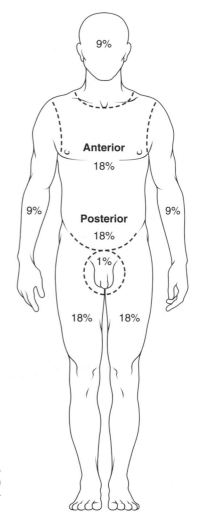

Figure 17-2. Rapid estimation of burn extent can be determined by the rule of nines. Only partial-thickness (second-degree) and full-thickness (third-degree) burns are considered for percentage area determination.

and full-thickness burns on initial presentation of a patient to a wound care facility. Often these two types of burns are treated in the same manner and require grafting for final coverage of the damaged area.

- *Deep thermal burns (fourth-degree):* All soft tissue is burned away in these burns, leaving exposed bone.

Extent of the Burn

Proper estimation of the extent of body surface area affected is crucial to burn management. Only partial-thickness (second-degree) and full-thickness (third-degree) injuries are considered in the calculation. The "rule of nines" is adequate for initially estimating burn size in adults (Fig. 17-2). Surface anatomy can be divided into areas that represent 9% or multiples of 9% of the body surface. The head and each arm constitute a 9% surface area apiece, whereas one leg is 18%. The entire surface area of the thorax and abdomen combined, anterior and posterior, is 36%.

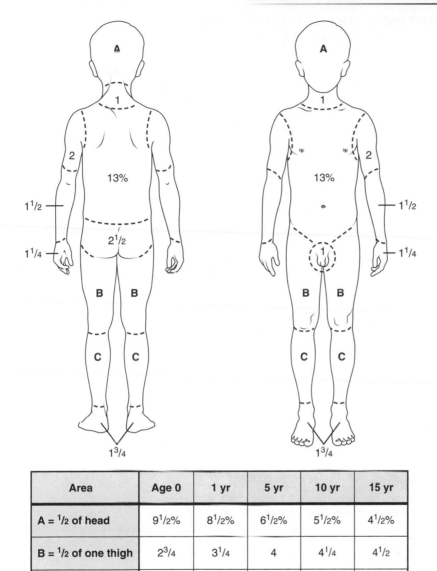

Area	Age 0	1 yr	5 yr	10 yr	15 yr
A = $^1/_2$ of head	$9^1/_2$%	$8^1/_2$%	$6^1/_2$%	$5^1/_2$%	$4^1/_2$%
B = $^1/_2$ of one thigh	$2^3/_4$	$3^1/_4$	4	$4^1/_4$	$4^1/_2$
C = $^1/_2$ of one leg	$2^1/_2$	$2^1/_2$	$2^3/_4$	3	$3^1/_4$

Figure 17-3. Estimation of burn size in children. The relative area sizes change significantly with age.

Greater precision in estimating burn size can be obtained by using standard, more detailed charts that subdivide the anatomic parts. These diagrams also take into account the variations in surface area that occur with age (Fig. 17-3). In young children, the surface area of the head constitutes a much greater area relative to the rest of the body than it does in adults. As an individual grows, the lower extremities become proportionately larger, whereas the trunk and arm proportions stay relatively the same throughout life. Final surface area proportions are not reached until after age 15.

GUIDELINES FOR HOSPITALIZATION AND OUTPATIENT MANAGEMENT

Box 17-1 lists suggested criteria for hospital management of burns. Patients not meeting these criteria can be considered victims of minor, partial-thickness burns and can be treated as outpatients. Opinions of different authorities vary on what constitutes an appropriate burn size that can be treated without having to admit the patient to a hospital. The total extent of burn limit for outpatient management varies from 10% to 15% of the area that has sustained a superficial burn.[6,13,15] Superficial partial-thickness burns can vary from 3% to 5%, and full-thickness can vary from 1% to 3%. Highly motivated, responsible adults with good support systems are likely to do well on an outpatient basis with burns approaching the more extensive ranges.

Children are managed best on an inpatient basis with any partial-thickness burn that is greater than 10%. Pain relief, wound cleansing, débridement, and dressings are easier to manage in the hands of experienced personnel. After the parents recover from the trauma, they can be educated properly in the care of the burn before the child is discharged. Except for the most trivial burn, children younger than 2 years should be managed in the hospital. On the other end of the age scale, it is recommended that patients older than age 65 be considered for similar treatment.

As previously discussed, burns in crucial anatomic locations, such as the hands, feet, face, and perineum, are managed best in an inpatient setting. Full-thickness burns of greater than 3% of the body surface area require surgical management and grafting. Even smaller full-thickness burns, if initially treated outside the hospital, need to be referred to a specialist for continued management and possible later skin grafting.

If there is any suspicion of inhalational or airway injury, no matter how small or superficial the burn, the patient must be admitted for observation. Inhalational injury can be insidious, and overt signs and symptoms often do not appear for several hours postexposure.[4] Finally, the decision to treat patients in the hospital often is determined by the extent of underlying disease, alcohol or drug abuse, and suspicion of potential child abuse.

TREATMENT OF MINOR BURNS

Most burns that are treated on an outpatient basis are epidermal or superficial partial-thickness burns. Because these burns tend to have an overwhelmingly favorable outcome regardless of treatment, some of the controversies over management are not crucial. For the sake of completeness, however, these controversies are mentioned in context with each management step.

BOX 17-1	**Guidelines for Hospital Admission of Burn Victims**

1. Partial-thickness burns >15% surface area (>10% surface area of child)
2. Full-thickness burns >3% surface area
3. Suspected inhalational injury
4. Age <2 or >65 years
5. Partial-thickness or full-thickness burns of hands, face, perineum, or feet
6. Electrical burns
7. Severe underlying systemic disease
8. Acute alcohol or drug abuse
9. Suspected child abuse

Epidermal Burns (First-Degree)

Epidermal, or first-degree, burns usually are called to the attention of medical care personnel only if the burns are extensive or extremely painful. A gentle cleansing with a nonirritating soap, such as Ivory Flakes or Dreft, mixed in a solution of cool saline is recommended. Diluted (with 2 to 4 parts cool saline) chlorhexidine (Hibiclens) also can be used.[1] For symptom relief at home, the patient can apply many commercial preparations containing at least 60% aloe vera. Not only does aloe vera have some antimicrobial activity, it also provides local pain relief.[12,13] Analgesia can be supplemented with aspirin, ibuprofen, acetaminophen, or codeine for 48 to 72 hours, after which the acute pain eventually subsides.

Epidermal burns usually heal within 5 to 7 days after going through epidermal desquamation. Occasionally, epidermal burns convert to superficial-thickness injuries, with blistering 12 to 24 hours after heat exposure. If this conversion occurs, the patient should return to a medical care facility or contact the primary care physician.

Superficial Partial-Thickness Burns (Superficial Second-Degree)

Cleansing

Partial-thickness burns also are managed best by an initial cleansing with a nonirritating soap (e.g., Dreft) or with chlorhexidine (Hibiclens) diluted in 2 to 4 parts of cool saline. Ice chips can be mixed into the solution to provide a cooling effect. Hair can be clipped but should not be shaved with a razor in the burn site in order to prevent any further damage to the remaining dermal appendages from which new epidermis arises.[16] To clean and débride effectively a partial-thickness burn, which is extremely sensitive to touch or manipulation, a parenteral narcotic often is recommended for the patient.

Blisters and Débridement

When cleansing has taken place, the next step is débridement (Fig. 17-4). Necrotic and partially sloughed epidermis and dermis are removed using forceps and tissue scissors. This skin is dead and insensitive; therefore local anesthetics are not required. The dead tissue is incised with scissors at the edge of viable epidermis, taking care not to cut into sensitive intact skin. A controversy in burn management is whether to remove intact blisters. Proponents for blister removal point to the ideal culture media that blister fluid represents with a concomitant risk of burn infection.[13] There is clinical and experimental evidence, however, that leaving blisters intact has several beneficial effects on burn wounds.[17-19] Intact blisters tend to prevent capillary stasis and retard necrosis within burn injury sites and decrease desiccation of the burn wound. It also is believed that the retention of blisters aids in the control of pain, a benefit that is especially important over joint surfaces, where pain can limit active movement, leading to potential joint stiffness.[20] As a general rule, large confluent blisters are likely to break easily and should be removed. Small intact blisters on the hands, feet, and over joints, should be left intact. It can be argued that blisters on noncompliant patients should be removed to prevent infection from neglect or improper home care.

Burn Dressing

Preferences for burn dressing vary widely among practitioners. Topical treatments range from no agent at all to a variety of topical antibiotics and several newer synthetic wound coverings. Because the eventual outcome of limited superficial partial-thickness burns is uniformly good, there is no clear preference for one agent or dressing over another.

Uncomplicated partial-thickness burns of the head and neck, for practical reasons, are best left open during treatment. Gentle cleansing one to two times daily, followed

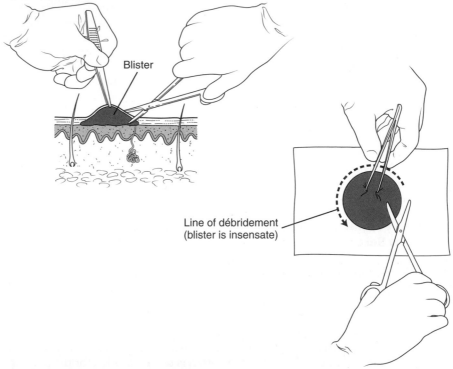

Figure 17-4. Blister debridement *(side view):* Hold dead blister skin with forceps and *(top view)* trim dead skin away at border of intact skin.

by the application of an antibacterial ointment such as bacitracin or Polysporin, leads to complete healing in 2 to 3 weeks.

Most other partial-thickness and full-thickness burns are treated with burn dressings (Fig. 17-5).[21] After cleansing and débridement, the burned area is covered with an antibacterial ointment with a gloved finger or sterile applicator. Petroleum-based ointments, such as bacitracin or polymyxin B sulfate/bacitracin (Polysporin), are preferred for ease of application, enhanced wound healing, and good suppression of bacterial colonization.[13] Ointment is followed by a single layer of fine-mesh gauze or a nonadherent material, such as Adaptic. A nonadherent base is important to protect fragile epidermal and dermal cells during dressing changes. Gauze "fluffs," created by the unfolding of gauze 4 × 4 sponges, are packed over the fine-mesh gauze layer. The fluffs absorb copious drainage created by the fresh wound. The dressing is anchored with a gauze bandage roll and tape strips.

Silver sulfadiazine (Silvadene) is the most commonly used burn product, but it is impractical for open treatment and can form a pseudomembrane over partial-thickness burns that is difficult and painful to remove. It cannot be used in patients with sensitivity to other sulfa drugs, and transient leukopenia has been reported with this agent.[22] Silver sulfadiazine has a long record of effectiveness in large burns but has been challenged as the agent of choice for minor burns.[23] In a large literature review, there was not enough evidence to support or refute the use of silver sulfadiazine as a treatment for minor, ambulatory burns.[24] At the burn center at the University of Cincinnati, petrolatum-based antibacterial agents are preferred over silver sulfadiazine for the treatment of minor burns.

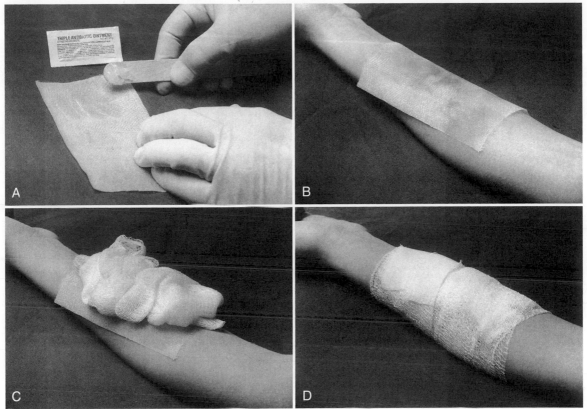

Figure 17-5. Burn dressing application. **A,** Petroleum-based antibiotic ointment is applied to fine mesh gauze. **B,** The impregnated gauze is placed over burn area. **C,** Gauze "fluffs" made from sponges are added to the base to absorb burn wound exudate. **D,** The dressing is completed with a gauze bandage wrap and strips of adhesive tape.

The interval between dressing changes varies among practitioners. Many burn authorities recommend twice-daily changes to maintain the effectiveness of the antibacterial ointment or cream. In practicality, once-daily changes are probably sufficient for limited partial-thickness burns. Patients are sent home with specific instructions and burn supplies as listed. The follow-up interval varies based on the compliance and motivation of the patient and the extent and location of the burn. Burns of the hand need close follow-up with a visit to a caregiver within 48 to 72 hours of the injury. Further visits are individualized.

Synthetic dressings offer another alternative for patients with limited partial-thickness burns. Many products are on the market, including DuoDerm, Opsite, Vigilon, and Biobrane. These dressings can be applied to fresh burns that have been cleaned and débrided of dead skin and any debris.[25] The dressing is cut in a customized manner to correspond to the burn site with approximately a 1-cm to 2-cm marginal overlap. An outer gauze wrap is applied to maintain dressing adherence and to absorb excessive exudate. These dressings afford good pain relief and can be left on for the duration of the healing. The dressings are time-consuming and difficult to apply, however. They can dry, crack, and peel at the edges.[26] These dressings are not suitable for covering joints or large areas. Use of these dressings should be in consultation and agreement with the caregiver responsible for follow-up and ongoing care when the patient leaves the emergency department.

Home Management and Follow-up

Burn supplies, including gauze sponges, gauze wrap, antibacterial soap, and a sterile tongue depressor, are dispensed or prescribed along with written and verbal instructions on how to use them. A small jar or tube of topical antimicrobial agent also is dispensed or prescribed. The patient is instructed to remove the first dressing the morning after his or her first wound care visit. The burned area is washed gently with the soap and two or three of the sterile sponges that have been provided. A topical agent is spread over the wound, and gauze wrapping is applied. Some authorities believe that the first dressing can remain in place for 2 or 3 days. At the University of Cincinnati burn center, it is believed that once- or twice-a-day changes prevent the exudate buildup and crusting that can disrupt epithelialization when infrequent dressing changes are made. There is no clear evidence to support any specific dressing change interval for minor burns.

All minor burn victims are seen in follow-up 48 hours after initial treatment. From that time on, individualized treatment regimens are prescribed. Strict elevation of the burned part is essential to proper healing. The use of slings for upper extremity and hand burns can accomplish this goal while the patient is in an upright position. Gentle but frequent motion of joints within the burn-injured anatomic parts also is mandatory. Pain often deters a patient from this activity, so appropriate oral medication, such as aspirin, ibuprofen, acetaminophen, or codeine, may be required early during convalescence. Usually, however, if the patient thoroughly understands the need for joint motion, cooperation with burn care personnel quickly follows despite some wound discomfort.

Deep Partial-Thickness and Full-Thickness Burns

Full-thickness burns that cover less than 3% of the body surface area and that are in a noncritical site (hand or face) can be treated in the manner described previously for partial-thickness burns. Before proceeding, however, it is best to discuss the case with a consultant. These patients require close follow-up care, and initial treatment decisions are best made in concert with a consultant.

Tetanus and Antibiotic Prophylaxis

Finally, tetanus prophylaxis and the possibility of wound infection need to be considered. Tetanus toxoid and tetanus immune globulin should be given to all burn patients in accordance with the recommendations in Chapter 21. Currently, no studies support the use of prophylactic oral or parenteral antibiotics in minor superficial burns.[18,27,28] Control and antibiotic-treated groups consistently yield the same infection rate of approximately 3% to 4%. Should a burn wound infection develop, it is best managed with local wound care and appropriate antibiotics at that time.[29]

References

1. Baxter CR, Waeckerle JF: Emergency treatment of burn injury, *Ann Emerg Med* 17:1305–1315, 1988.
2. Lawson-Smith P, Jansen EC, Hyldegaard O: Effect of hyperbaric oxygen therapy on whole blood cyanide concentrations in carbon monoxide intoxicated patients from fire accidents, *Scand J Trauma Resusc Emerg Med* 18:32, 2010.
3. Trunkey D: Inhalation injury, *Surg Clin North Am* 58:1133–1140, 1978.
4. Achauer B, Allyn PA, Furnas DW, Bartlett RH: Pulmonary complications of burns, *Ann Surg* 177: 311–319, 1973.
5. Gruber RP, Laub DR, Vistness LM: The effect of hydrotherapy on the clinical course and pH of experimental cutaneous chemical burns, *Plast Reconstr Surg* 55:200–203, 1975.

6. Cone JB: Minor burns: standards for outpatient treatment, *Consultant* 27:37–42, 1987.

7. Davies J: Prompt cooling of burned areas: a review of benefits and the effector mechanisms, *Burns* 9:1–6, 1983.

8. Pushkar N, Sandorminsky B: Cold treatment of burns, *Burns* 9:101–110, 1983.

9. Saranto J, Rubayi S, Zawacki B: Blisters, cooling, antithromboxanes, and healing in experimental zone-of-stasis burns, *J Trauma* 23:927–933, 1983.

10. Raine TJ, Heggers JR, Robson M, et al: Cooling the burned wound to maintain microcirculation, *J Trauma* 21:394–397, 1981.

11. McCormack RA, La Hei ER, Martin HCO: First-aid management of minor burns in children: a prospective study of children presenting to the Children's Hospital at Westmead, Sydney, *Med J Aust* 178:31–33, 2003.

12. Griglak MJ: Thermal injury, *Emerg Clin North Am* 10:369–383, 1992.

13. Heimbach D, Engrav L, Marvin J: Minor burns, *Postgrad Med* 69:22–32, 1981.

14. Sances A Jr, Larson SJ, Myklebust J, Cusick JF: Electrical injuries, *Surg Gynecol Obstet* 149:97–108, 1979.

15. Hudsith J, Rayatt S: First aid and treatment of minor burns, *BMJ* 328:1487–1489, 2004.

16. Shuck J: Outpatient management of the burned patient, *Surg Clin North Am* 58:108–117, 1978.

17. Moserova J, Runtova M, Broz L: The possible role of blisters in dermal burns, *Acta Chir Plast* 25:51–53, 1983.

18. Moylan J: Outpatient treatment of burns, *Postgrad Med* 73:235–242, 1983.

19. Zawacki B: Reversal of capillary stasis and prevention of necrosis in burns, *Ann Surg* 180:98–102, 1974.

20. Swain AH, Azadian BS, Wakeley C, Shakespeare PG: Management of blisters in burns, *BMJ* 295:181, 1987.

21. Greenhalgh DG: Topical antimicrobial agents for burn wounds, *Clin Plast Surg* 36:569–606, 2009.

22. Subrahmanyam M: A prospective randomized clinical and histological study of superficial burn wound healing with honey and silver sulfadiazene, *Burns* 24:157–161, 1998.

23. Chung YJ, Herbert ME: Myth: silver sulfadiazine is the best treatment for minor burns, *West J Med* 175:205–206, 2001.

24. Miller AC, Rashid RM, Falzon L, et al: Silver sulfadiazine for the treatment of partial-thickness burns and venous stasis ulcers, *Am Acad Dermatol* 10:e1–e7, 2010.

25. Curreri PW, Desai MH, Bartlett RH, et al: Safety and efficacy of a new synthetic burn dressing, *Arch Surg* 115:925–927, 1980.

26. Warren R, Snelling C: Clinical evaluation of the Hydron gel burn dressing, *Plast Reconstr Surg* 66:361–368, 1980.

27. Boss WK, Brand DA, Acampora D, et al: Effectiveness of prophylactic antibiotics in the outpatient treatment of burns, *J Trauma* 25:224–227, 1985.

28. Timmons M: Are systemic prophylactic antibiotics necessary for burns? *Ann R Coll Surg Engl* 65:80–81, 1983.

29. Richards R, Mahlangu G: Therapy for burn wound infection, *J Clin Hosp Pharm* 6:223–243, 1981.

CHAPTER 18
Cutaneous and Superficial Abscesses

Key Practice Points

- In recent years, there has been a threefold increase in superficial soft tissue infections (SSTI) including abscesses. The rise in community-acquired methicillin-resistant *Staphylococcus aureus* (CA-MRSA) is behind that increase.
- Abscesses can begin as solid nodules—furuncles—that suppurate and form a pus-filled mass. Abscesses are fluctuant and soft to palpation because of the pus-filled center.
- CA-MRSA is now found in 50% to 80% of abscesses.
- Breast abscesses can be complicated because of the involvement of the occluded periareolar ducts, and they might require consultation for treatment.
- Bartholin's gland abscesses can be associated with sexually transmitted diseases that need to be treated at the time of drainage.
- Buttock abscesses can be drained by emergency caregivers. Perianal and perirectal abscesses are best managed by consultants.
- The decision to drain an abscess requires the presence of pus. If there is doubt, needle aspiration or ultrasound examination can resolve the issue.
- When pus is not present, the patient is treated with antibiotics that include coverage for CA-MRSA. Treatment continues until the lesion heals or becomes an abscess.
- The most common mistake in abscess drainage is making the incision too small. It should be at least two thirds of the size of the abscess cavity.
- Whereas simple abscesses caused by CA-MRSA will heal with drainage alone, the role of antibiotics has not been completely defined. Coverage is recommended for those with risk factors, which include associated cellulitis, immunosuppression, fever, and so forth.
- After initial incision and drainage, the patient returns in 2 to 3 days for packing removal and reevaluation.
- Uncomplicated, properly drained abscesses, including those caused by CA-MRSA, resolve without antibiotics. Antibiotics are recommended for abscesses with surrounding cellulitis, toxicity, diabetes, immuno-compromise, location on the face, and cardiac valve disease.

Cutaneous and other superficial abscesses commonly are diagnosed and treated in emergency departments (EDs). From 1993 to 2005 there was a threefold increase in superficial soft tissue infections (SSTI) presenting to EDs.[1] The increase is largely due to the emergence of community-acquired methicillin-resistant *Staphylococcus aureus* (CA-MRSA).[2] The majority of abscesses and other SSTIs that present to EDs are now due to CA-MRSA. In some EDs, the rate of CA-MRSA SSTIs exceeds 80%.[2] Although drainage is the key therapeutic intervention for all abscesses, significant differences between types and locations exist and necessitate individualized treatment. Most cases, including those caused by CA-MRSA, can be managed in the ED with routine outpatient follow-up care. A few cases require specialist consultation, however, for possible operative intervention or inpatient management.

CLINICAL PRESENTATIONS

Cutaneous Abscesses

A cutaneous abscess is defined as a "localized collection of pus causing a fluctuant soft tissue swelling surrounded by firm granulation tissue and erythema."[1] Abscesses can begin as furuncles, which are firm, red, tender solid nodules that can become abscesses if not treated with antibiotics. Cutaneous abscesses can occur on any body surface but tend to be more common in certain areas.[3] The most common sites are the head, neck, axillae, and buttock and perineal areas. Carbuncles are deep abscesses, with multiple loculations, that occur at the nape of the neck, chin, back, and thighs.

Any interruption of the protective layers of the skin, even trivial, with subsequent invasion of exogenous or endogenous microflora, can lead to abscess formation. Abscesses can also be the result of an obstruction of the apocrine and sebaceous glands. Sebaceous glands are widely distributed over the body, and apocrine glands are found most commonly in axillae and anogenital regions. These glands frequently form cysts that are prone to abscess formation. CA-MRSA now makes up the majority of soft tissue abscesses, up to 80% depending on the local microbiology.[2] Other organisms include methicillin-sensitive *S. aureus* (MSSA), *Proteus mirabilis*, and group A streptococci. It is important to know what the local sensitivities to antibiotics are so that appropriate antibiotics can be selected.

Abscesses caused by CA-MRSA can be characterized by an abscess-like lesion but with a central black eschar. Satellite lesions can also occur. Certain populations are at higher risk for CA-MRSA. They are children, athletes, those who have contact with a CA-MRSA patient, urban underserved individuals, incarcerated people, the military, those with HIV, men who have sex with men, and animal handlers.[2] Studies have shown that simple abscesses without surrounding cellulitis or other complicating factors can be treated with incision and drainage alone.[4] However, the role of antibiotics has yet to be completely defined.[5]

Of special note are abscesses that arise on the upper lip and nose. Infections in these sites drain through the facial and angular emissary veins to the cavernous sinus. As discussed in the following section, antibiotics are indicated in the treatment of these lesions.

Hidradenitis Suppurativa

A common and difficult condition to manage that predisposes to abscess formation is hidradenitis suppurativa, which is a chronic, relapsing, inflammatory involvement of apocrine glands of the axillae and pubic regions.[6] Abscess formation is followed by extensive, excessive scarring. The microbiology of these infections is complex. Coagulase-negative *Staphylococcus* and *S. aureus* are the most common organisms.[7] The rate of CA-MRSA has yet to be determined but is highly likely to be causal in some abscesses.

Anaerobes are also present. Recurrent abscess formation also predisposes to fistula tracks, skin and subcutaneous induration, and inflammation in various stages of progression. Emergency management is limited to incision and drainage of the discrete abscesses. These patients require long-term care and a program of management best coordinated and administered by specialists (e.g., dermatologists or surgeons). A strong relationship between hidradenitis and smoking has been found, and patients should be strongly encouraged to stop smoking.[7]

Breast Abscesses

Although breast abscesses commonly are associated with the postpartum period, more than 90% occur outside of that period.[8] Postpartum mastitis, which can occur in nursing mothers 2 to 6 weeks after delivery, predisposes to abscess formation. Mastitis is caused by an invasion of *S. aureus* through sore, abraded nipples. Like other SSTIs, postpartum infections are increasingly a result of CA-MRSA.[9] Other organisms are MSSA, anaerobes, and mixed flora. These patients are often quite sick from extensive local involvement, pain, chills, and fever. Initial treatment of mastitis without abscess includes ice packs, breast support, analgesics, and antistaphylococus antibiotics. Breast feeding can continue and is beneficial.

Nonpuerperal abscesses can occur in superficial and deep tissues of the breast. Superficial abscesses can be cutaneous or periareolar. Periareolar abscesses, the most common breast abscess, arise from occluded ducts and are associated with the multiple organisms listed previously. These abscesses involve mammary and ductal tissue.

Deep breast abscesses are either intramammary or retromammary. As is the case for periareolar abscesses, fluctuance can be difficult to detect. Fluctuance also is difficult to diagnose when overlying cellulitis is deep and extensive. In these cases, needle aspiration or ultrasound may be required to ensure the proper treatment (i.e., incision and drainage). Because of the complexity of breast abscesses, and the frequent involvement of ductal tissue, consultation should be considered.

Bartholin's Gland Abscesses

Bartholin's glands, located in the posterior portion of the vestibule of the vagina, can form cysts from ductal occlusion. These cysts can go on to form abscesses. In addition to the abscess, the labium usually is inflamed and tender. Studies have cultured a wide range of organisms from these abscesses. These include *Neisseria, Chlamydia,* gram positives, gram negatives, and anaerobes. The most recent study, however, did not show any primary sexually transmitted disease (STD) organisms.[10] Despite that fact, it is still considered necessary to culture the cervix for those organisms or to treat for them empirically.

Pilonidal Abscesses

A common abscess presenting to EDs can arise from the sacrococcygeal pilonidal sinus in the midline of the superior buttock divide at the base of the coccyx.[11] Patients often present with painful induration of the buttock crease. Fluctuance may not be appreciated; needle aspiration or ultrasound is sometimes necessary to diagnose purulence. Cultures reveal gram-negative enteric organisms and anaerobes. These abscesses often recur unless the sinuses are excised after initial drainage.

Buttock and Perianal Abscesses

Buttock abscesses are common but must be clinically distinguished from perianal and perirectal infections (Fig. 18-1). Buttock abscesses occur cutaneously and do not involve the anus. They can be incised and drained by an emergency caregiver. Perianal abscesses

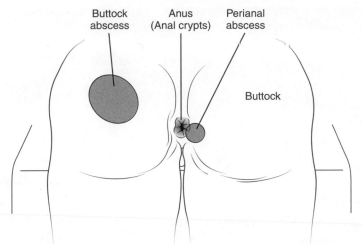

Figure 18-1. View of buttocks and anus. A buttock abscess is located away from anus. Perianal abscesses involve the anal crypts and anus.

arise from anal crypts and impinge on the anal sphincter. A consultant surgeon is usually involved in the care of these patients. In contrast to patients with buttock abscesses, rectal examination is painful for patients with perianal abscesses. Perianal abscesses often are associated with fistula in ano. The presence of a perianal abscess also might point to other serious, related abscesses and infections of the ischiorectal, intersphincteric, and pelvirectal areas. Patients with these deeper abscesses complain of deep rectal or pelvic pain. They often have fever and appear toxic, as manifested by diaphoresis and tachycardia. A rectal examination reveals marked tenderness of the anal sphincter and rectum. Masses can be palpated with the examining finger. This condition requires urgent intervention by a consultant in an operative setting. Until recently, the predominant organisms cultured from perirectal abscesses were gram negatives and anaerobes with some gram positives.[12] Common organisms include *Escherichia coli, Bacteroides,* and *Streptococcus* species. Recently, CA-MRSA has been cultured in up to 20% of cases.[13,14]

Parenteral Drug SSTI
A common problem seen by emergency physicians is abscess formation in parenteral drug users. Not only are the patients at risk for bacterial tissue invasion, but also chemical irritants can provoke intense and extensive involvement. These abscesses are often extensive and involve the thighs, buttocks, or forearms. Parenteral drug users have a high incidence of other infectious complications, such as hepatitis, endocarditis, and human immunodeficiency virus–related disorders. Local complications include soft tissue necrosis, intraarterial injection, septic arthritis, and osteomyelitis. Common organisms include streptococci, staphylococci (MSSA, MRSA), and anaerobes.[15] Caregivers are urged to observe strict blood and body fluid precautions when draining the patient's abscesses.

MANAGEMENT OF ABSCESSES
When confronted with a suspected abscess, palpation does not always reveal fluctuance. Abscesses on the back of the neck, sacrococcygeal area, buttocks, and thighs can be deep or accompanied by significant overlying tissue induration. Whenever an abscess is suspected but is clinically not evident, needle aspiration can be performed with an 18-G needle attached to a 5-mL or 10-mL syringe.

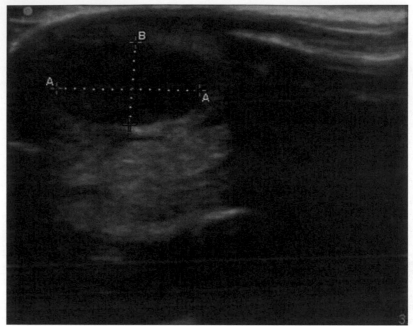

Figure 18-2. Abscess cavity as viewed by ultrasound.

With the emergence of ultrasound as a diagnostic tool in the ED, this technique can be used to diagnose pus accumulation in cases in which aspiration has failed, but the clinical setting is consistent with abscess formation[16] (Fig. 18-2). Ultrasound can guide needle aspiration to confirm the presence and location of the abscess cavity. Drainage is facilitated, and ultrasound can be used in follow-up to confirm resolution.

When pus is not aspirated, the inflammatory mass, or furuncle, has not suppurated. Attempts at incision and drainage are not indicated. In this setting, the patient is placed on antibiotics and twice-daily warm compresses or soaks. The furuncle either heals or goes on to form pus that requires drainage. The patient is advised of either possibility and is provided with appropriate follow-up, even if antibiotics are administered. Usually, within 48 to 72 hours, the furuncle "declares" itself (i.e., begins resolution or suppurates). For choice of antibiotics, see the section in the following text regarding antibiotic use.

In patients with cardiac valvular disease, prophylactic antibiotics as recommended by the American Heart Association should be administered before incision and drainage.[17] Antibiotic prophylaxis is also recommended in patients with implanted orthopedic or other medical devices. Cefazolin, 2 g intravenously, is recommended to be administered before the procedure. In β-lactam–allergic patients, 900 mg of clindamycin intravenously or 1 g of azithromycin intravenously is an appropriate choice.

Technique for Incision and Drainage

- When the presence of pus has been established, the abscess site is briefly cleaned with a wound cleansing solution, such as povidone-iodine or chlorhexidine. Wound cleansing of these obviously contaminated sites is performed to render the field clear of gross contaminants and to prevent extraneous microflora from contaminating any wound cultures should they be indicated.

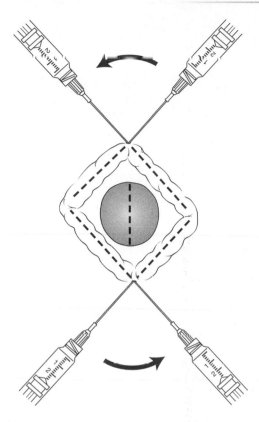

Figure 18-3. Field block approach to local anesthesia for abscess. Note: Wait 5 to 10 minutes following block for full anesthesia to occur.

- Incision and drainage manipulations are painful. For small abscesses (<5 cm in diameter), a field block followed by injection of the abscess roof often suffices for pain control (Fig. 18-3). Before administering the local block, parenteral narcotics can bring considerable relief to the patient. Intramuscular or intravenous morphine or hydromorphone allow the patient to be more comfortable for the local anesthetic, which can be very painful to the sensitive tissue surrounding an abscess. For larger abscesses or those in difficult areas such as the breast or the perineum, conscious sedation, as described in Chapter 6, is effective. If formal conscious sedation is not necessary or feasible, a parenteral dose of morphine, meperidine (Demerol), or hydromorphone (Dilaudid) can be given 15 to 30 minutes before the procedure.
- The instruments and items needed to drain an abscess include a knife handle and a no. 11 blade, a hemostat, gauze packing, and an irrigation syringe mated to a 16-G or 14-G plastic intravenous catheter. When the field of local anesthesia is created, an incision that is the full length of the fluctuance or, at minimum, two thirds of the diameter of the abscess cavity itself is made (Fig. 18-4). A common mistake is to make a small, stablike incision. Wide incisions are necessary to provide for adequate cavity probing and loculation disruption, irrigation, and packing placement.
- After the incision is made, the operator gently probes the abscess cavity with either a hemostat or a finger. When all of the abscess cavity surfaces have been explored and loculations have been broken up, irrigation with saline is performed through the catheter until all purulence is evacuated. Drainage is considered adequate when the saline effluent is free from pus and appears blood tinged.

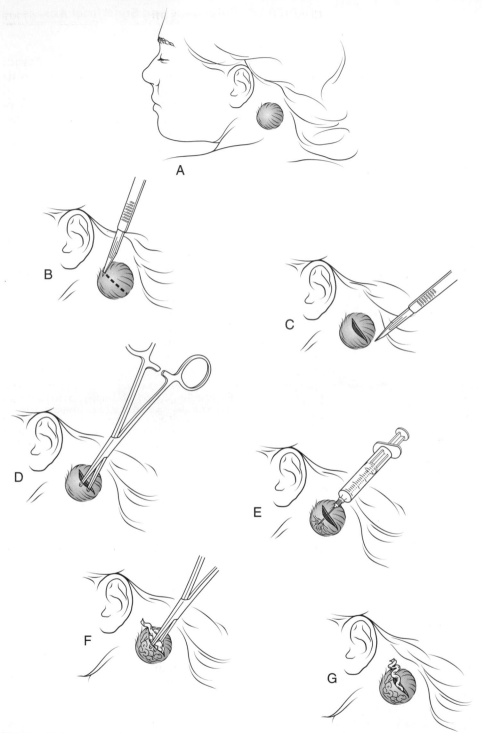

Figure 18-4. Procedure for abscess drainage. **A,** Typical cutaneous abscess. **B,** A scalpel with no. 11 blade is used to "lance" fluctuant mass. **C,** The incision should be generous and at least two thirds of the diameter of the cavity. **D,** A hemostat is used to probe the cavity and gently break up loculations. **E,** The cavity is irrigated until the effluent is clear of purulence. **F,** Gauze tape is used to pack the cavity. Caution is taken not to overpack and obstruct subsequent flow and drainage of remaining purulence. **G,** A 2- to 3-inch tail is left to prevent incision site closure and to aid in packing removal at a later time (2 to 3 days postprocedure).

- The next step in the procedure is to pack the abscess cavity gently and loosely with plain or medicated ribbon gauze. For small abscesses drained in the ED, ¼-inch-wide gauze strips are adequate. The purpose of the gauze packing is to promote continued drainage from the abscess cavity. Excessive packing of the cavity can create the opposite of the intended outcome. Packing at the incision opening can become encrusted with dried purulence, causing an iatrogenic obstruction to further drainage.
- A bulky dressing, with gauze sponges or layers, is placed over the site to absorb the inevitable continued purulent drainage. This dressing remains in place for 48 to 72 hours, at which time it is removed and the abscess is inspected.

Special Treatment Settings

Cutaneous abscesses caused by sebaceous cysts are drained in the manner described previously. These abscesses recur, however, as long as the cyst remains. After drainage, the abscess cavity should be allowed to heal completely. The cyst can be removed easily in its entirety when it is not inflamed. Attempts to remove the cyst at the time of abscess intervention are met only with failure. The cyst wall, at that time, is friable and easily tears. Even if a small fragment of the wall is left behind, a new cyst forms with the resultant return in risk for new abscess formation. After incision and drainage, patients should be referred for later cyst removal after all inflammation has subsided.

Because of the cosmetic concerns involved in the treatment of facial abscesses, if possible, drainage can be accomplished through the intraoral mucosal surface. When draining a facial abscess on the cutaneous surface, any incision has to conform to the tension lines as discussed in Chapter 3. Some facial abscesses may require consultation.

Uncomplicated superficial breast abscesses can be incised and drained as described previously. It is important, however, to make the skin incision in a radial orientation using the nipple as the "hub." Periareolar, intramammary, and deep breast abscesses can be difficult to drain and often are best drained under general anesthesia by a consultant in an operative setting.

The drainage of Bartholin's abscesses is achieved using a specially designed Word catheter[18] (Fig. 18-5). To avoid excessive bleeding during the procedure, the drainage incision is made on the medial wall of the abscess closest to the introitus. Incisions carried out laterally on the labial surface tend to bleed secondary to the vasodilation in that area caused by the inflammatory response to the infection. When the incision is made and irrigation is completed, the catheter is inserted and inflated. In contrast to other abscesses, the incision for Bartholin's abscesses is smaller so that the catheter, which has a narrow diameter, remains secure and does not fall out prematurely. Sitz baths can begin immediately for comfort and to encourage drainage. The catheter is left in for 4 to 6 weeks to allow epithelialization of the drainage track and to lessen the risk of recurrence.

Pilonidal abscesses are drained through generous incisions and are packed in the standard manner. These patients are referred for definitive treatment by a consultant, particularly if recurrence has become a problem. Buttock abscesses also are treated as described earlier. Caution is urged in attempting to drain a perianal abscess. These abscesses are exceedingly painful to manipulate and can indicate deeper involvement within the pelvirectal spaces. Consultation should be considered for these abscesses.

FOLLOW-UP CARE

Most small cutaneous abscesses treated in the ED require a single packing that stays in place 2 to 3 days. On the first return follow-up visit, the dressing and packing are removed. With successful drainage, the patient reports significant pain relief, and there is minimal continued drainage. For these patients, a regimen of daily wound soakings

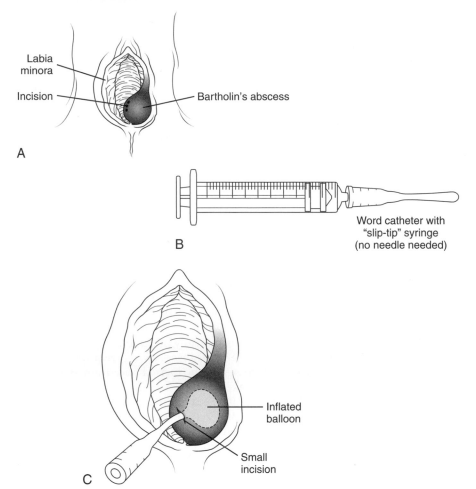

Figure 18-5. **A,** Location of Bartholin's abscess and medial location of incision. **B,** Example of Word catheter. **C,** Word catheter insertion with balloon inflated.

for 20 to 30 minutes for approximately 5 to 7 days suffices to maintain any further drainage until the abscess heals. Abscess cavities heal within 1 to 2 weeks. If the abscess is large and there is continued drainage, repacking can be performed at 2- to 3-day intervals as necessary. If the patient complains of unremitting pain and discomfort at the drainage site on the first return visit, an undrained cavity or loculation should be considered.

ANTIBIOTIC USE IN ABSCESS CARE

For common, uncomplicated cutaneous abscesses, incision and drainage is curative, including those caused by CA-MRSA.[2,19] Antibiotics offer no advantage in immunocompetent patients.[20-22] Under certain conditions, however, antibiotics are recommended, for example, when the abscess is surrounded by cellulitis that extends well beyond the margins, or when diabetes, immunosuppression, signs of toxicity (fever, tachycardia), or face and valvular disease are present. There is some recent data that indicate treatment of uncomplicated abscesses may not change the immediate outcome, but administration of antibiotics could lower the recurrence rate.[23] Because of the high incidence of CA-MRSA in abscesses, the choice of antibiotics should include coverage for that organism. Local sensitivities can vary and can affect that choice. If an initial intravenous antibiotic is considered necessary, vancomycin, daptomycin, linezolid, and tigecycline can be used. Oral therapy choices include TMP/SMX, doxycycline, clindamycin, and linezolid. At the University of Cincinnati, when empirical oral antibiotics are prescribed for a complicated abscess, TMP/SMX plus cephalexin or clindamycin is administered for 7 days. Linezolid alone can be used as well. The rationale is to ensure that coverage is effective against both CA-MRSA and MSSA.

References

1. Pallin D, Egan J, Pelletier A, et al: Increased US emergency department visits for skin and soft tissue infections, and changes in antibiotic choices, during the emergence of community-associated methicillin-resistant *Staphylococcus aureus, Ann Emerg Med* 51:291–298, 2008.
2. David MZ, Daum RS: Community-associated methicillin-resistant *Staphylococcus aureus*: epidemiology and clinical consequences of an emerging epidemic, *Clin Microbiol Rev* 23:616–687, 2010.
3. Meislin HW, Lerner SA, Graves MH, et al: Cutaneous abscesses: anaerobic and aerobic bacteriology and outpatient management, *Ann Intern Med* 87:145–149, 1977.
4. Rajendran PM, Young D, Maurer T: Randomized, double-blind, placebo-controlled trial of cephalexin for treatment of uncomplicated skin abscesses in a population at risk for community-acquired methicillin-resistant *Staphylococcus aureus* infection, *Antimicrob Agents Chemother* 51:4044–4048, 2007.
5. Liu C, Bayer A, Cosgrove SE, et al: Clinical practice guidelines by the Infectious Disease Society of America for the treatment of methicillin-resistant *Staphylococcus aureus* infections in adults and children: executive summary, *Clin Infect Dis* 52:285–292, 2011.
6. Paletta C, Jurkiewicz MJ: Hidradenitis suppurativa, *Clin Plast Surg* 14:383–390, 1987.
7. Slade DEM, Powell BW, Mortimer PS: Hidranitis suppurativa: pathogenesis and management, *Bri J Plast Surg* 56:451–461, 2003.
8. Scholefield JH, Duncan JL, Rogers K: Review of a hospital experience of breast abscesses, *Br J Surg* 74: 469–470, 1987.
9. Berens P, Swaim L, Peterson B: Incidence of methicillin-resistant *Staphylococcus aureus* in postpartum breast abscesses, *Breastfeed Med* 5:113–115, 2010.
10. Bhide A, Nama V, Patel S, et al: Microbiology of cysts/abscesses of Bartholin's gland: review of empirical antibiotic therapy against microbial culture, *J Obstet Gynecol* 30:701–703, 2010.
11. Khalil PN, Brand D, Siebeck M, et al: Aspiration and injection-based technique for incision and drainage of sacrococcygeal pilonidal abscess, *J Emer Med* 36:60–63, 2009.
12. Marcus RH, Stine RJ, Cohen MA: Perirectal abscess, *Ann Emer Med* 25:597–603, 1995.
13. Brown SR, Horton JD, Davis KG: Perirectal abscess infections related to MRSA: a prevalent and under-recognized pathogen, *J Surg Ed* 66:264–266, 2009.
14. Ulug M, Gedik E, Girgin S: The evaluation of bacteriology in perianal abscesses of 81 adult patients, *Braz J Infect Dis* 14:225–229, 2010.
15. Buckland A, Barton R, McCombe D: Upper limb morbidity as a direct consequence of intravenous drug abuse, *Hand Surg* 13:73–78, 2008.
16. Blaivas M: Ultrasound-guided breast abscess aspiration in a difficult case, *Acad Emerg Med* 8:398–401, 2001.
17. Sanford JP, Gilbert DN, Sande MA, editors: *Guide to antimicrobial therapy*, Dallas, 2010, Antimicrobial Therapy.
18. Word B: Office treatment of cysts and abscess of Bartholin's gland duct, *South Med J* 61:514–518, 1968.
19. Elston DM: Methicillin-sensitive and methicillin-resistant *Staphylococcus aureus*: management principles and selection of antibiotic therapy, *Dermatol Clin* 25:157–164, 2997.
20. Blick PWH, Flowers MW, Marsden AK, et al: Antibiotics in surgical treatment of acute abscesses, *BMJ* 28:111–112, 1980.
21. Llera JL, Levy RC: Treatment of cutaneous abscess: a double-blind clinical study, *Ann Emerg Med* 14: 15–19, 1985.
22. Macfie J, Harvey J: The treatment of acute superficial abscesses: a prospective clinical trial, *Br J Surg* 64:264–266, 1977.
23. Newland JG, Herigon JC: Antibiotics provide no additional benefit to surgical management of paediatric skin abscesses, *Evidence-Based Med* 15:138–139, 2010.

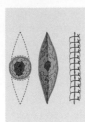

CHAPTER 19

Complicated, Chronic, and Aging Skin Wounds

Key Practice Points

- Deep cutaneous and necrotizing infections are often heralded by severe pain before skin signs appear.
- Microorganisms responsible for deep infections can include community-associated methicillin-resistant *Staphylococcus aureus* (CA-MRSA), group A *Streptococcus,* and clostridia, in addition to a variety of gram-positive, gram-negative, and anaerobic bacteria.
- Treatment of severe, deep necrotizing infection requires a combination of surgical débridement and broad-spectrum antibiotics.
- Sutured wounds have a low infection rate. Infection is recognized by increasing pain, cloudy or purulent discharge, and palpable tenderness.
- If a sutured wound becomes infected, *all* of the sutures have to be removed. Attempts to maintain some sutures will lead to continued infection even if antibiotics are prescribed.
- Chronic skin ulcers are most often caused by diabetes, peripheral arterial or venous disease, and pressure.
- The main responsibility of an emergency caregiver when confronted with a chronic skin ulcer is to assess for life-threatening or limb-threatening emergencies.
- The goals of the emergency caregiver are to begin the process of reducing necrotic tissue load and to disinfect the wound to prepare for the growth of granulation tissue.
- Reduction of tissue load can begin with wet-to-dry dressings, and disinfection can begin with antibiotic therapy.
- Skin tears most often occur in aging skin or skin compromised by drugs such as corticosteroids.
- Skin tears are often best closed with wound tapes or wound adhesives. Compromised skin does not hold sutures well.
- Like skin ulcers, skin tears that have led to tissue loss should be referred to specialists in chronic wound care.

Although acute wounds and lacerations compose the bulk of wound care problems that present to emergency and urgent care facilities, the patients with complicated and chronic wounds can present a variety of challenges. Rarely, a small, even trivial, wound can become infected with bacteria that cause deep cutaneous and necrotizing infections. These wounds require rapid, aggressive diagnosis and intervention.

Despite the best efforts to cleanse and repair lacerations, a few patients return with symptoms and signs of infection. The diagnosis of infection has to be confirmed and followed by the steps needed to treat the Infection and to promote healing.

Patients with chronic skin ulceration, a condition that affects more than 2 million people in the United States annually, can require emergency care.[1] The goals of that care are limited but important. Professionals best perform the ongoing care, with eventual healing occurring, in a setting designed for and with expertise in chronic wound care.

Finally, a challenging wound care problem is skin tears in aged patients or skin affected by drugs such as corticosteroids. Sutures do not hold well and can tear through compromised skin. Treatment choices include wound tapes and wound adhesives. If there is tissue loss, these patients, like those with skin ulcers, should be referred to care-givers with experience in complicated wounds.

DEEP CUTANEOUS AND NECROTIZING INFECTIONS

The most feared complication of a laceration, puncture, or other traumatic wound is a deep cutaneous and necrotizing soft tissue infection. This complication is rare. These infections are more likely to occur in older patients with diabetes, vascular com-promise, and other chronic, debilitating illnesses.[2] For these patients, deep infections are caused by a variety of gram-positive, gram-negative, and anaerobic organisms. The lower extremity is the most commonly affected site. The perineum and surgical inci-sions also are vulnerable to these infections.[3] The overlying skin becomes discolored and swollen and can evolve into blebs and exudative lesions. These patients require extensive evaluation, including radiographs of the involved site. Broad-spectrum anti-biotics are administered. A surgical consultation is obtained as soon as possible if the infected area is life threatening or limb threatening.

In a young, healthy patient with a minor wound, the most important feature of a developing deep necrotizing and fascial infection is pain out of proportion to clinical findings.[4] Patients may or may not present to a care facility at the time of the wounding. Within hours, however, they begin to complain of severe pain at the wound site. The surrounding skin and soft tissue are minimally involved. The most likely organisms to be present in this setting are beta-hemolytic streptococci or the clostridia. These infected wounds can progress to full toxic streptococcal syndrome or gas gangrene.

Because these infections are rare, they often are not recognized until skin changes occur and the patient exhibits systemic symptoms, including tachycardia, tachypnea, acidosis, and eventually hemodynamic instability. A high index of suspicion and a will-ingness to act early in the course may lessen the severity and improve the outcome.

Evaluation and Treatment

Whenever a deep, necrotizing infection is suspected after a laceration or other wound occurs, the following diagnostic and treatment steps are performed:

- Complete hematologic tests, including clotting studies, and biochemical profiles are obtained.
- Oxygen saturation is determined and oxygen supplementation is begun if indicated.
- Intravenous fluids are begun with normal saline or lactated Ringer's solution.
- Radiographs of the involved area are taken to assess for foreign-body or gas formation.
- A Gram stain is performed on any exudates or bleb fluid to determine the presence of organisms. Gram-positive rods can be present in clostridial infections, and gram-positive cocci are indicative of beta-hemolytic streptococci.
- Broad-spectrum antibiotics, such as piperacillin/tazobactam, or clindamycin/genta-micin, are administered. In cases in which the diagnosis of clostridia is confirmed,

high-dose penicillin is given. It is important to note that prompt administration of antibiotics can improve outcome.[5]

- A surgical consultation is obtained. Immediate surgical intervention may be necessary as a limb-saving or lifesaving measure.
- In cases of suspected or confirmed clostridial myonecrosis or gas gangrene, hyperbaric oxygen has been shown to be an effective adjunct. If available, consultation with an hyperbaric oxygen specialist is recommended.[2]

INFECTIONS OF LACERATION REPAIR

Approximately 3% to 6% of wounds and lacerations treated in an emergency department (ED) become infected.[6] Signs of infection include increasing pain and tenderness of the wounded area, redness spreading away from the wound edges, and discharge or pus formation. Most patients return to the original facility or caregiver for treatment.

Before any action is taken, the diagnosis of infection needs to be confirmed. Patients react differently to healing wounds. Normal discomfort for most can be very painful for others. All wounds exude a small amount of thin, bloody material for 1 or 2 days. A narrow margin of erythema is normal. When to declare these findings abnormal and consistent with infection can be a judgment call. Sometimes, when the diagnosis is unclear, the patient can be reexamined in 24 hours. If a true infection is present, it becomes apparent in the next 24 to 48 hours. Some clinicians place the patient on antibiotics during that period in an attempt to stop an early infection. If an infection has become established, however, antibiotics are unlikely to suppress it while the sutures are still in place.

Management of Infected Lacerations

When an infection has been diagnosed, the following guidelines are suggested:

- *Removal of sutures:* Sutures act as foreign bodies. In the face of infection, all sutures, including deep and skin closure sutures, must be removed. Attempts to remove only some of the sutures or every other one only prolong the infection.
- *Cleaning and irrigation:* When sutures are removed, the wound is drained and irrigated to remove any collection of pus or infected exudates.
- *Wound exploration:* The wound is explored for retained foreign material or debris.
- *Antibiotic therapy:* Because most infections are caused by *Staphylococcus aureus* or streptococci, a first-generation cephalosporin, cephalexin, can be administered for 7 to 10 days. If there is significant cellulitis, therapy can be started with a dose of intravenous cefazolin. In the event of allergy to β-lactam antibiotics, clindamycin or a macrolide can be substituted. If CA-MRSA is suspected, trimethoprim/sulfamethoxazole (TMP/SMX) or tetracyline can be substituted or added. Local sensitivities to CA-MRSA can dictate the appropriate antibiotic.
- *Home care:* The wound is cleansed daily with soap and water. Hydrogen peroxide can be added or used alone. Cotton swabs or small sterile sponges can be used to remove debris and exudates until the infection is brought under control. The wound is covered with a gauze pad and tape between cleanings.
- *Consultation:* Wounds in cosmetically unimportant locations can be left to heal by secondary intention. If cosmesis is a concern, the patient can be referred to a plastic surgeon for further care.

CHRONIC SKIN ULCERATIONS

Although no statistics define the numbers of patients presenting to the ED with skin ulcers, it is a frequent occurrence, particularly in EDs serving socially and economically disadvantaged groups. Skin ulcers stem from specific systemic or regional disorders. The most common are vascular diseases, diabetes, and neurologic disorders.[7]

Cofactors include chronic systemic disease, prolonged bed rest, malnutrition, body size, suboptimal care, weight-bearing surfaces, and patient neglect. The net result of the combined pathophysiologic process is localized loss of integrity of the epidermis, dermis, and subcutaneous tissue secondary to ischemia. If unchecked, the ulcerative process can involve deep fascia, muscle, and bone. Skin ulcers most likely to be encountered by the ED physician include ulcers caused by pressure, venous stasis, arterial insufficiency, and diabetes.[2]

The ischium, sacrum, and trochanter of the hip account for 60% of pressure ulcers; 17% occur in the foot area.[8] These ulcers almost always occur in chronically debilitated, bedridden patients and neurologically impaired patients, such as quadriplegics and paraplegics.

Chronic venous insufficiency is the setting for venous ulceration. Venous ulcers are most common over the inner aspect of the distal leg and ankle. Most ulcers lie along the saphenous vein system. Edema of the lower extremity and stasis dermatitis can precede ulcer formation. Venous ulcers are shallow and tender and have variably shaped borders.

The hallmark of arterial ulcers is resting pain.[2] These ulcers are most common over the lateral ankle, toes, and base of the fifth metatarsal head and heel and ball of the foot. The other signs of arterial insufficiency are usually present, including pale atrophic skin, hair loss, and nail dystrophy. A history of claudication is common, and peripheral pulses are either weak or absent.

Most diabetic ulcers occur in the forefoot and toes.[9] The ulcerated foot is classified as ischemic or neurotrophic. Clinically, if the ankle pulses are present and there are good signs of arterial profusion, the ulcer is neurotrophic in origin. By comparison, ischemic ulcers present with diminished pulses in pale and atrophic tissue.

Evaluation of Chronic Ulcerations

The first duty of the ED physician in evaluating a patient with a chronic skin ulcer is to assess for a life-threatening or limb-threatening condition. Patients presenting to the ED with skin ulcerations often do so because of changes in their general medical condition, rather than for the ulcer itself.[2] The four major threats to life and limb that should be considered are venous thrombosis, acute arterial occlusion, severe (systemic or regional) infection, and metabolic abnormalities. For patients with systemic symptoms or potential life threats, the initial stabilization steps consist of providing oxygen supplementation, establishing intravenous access, and placing the patient on a cardiac monitor. Evaluation includes obtaining hematologic and metabolic profiles, an electrocardiogram, and radiographs as needed. Specifically, the ulcer site is evaluated by radiograph to look for tissue gas or osteomyelitis.

When life-threatening and limb-threatening conditions have been considered, a more focused evaluation can be performed. An attempt should be made to define the cause of the ulcer and to determine its extent. Because ulcers occur most commonly in the lower extremities, the focus of the examination is mostly on the buttocks, legs, and feet.

The vascular and neurologic examination of the lower limbs necessitates the most attention. When arterial disease is suspected, femoral, popliteal, dorsalis pedis, and posterior tibial pulses should be examined. Further evidence of arterial disease includes bruits in the midabdominal, femoral, or popliteal regions. Capillary refill (<4 to 8 seconds in normal individuals) can be tested. An ankle systolic pressure of <60 mm Hg or an ankle-brachial index (the ratio of lower leg to arm blood pressure) <0.4 is highly indicative of severe arterial disease. Assessment of the venous system is more difficult and often requires specialized testing, such as Doppler ultrasound of the lower extremity venous system.

Management of Skin Ulcerations

When the general health of the patient has been addressed and the cause of the ulcer has been determined, specific ulcer therapy can be initiated. The goals of care for patients with ulcers are as follows[7]:

- To decrease the necrotic tissue load and to maintain wound cleanliness
- To disinfect the wound site
- To initiate stimulation of granulation tissue

The specific management recommendations for the infected, necrotic ulcer are as follows:

- *Cleansing:* All ulcers should be cleaned. At the initial ED visit, standard wound cleansing solutions, such as povidone-iodine and chlorhexidine, can be used. They should be diluted with saline before use.
- *Irrigation:* Probably more important than wound cleansing is saline irrigation under pressure. This technique has been shown effective in removing bacteria, loose debris, and exudates from ulcers. In the ED, a 20-mL or 50-mL syringe with an 18-G needle is an appropriate choice for irrigation.
- *Wet-to-dry dressings:* For all but the cleanest wounds with viable granulation tissue, the initial choice of dressing is the traditional wet-to-dry saline dressing.[2]
  - The ulcer cavity is packed with moistened saline gauze. This technique permits tissue and debris to embed in the gauze matrix as it dries. Removal of dried gauze effectively débrides the wound. The gauze is kept in place by a gauze bandage wrap (Kling).
  - This process is repeated at least two or three times daily. Patients and families are instructed in this technique if they have the initiative and resources to assist in managing the procedures.
  - It is important to let the dressing dry completely and be removed without moistening. The gauze attaches to and lifts up the necrotic tissue debris only if dry.
  - Wet-to-dry dressings are continued for several days until the exudate and debris are significantly reduced, and granulation tissue appears.
- *Discharge:* The patient is given specific instructions on discharge.
  - In addition to the frequent dressing changes, the patient should elevate the affected extremity as much as possible. Continued dependency of the extremity encourages unnecessary edema and retards healing.
  - As previously mentioned, antibiotics can be prescribed for the patient. Amoxicillin/clavulanate, ciprofloxacin, cephalexin, and clindamycin have shown efficacy in treating chronic wounds and ulcers.[9]
  - The patient should be returned to the care of a physician who has chronic wound care support and ability. Only after the wound has been débrided and rendered infection free can other interventions be applied to continue ulcer healing.

Ultimately, patients with chronic ulcers can benefit from a variety of newer synthetic dressings, wound vacs, Unna boots, skin grafting, wound growth factors, and hyperbaric medicine.[10] These options can be tailored to the individual case. Ideally, patients should be referred to specialized wound care centers, which often are associated with hyperbaric medicine facilities.

SKIN TEARS IN AGED OR COMPROMISED SKIN

Skin tears and pretibial lacerations most often occur in the elderly and in patients being treated with corticosteroids. The majority (80%) of skin tears occur in the upper extremity, the forearm, and 20% of skin tears occur in the pretibial area.[11] Aging and corticosteroids reduce the amount and strength of elastin in the dermis.[12] The skin is dry, wrinkles, and sags. It is very friable and is susceptible to minor wounding forces. It also does not hold sutures well. Sutures increase the risk for wound edge necrosis and delayed healing.[13]

There are multiple categorizations of skin tears, but they fall into three general types described by Payne and Martin[14]:

- *Type 1:* Skin tears without loss of tissue: linear lacerations or flaps that, when unfurled, fill the wound defect.
- *Type 2:* Wound, usually a flap, with ≤25% loss of tissue. The flap cannot completely cover the defect.
- *Type 3:* Wound avulsion with complete loss of tissue and a remaining defect.

Repair of Skin Tears: General Principles
- Any necrotic tissue should be carefully débrided. When in doubt, retain the tissue for closure to provide for more coverage. The tissue can always be removed later.
- Hematoma in the wound is removed to prevent interference with wound closure. Hematomas can particularly interfere with attachment of a flap to its base.
- Fat is débrided from the underside of a flap and/or base also to prevent closure and coverage of the defect.
- If anesthetic is required for débridement, use lidocaine 1% or 2% without epinephrine to prevent excessive vasoconstriction in thin, compromised skin.
- Cleansing of skin tears before closure is performed with 0.9% saline or a non-toxic wound cleanser. The saline or cleanser is best delivered by gentle irrigation (Fig. 19-1).
- Laceration and flap edges are never closed under tension. Tension can interfere with blood flow and can cause tissue necrosis.
- Because skin tears can take up to 21 days to heal, after initial wound care, the patient should be referred to a physician or center with experience in skin tears or chronic wound care.[15]

Repair of Type 1 Skin Tears: Lacerations
- Observe General Principles listed previously.
- Gently appose wound edges and apply wound tapes.
- As an alternative, wound adhesive can be used in lacerations under low tension[16] (see Fig. 19-1).
- Wound adhesive is painted on the apposed wound edges with a 1-cm to 2-cm border. Two to three layers are laid down letting each layer dry before applying the next.
- Closed lacerations do not require dressings. If protection is needed, then a gauze wrap can be applied. Be sure that the wound adhesive is completely dry before applying a gauze wrap.

Repair of Type 1 Skin Tears: Flaps
Without Tissue Loss
- Observe General Principles described previously including the principles for hematoma and fat removal.
- Using a gloved finger or saline-moistened gauze pad, push and flatten flap until it fills the defect caused by the wound.
- Apply wound tapes to the wound edges for closure.
- As an alternative, wound adhesive can be used as well. It is applied as described previously for lacerations. Gentle traction on the flap tip with the physician's fingers may keep the flap in place during adhesive application. The flap tip can be anchored with a wound tape.

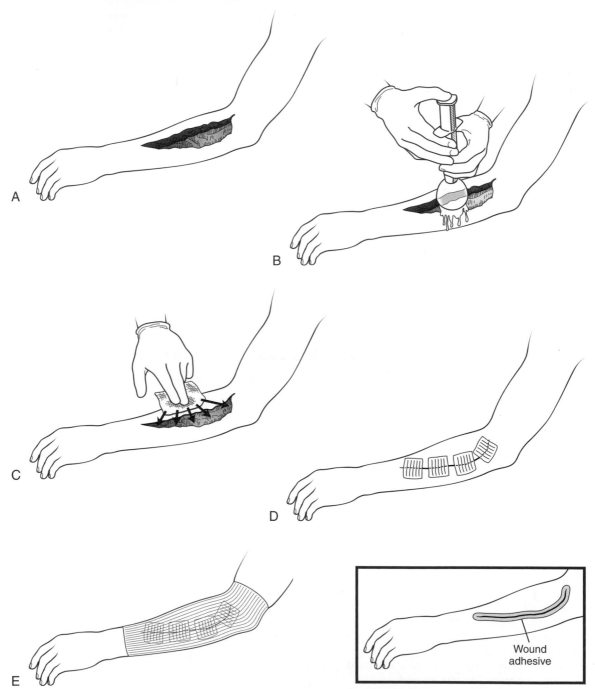

Figure 19-1. Closure of a type 1 skin tear laceration. **A,** Example of skin tear laceration. **B,** Cleanse wound irrigation using saline or povidone-iodine diluted 10:1 with saline. **C,** Gently appose skin flap with gauze pads. **D,** Apply wound tapes as illustrated. **E,** Cover wound with nonadherent gauze wrap or tube gauze. *Inset,* Wound adhesive is an alternative to wound tapes. Leave open to air after application. Do not cover with gauze. (From Singer AJ, Dagum AB: Current management of acute wounds, *N Engl J Med* 359:1037–1046, 2008.)

- Closed lacerations do not require dressings. If protection is needed, then a gauze wrap can be applied. Be sure that the wound adhesive is completely dry before applying a gauze wrap.

Repair of Type 2 Skin Tears: Flap Formation with Partial Tissue Loss (Usually <25%)

- Observe General Principles described previously.
- Using a gloved finger or saline-moistened gauze pad, push and flatten flap until it fills the as much of the defect as possible.
- Apply wound tapes to close wound edges that can be brought together.
- Cover the flap and defect with a nonadherent dressing such as Adaptic, and cover with gauze pads and a gauze wrap. Do not use ointments. Hydrocolloid or hydrogel nonadherent dressings can be used as well.
- Refer the patient to a specialist in wound care or a wound care center to continue management of the wound, particularly of the defect.

Repair of Type 3 Skin Tears: Complete Avulsion or Loss of Tissue with Remaining Defect

- Gently débride defect and wound edges of necrotic tissue, hematoma, and fat. Use lidocaine anesthetic as described previously.
- Cover the defect with a nonadherent dressing such as Adaptic, and cover with gauze pads and a gauze wrap. Do not use ointments. Hydrocolloid or hydrogel nonadherent dressings can be used as well.
- Refer the patient to a specialist in wound care or a wound care center to continue management of the wound, particularly of the defect.

References

1. Fletcher J: Measuring the prevalence and incidence of chronic wounds, *Prof Nurse* 18:384–388, 2003.
2. Trott AT: Chronic skin ulcers, *Emerg Clin North Am* 10:823–845, 1992.
3. Stone DR, Gorbach SL: Necrotizing fasciitis: the changing spectrum, *Infect Dis Dermatol* 15:213–216, 1997.
4. Kaul R, McGeer A, Low DE, et al: Population-based surveillance for group A streptococcal necrotizing fasciitis: clinical features, prognostic indicators, and microbiologic analysis of seventy-seven cases, *Am J Med* 103:18–24, 1997.
5. Kumar A, Roberts D, Wood KE, et al: Duration of hypotension before initiation of effective antimicrobial therapy is the critical determinant of survival in human septic shock, *Crit Care Med* 34:1589–1596, 2006.
6. Cummings P, Del Beccaro MA: Antibiotics to prevent infection of simple wounds: a meta-analysis of randomized studies, *Am J Emerg Med* 13:396–400, 1995.
7. O'Meara SM, Cullum NA, Majid M, et al: Systematic review of antimicrobial agents used for chronic wounds, *Br J Surg* 88:4–21, 2001.
8. Phillips TJ: Chronic cutaneous ulcers: etiology and epidemiology, *J Invest Dermatol* 102:S38–S41, 1994.
9. Ramasastry SS: Chronic problem wounds, *Clin Plast Surg* 25:367–396, 1998.
10. Dieter S: Debridement for chronic wounds, *Adv Nurse Pract* 9:65–66, 2001.
11. Bradley L: The conservative management of pre-tibial lacerations, *Nurs Times* 98:62–69, 2002.
12. Battersby L: *Exploring the best practice in management of skin tears in older people.* www.nursingtimes.net/exploring-best-practice-in-the-management-of-skin-tears-in-older-people/5000502.article. Accessed April 23, 2009.
13. Sutton R, Pritty P: Use of sutures or adhesive tapes for primary closure of pretibial lacerations, *Br Med J* 290:1627, 1985.
14. Payne RL, Martin ML: Defining and classifying skin tears: need for a common language, *Ostomy Wound Manag* 39:16–26, 1993.
15. Murray E: *Guidelines for the management of skin tears*, Sydney, 2005, St Vincents & Mater Health Sydney Nursing Monograph, pp 31–36.
16. Xu X, Lau K, Taira BR, et al: The current management of skin tears, *Am J Emerg Med* 27:729–733, 2009.

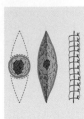

CHAPTER 20
Wound Dressing and Bandaging Techniques

Key Practice Points

- Wounds heal faster and with less pain when a moist environment is created by an ointment or a dressing.
- Neat, well-applied dressings inspire the patient to be confident in the physician and in the prognosis for healing.
- A basic wound dressing has four parts: antibiotic ointment, a nonadherent base, absorbent gauze sponges (gauze wrap if needed), and wound tape.
- Antibiotic ointments can enhance the moist environment; however, studies have not conclusively shown that ointments reduce wound infection.
- Uncomplicated facial and scalp wounds do not require dressings. Antibiotic ointment should be applied two to three times daily to prevent dried coagulum buildup that can interfere with suture removal.
- Never wrap tape circumferentially completely around an extremity or finger. Circumferential tape can cause a tourniquet effect as the wound area undergoes natural swelling.
- The first dressing change after discharging the patient should be in 24 to 48 hours to check for infection and to clean away residual blood and wound exudate.
- Patients can shower between bandage changes, starting 24 to 48 hours following repair. Soaking baths, however, are discouraged.

This chapter discusses the general principles of wound dressing and some recommendations for dressing and bandaging. The recommendations depend on the type of wound, body location, and other factors. Specialized dressings for burns are discussed in Chapter 17.

WOUND DRESSING PRINCIPLES

The first decision to make after repairing a wound is whether to apply a dressing at all. Uncomplicated lacerations of the face and scalp are often left open. The head and face are extremely vascular, and wounds in these areas are resistant to infection. If the patient is careful and keeps the wound clean, a sutured laceration heals without event. These wounds need the regular application of a petrolatum-based antibacterial ointment to maintain a moist environment and to help prevent crusting that can interfere with suture removal.[1,2] The generally accepted practice for wounds and lacerations that are not on the head or the face is to apply a wound covering, although there is little evidence that a dressing improves the eventual scar appearance of sutured lacerations.

One study of uncovered surgical incisions that were sutured postoperatively could not document an increase in the rate of infection compared with dressed incisions.[3]

When the decision is made to apply a dressing, the following principles should be observed:

- *Moist Environment*

    The wound must remain moist. Experimental studies convincingly show that desiccation by exposure can delay epithelial layer formation significantly.[2,4] A moist environment has been shown to decrease the number of days to healing and reduces wound pain.[5]

    Figure 20-1 illustrates the pathways for epidermal healing in moist and dry environments. In an uncovered wound, epithelial cells are forced to find a pathway beneath dry coagulum/exudate and dermal remnants. In practice, synthetic dressings (e.g., Adaptic, Xeroform, Telfa, and Band-Aids) are nonadherent, porous coverings that allow for the drainage of exudate but do not permit excessive desiccation. Topical antibiotic ointments can provide a moist environment for unbandaged wounds.

- *Tidiness*

    A dressing must be neat and uncomplicated. Sloppy or poorly applied dressings and bandages do not convince a patient that good wound care has been delivered. Many small wounds are served best by one or two simple adhesive bandages (Band-Aid). This dressing remains one of the most versatile and appropriate wound coverings yet devised.

- *Nonadherent, Porous Base*

    The base of a dressing, the portion in direct contact with the wound surface, should not be adherent. Plain, fine-mesh gauze is an example of a dressing that sticks to wounds by becoming incorporated in the coagulum. When the gauze is removed, it can disrupt healing by disturbing the delicate epithelial covering. A good wound covering also has to allow for the passage of exudate so that excessive accumulation does not occur. Adaptic, Xeroform, and Telfa are examples of nonadherent materials.

- *Protection*

    Protection from contamination is best accomplished by ensuring that, in addition to the nonadherent base, the wound is well covered with gauze sponge material and an appropriate gauze wrap. Gauze sponges help meet the protection requirement of wound dressing. Most minor wounds and lacerations produce little exudate; a simple 2 × 2 or 4 × 4 gauze sponge, or even a Band-Aid, suffices for this purpose. Complicated or contaminated wounds with a potential for infection are likely to exude freely and

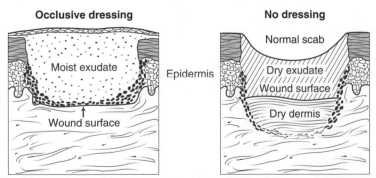

Figure 20-1. The different pathways necessary for epithelial cells to migrate to provide an epithelial cell covering of an open wound. The moist environment experimentally appears to provide for more rapid healing than a dry environment as seen in open, uncovered wounds.

copiously. In addition to several layers of gauze sponges, frequent dressing changes often are necessary.

• *Partial Immobilization*

Finally, dressings should protect the healing wound and should provide partial immobilization of the injured part. Many forces can disrupt a suture line, ranging from contact with clothing to accidental minor trauma to the wound. Gauze sponges in combination with gauze wrapping suffice for the purpose of wound protection. Occasionally, rigid splinting, particularly for lacerations over joints, is necessary. In general, excessive wrapping should be avoided, however, to prevent complete immobilization of a moving anatomic part, particularly the hand. Although rest for the injury is necessary, some movement is encouraged within the bandage. The goal is to prevent the stiffening of joints that can occur, especially in elderly patients.

Young children present a particularly difficult challenge in wound dressing. Their wounds heal rapidly and, in practice, seem to be resistant to infection. The principle of simplicity is important. A Band-Aid, when it can be used appropriately, is the dressing of choice for small wounds. If the Band-Aid is removed by the child, it can be replaced easily by the parent. Children are more likely to leave Band-Aids in place, because this dressing is recognized as a "badge" for other children to appreciate. When more complicated dressings have to be used on the hand, a "mitten-like" bandage that encompasses the entire hand is often recommended. If the laceration or wound is serious, older children generally seem to have an instinctive understanding that prevents them from removing dressings.

BASIC WOUND DRESSINGS

Unbandaged Wounds: Topical Antibiotics

Topical antibiotic ointments are currently recommended for facial wounds (e.g., lacerations, abrasions, burns) or any other wound, such as an abrasion, that is treated without bandaging. These ointments provide a moist wound healing environment in the absence of a bandage. They also reduce dry exudate, or scab, formation, which makes suture removal much easier. Suppression of infection and improved wound edge healing, particularly for flaps, are reasons to support the use of topical agents.[6-8] In an evidence-based review of the application of ointment to lacerations and other small wounds, however, all of the cited studies had significant weaknesses.[9] The question of whether ointment reduces wound infection remains unanswered.

Topical ointments should be thinly applied two to three times daily to maintain consistent coverage. Petrolatum-based antibacterial ointments (e.g., polymyxin B sulfate/neomycin [Neosporin] and silver sulfadiazine [Silvadene]) have been shown experimentally to encourage epithelialization effectively as compared with other ointments (e.g., nitrofurazone [Furacin] and Pharmadine, which contains povidone-iodine).[10] Neosporin is easier to apply to the face than silver sulfadiazine, which needs to be applied in a thick layer. Other agents that can be used for this purpose are polymyxin B sulfate/bacitracin (Polysporin) and zinc salt/polymyxin/neomycin (Bacitracin). If a patient is known to be sensitive to neomycin, plain petrolatum ointment can be used. Petrolatum-based topical antibiotic ointments should not be used on wounds closed with wound adhesive. The petrolatum will soften and disrupt the adhesive.

Bandaged Wounds

The basic wound covering consists of four materials:

• Antibacterial ointment
• Nonadherent base
• Absorbent gauze sponges (gauze wrapping if needed)
• Tape to secure the dressing

Dressing Application

After repair, an antibacterial ointment can be thinly and gently spread over the wound. Based on the preceding discussion, application of a topical agent for sutured lacerations can be considered optional. The main use of these ointments under bandages is to lessen dry exudate formation and to add to the moist environment of the dressing. Ointments can be applied at each bandage change. Neosporin, Polysporin, and Bacitracin are commonly used.

In a sterile fashion, the nonadherent base is cut to conform with the general wound area (Fig. 20-2). Depending on the potential for wound drainage and exudation, gauze sponges are placed over the base. On an extremity, a gauze wrap is applied, followed by tape. On flat surfaces where gauze wrapping is not appropriate, the tape is placed directly over the gauze sponges.

A common tape adhesive adjunct is tincture of benzoin. This substance is effective in keeping tape adherent to the skin for the duration of the dressing. Precautions have to be taken, however, so that benzoin is not spilled directly into the wound. Under experimental conditions, this compound has been shown to increase the potential for wound infection when it comes into direct contact with the raw wound surface.[11]

One of the most important precautions in dressing and bandaging is never to wrap tape circumferentially around an extremity or a digit (Fig. 20-3). If brought around the finger or wrist to adhere to itself, tape becomes a nonexpanding band that causes a tourniquet effect on the vascular blood supply to the distal regions of a hand or finger.

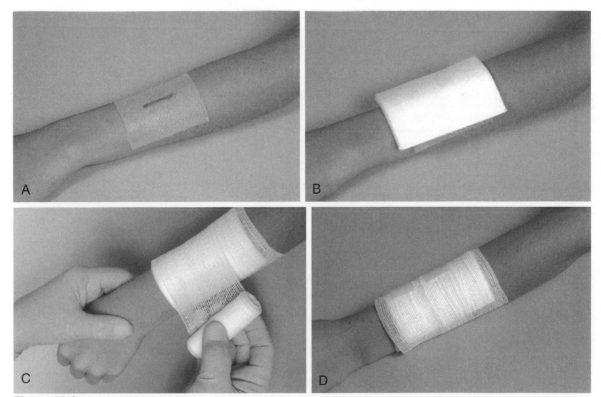

Figure 20-2. Basic components of a wound dressing. **A,** A nonadherent base over a layer of antibiotic ointment. **B,** Gauze sponge covering. **C,** Gauze wrap. **D,** Tape application to secure dressing.

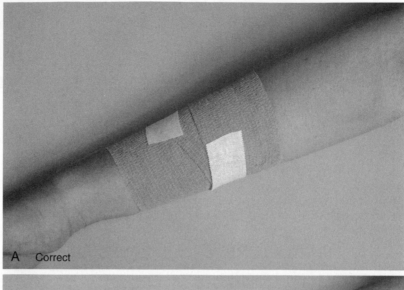

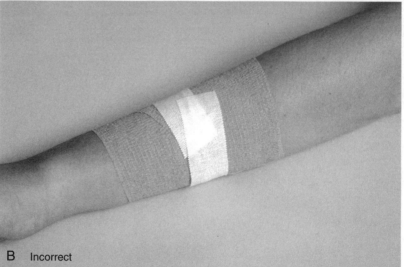

Figure 20-3. Technique for correct taping of a bandage. **A,** Correct: Tape does not overlap if it surrounds an extremity. **B,** Incorrect: Overlapping tape can cause unwanted constriction and distal edema.

Pressure builds as congestion and edema develop. This pressure can cause complete cessation of blood flow with attendant ischemic necrosis of the anatomic part. This tourniquet effect is one of the worst potential complications of wound care.

HOME CARE AND DRESSING CHANGE INTERVALS

Dressing change intervals vary considerably and can depend on the patient, wound characteristics, and home care plan. In general, dressings should be kept clean and dry. Because the initial dressing is placed while the wound might be oozing blood or exudate, and the dressing may thus be bulky, it is often useful to instruct the patient to change the dressing 24 to 48 hours after the repair. This change serves several

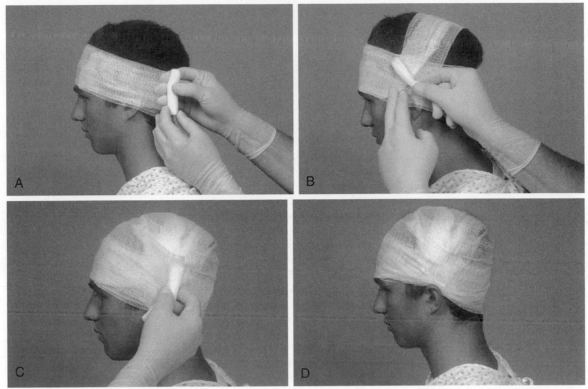

Figure 20-4. Technique for application of a scalp dressing. **A,** Dressing is begun by wrapping gauze around the midforehead and directly over the occipital protuberance. This beginning allows for stabilization of the scalp dressing. Attempts to wrap the dressing higher on the scalp lead to inevitable loosening of the dressing. **B,** If a recurrent portion of the dressing is necessary to cover lacerations or wounds on the top of the head, or vertex, the recurrent portion is begun as illustrated. **C,** The recurrent portion is brought back and forth over the area of concern. The recurrent portion is anchored by repeat circumferential wraps. **D,** View of a completed recurrent scalp dressing. If possible, lift gauze above ear.

purposes: The wound can be inspected for early signs of infection, the new dressing is free of exudate and blood, and the second dressing is less bulky than the original one. Dressing changes thereafter can be individualized based on the patient's ability to maintain the integrity and protective function of the dressing. The patient can shower between bandage changes after 24 to 48 hours following repair. Water can be allowed to run over the wound, but soaking baths are discouraged. See Chapter 22 for further home care information and instructions.

BODY AREA DRESSINGS

Scalp

Most simple sutured lacerations of the scalp can be left open to the air. A small amount of blood coagulum develops quickly along the suture line and acts as a wound covering. Because the scalp is extremely vascular and tends to bleed profusely when injured, however, a dressing occasionally needs to be applied to the area after repair is completed. Figure 20-4 shows the basic bandage and the method used to continue that wrapping as a recurrent dressing for wounds closer to the crown of the head. The initial gauze wrap should include the greatest diameter of the skull to prevent inadvertent slippage. The forehead just above the brow and the external occipital protuberance are the landmarks acting as center points for the wrap. Otherwise the dressing slips over the crown and falls off.

Great care must be taken not to cause excessive pressure on the ears when applying a scalp dressing. Whenever possible, the ears should be brought out from underneath the bandage to prevent the complication of an ischemic necrosis of the skin of the ear or of the cartilage skeleton.

Face

As mentioned previously, facial lacerations can be left uncovered after repair. Small, uncomplicated lacerations of the ear, eyelid, nose, and lip are included in this recommendation. The patient can apply a thin film of an antibacterial ointment (e.g., Neosporin) daily. The antibiotic nature of this ointment is of questionable value at best, but the ointment base is useful in preventing the crusting of coagulum around the wound. When crusting is prevented, sutures are removed much more easily with minimal wound disruption. When a facial wound needs a covering to protect it from the environment, Band-Aids are recommended. Bulky bandages of the face are poorly tolerated by patients and tend to come off quickly.

Ear and Mastoid

Complicated ear injuries that are at risk for forming perichondral hematomas require a more involved dressing that applies pressure evenly over all of the contours of the ear. One or two 4 × 4 gauze sponges are cut in the contoured fashion shown in Figure 20-5. The sponges are placed around and behind the ear to provide support and a "bed" for the cartilaginous skeleton. The area within the helix is filled with petrolatum gauze and is "molded" over the antihelix, antitragus, and external canal. Two intact sponges are placed over the entire ear, and a 3- or 4-inch gauze bandage is brought around the head and over the ear several times. After the bandage is taped, it is tightened by placing a gauze tie just anterior to the ear. The net effect is to provide even pressure over the ear without compromising the blood supply.

Neck

The neck is an uncommon site for lacerations and other wounds. Dressings need to be secured effectively without compromising the airway or venous return through the jugular system. Simple wrapping with a gauze bandage over the dressing base suffices in most cases. For wounds of the posterior neck in the region of the occiput, the gauze bandage can be wrapped around the head and the neck to provide for adequate coverage and security (Fig. 20-6).

Shoulder

The shoulder can be a difficult area to dress, especially if the wound is large, is in the axilla, or is directly over the articular surfaces. The dressing illustrated in Figure 20-7 takes advantage of the trunk to anchor the shoulder portion. The wrap is brought alternately around the trunk and the shoulder/upper arm until it is complete. This dressing configuration also is useful for the upper arm, an area in which bandages tend to slip down with arm motion and gravity. A schematic of the shoulder dressing is illustrated in Figure 20-8.

Trunk

Most wounds on the trunk can be covered with the standard base described previously, and these wounds can be taped over benzoin. Larger wounds, such as burns, need larger bandages. The dressing described earlier to cover the shoulder can be extended

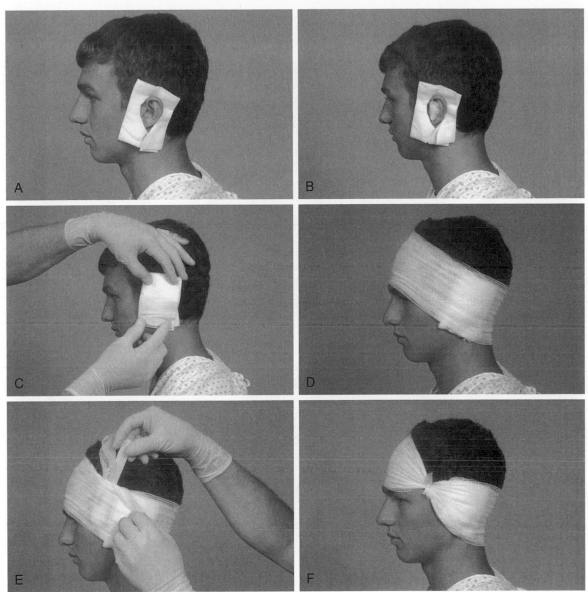

Figure 20-5. Technique for application of a mastoid dressing. **A,** With bandage scissors, cut a center portion out of two or three 4 × 4 gauze sponges so that they fit behind the cartilaginous skeleton of the ear. It is important that the cartilaginous skeleton is well supported and is not "crushed" against the scalp. **B,** Petrolatum gauze packing is placed and molded within the cartilaginous skeleton. **C,** Fresh sponges are placed over the molded petrolatum gauze. **D,** Circumferential gauze wrapping is placed from the midforehead directly over the external occipital protuberance. This portion is secured with tape. **E,** A gauze tie is inserted anterior to the affected ear using a tongue blade. **F,** This gauze is tied firmly in a square knot to provide even pressure over the ear, and the final appearance of the mastoid dressing is shown here.

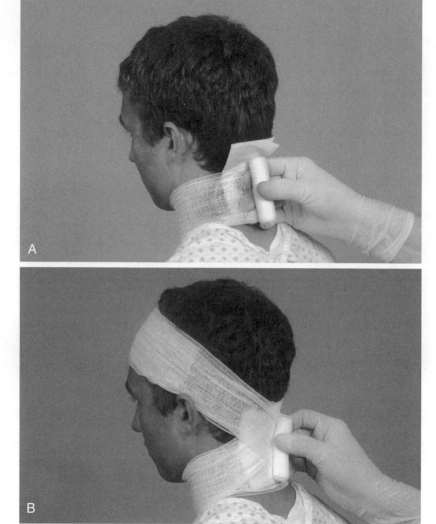

Figure 20-6. Technique for application of dressing of the posterior neck area. **A,** After placement of 4 × 4 sponges, gauze wrapping is brought gently around the neck to secure the gauze. **B,** In a recurrent manner, the dressing is continued around the frontal area and neck in a figure-eight fashion to secure the dressing completely. The ear is clear of the dressing.

downward over the trunk, and this dressing does not slip toward the abdomen. Another method to dress the trunk is illustrated in Figure 20-9.

Groin, Hip, and Thigh

The groin, hip, and thigh also are difficult regions to cover properly. The technique illustrated in Figure 20-10 is an all-purpose covering that protects most large wounds in those areas. Similar to the method for covering the shoulder, the gauze wrap is brought alternately around the trunk and thigh until it is complete.

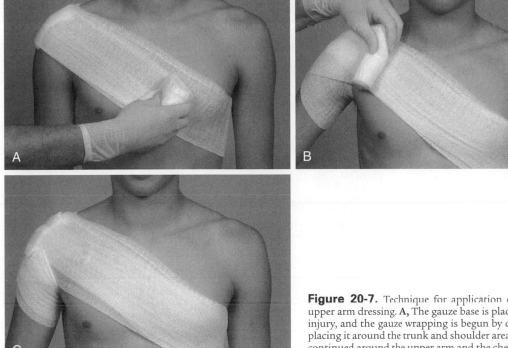

Figure 20-7. Technique for application of shoulder and upper arm dressing. **A,** The gauze base is placed in the area of injury, and the gauze wrapping is begun by circumferentially placing it around the trunk and shoulder area. **B,** The gauze is continued around the upper arm and the chest in an alternating manner. **C,** Final appearance of a shoulder dressing.

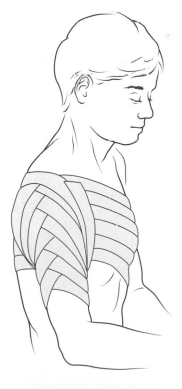

Figure 20-8. A schematic of the shoulder dressing is presented for clarification.

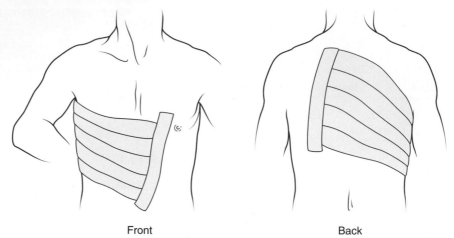

Front   Back

Figure 20-9. Technique for application of a truncal dressing. Gauze wrapping is brought around the hemithorax and is secured with benzoin and tape.

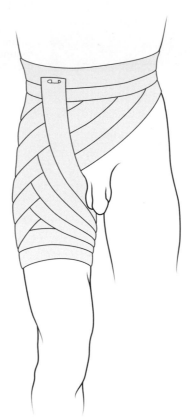

Figure 20-10. Technique for dressing the groin and upper thigh area. Similar to the shoulder dressing, the gauze is brought in an alternating manner first around the trunk and then the thigh.

Hand and Finger

Fingers can be bandaged in one of two ways: gauze wrapping or tube gauze application. After applying ointment and a nonadherent base, 2 × 2 sponges are placed over the actual wound. One or two layers of a 2-inch gauze bandage are placed over the finger (Fig. 20-11). The bandage is then turned to wrap the entire finger circumferentially from the finger base to the tip and back to the base again. To complete the bandaging, the gauze is carried in a figure-eight pattern down around the palm and finally is anchored at the wrist. Gauze bandaging of the finger alone tends to be inadequate, and the dressing can come off prematurely. The basic technique of tube gauze bandages is illustrated in Figure 20-12.

Injuries of the hand itself are bandaged as shown in Figure 20-13. Depending on the size of the hand, 2- or 3-inch gauze wrapping is placed over the nonadherent base and sponge covering. The gauze wrap includes the wrist to ensure proper anchoring. When two or more fingers are incorporated in a hand dressing, they have to be separated by gauze or sponge strips to prevent skin-to-skin contact and subsequent maceration.

Elbow and Knee

The elbow and knee can be wrapped circumferentially with 4-inch gauze. Although the dressing is adequate, it limits motion of the joint. When placed with the joint in some flexion, the figure-eight technique allows for more freedom of movement (Fig. 20-14). Incorporated into the bandaging are 4 × 8 gauze sponges that are placed over the extensor surfaces. These large sponges allow for "travel" as the joint is flexed and extended.

Ankle, Heel, and Foot

Ankle and foot dressings are straightforward. The gauze bandage wrapping is in the same figure-eight style used for the knee and elbow. When the foot is bandaged, the ankle always is included as the anchoring point.

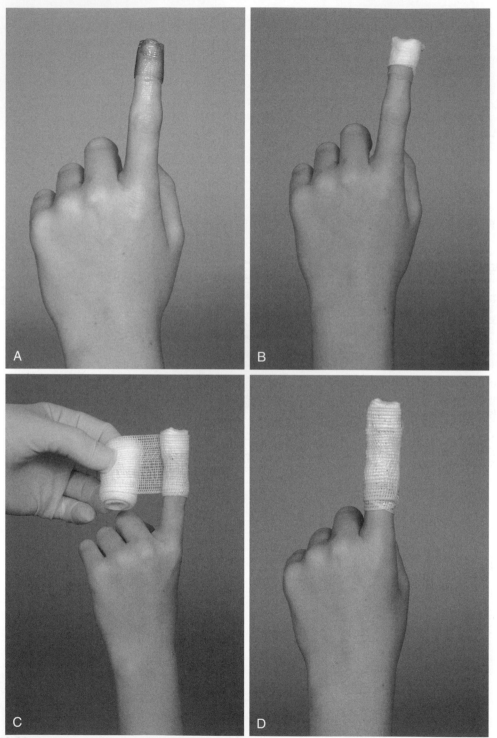

Figure 20-11. Technique for dressing a finger and fingertip. **A,** The dressing begins with a nonadherent base to cover the wound. **B,** A small 2 × 2 gauze sponge is molded over the tip. **C,** A 2-inch gauze bandage is wrapped around the finger, from tip to base. **D,** The dressing is secured with adhesive tape. Do not apply tape circumferentially to avoid digital edema and vascular compromise.

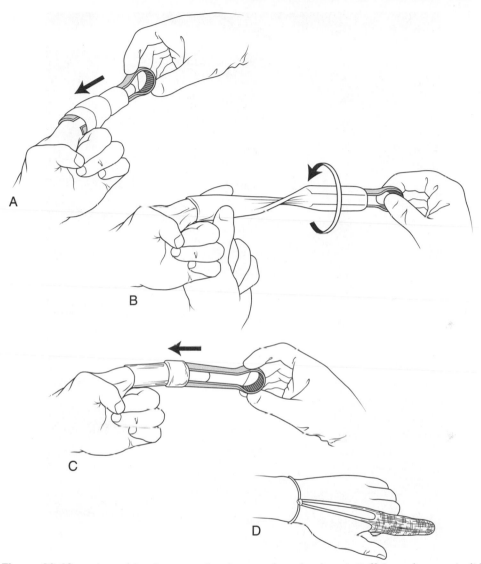

Figure 20-12. Technique for placement of a tube gauze finger bandage. **A,** Sufficient tube gauze is slid onto the applicator and is then brought over the finger. **B,** The first layer of tube gauze is secured as the applicator is brought distally from the finger and is rotated 180 degrees. **C,** The next layer of tube gauze is placed by the applicator over the digit. **D,** This process is repeated until an adequate number of layers of tube gauze have been applied.

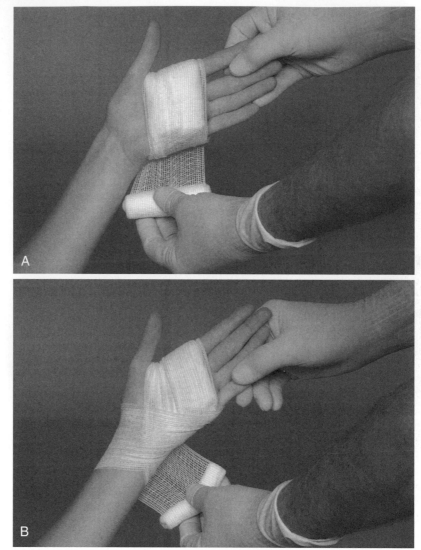

Figure 20-13. Technique for placing a dressing on the palmar or dorsal surface of the hand. **A,** The non-adherent base and 4 × 4 gauze sponges are placed on the palm or dorsum of the hand. The gauze wrapping is begun by securing this dressing base. **B,** The dressing is completed by alternate wrapping of the palm and the wrist with the gauze wrap. Tape is applied in a noncircumferential manner to complete the dressing.

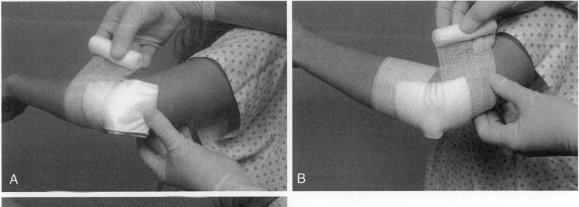

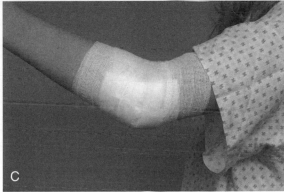

Figure 20-14. Technique for elbow or knee dressing. **A,** The gauze sponge is placed over the extensor surface of the knee or elbow and is secured with the beginnings of a gauze wrap. **B,** The gauze wrap is brought over to the opposite side of the gauze dressing base. **C,** An example of a completed dressing. Most elbow and knee dressings are fashioned with the knee or elbow in a slightly flexed position to provide for better patient mobility.

References

1. Stuzin J, Engrav LH, Buehler PK: Emergency treatment of facial lacerations, *Postgrad Med* 71:81–83, 1982.
2. Korting HC, Schollmann C, White RJ: Management of minor acute cutaneous wounds: importance of wound healing in a moist environment, *J Eur Acad Dermatol* 25:130–137, 2011.
3. Howells C, Young H: A study of completely undressed surgical wounds, *Br J Surg* 53:436–439, 1966.
4. Hinman C, Maibach H: Effect of air exposure and occlusion on experimental human skin wounds, *Nature* 200:377–378, 1963.
5. Beam JW: Management of superficial to partial-thickness wounds, *J Athl Train* 42:422–424, 2007.
6. Dire DJ, Coppola M, Dwyer DA, et al: Prospective evaluation of topical antibiotics for preventing infections of soft-tissue wounds repaired in the ED, *Acad Emerg Med* 2:4–10, 1995.
7. Leyden JJ, Sulzberger MB: Topical antibiotics and minor skin trauma, *Am Fam Physician* 23:121–125, 1981.
8. Singer AJ, Dagum AB: Current management of acute cutaneous wounds, *N Engl J Med* 359:1037–1046, 2008.
9. Zyl Van, Abbott D, Andrews D, et al: Routine use of antibiotic ointment and wound healing, *Emerg Med J* 19:556, 2002.
10. Eaglestein WH, Mertz PM: Effect of topical medicaments on the rate of repair of superficial wounds. In Dineen P, editor: *The surgical wound*, Philadelphia, 1981, Lea & Febiger.
11. Panek P, Prusak MP, Bolt D, et al: Potentiation of wound infection by adhesive adjuncts, *Am Surg* 38:343–345, 1972.

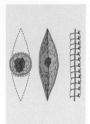

CHAPTER 21

Tetanus Immunity and Antibiotic Wound Prophylaxis

Key Practice Points

- All patients with abrasions, lacerations, burns, or other wounds require a tetanus immunization history.
- Tetanus occurs almost exclusively in patients with incomplete primary immunization.
- Tetanus prophylaxis for wounds provides an opportunity to boost immunity for pertussis and diphtheria with Tdap (combined tetanus, diphtheria, and pertussis) vaccines.
- Tetanus immune globulin (TIG) can be administered to patients with a true allergy to tetanus toxoid or patients who have not completed primary immunization, but TIG does not confer immunity for future wounds.
- Local pain and swelling are the most common reactions to tetanus prophylaxis, either Td or Tdap.
- Uncomplicated lacerations in otherwise healthy patients usually do not need prophylactic antibiotics.
- Although there is no clear scientific evidence, prophylactic antibiotics are recommended for complicated wounds, mammalian bites, impaired host defenses, and so forth (see text).
- Antibiotics should be started at the time of wound care to maximize their effect.
- In recent years, community-acquired methicllin-resistant *Staphylococcus aureus* (CA-MRSA) has become an important cause of wound infection.

Two issues of prophylaxis arise for virtually all patients with wounds and lacerations. A careful history is taken to establish the tetanus immune status of every patient. Although nurses in most emergency departments (EDs) are required to document immune status in their notes, the ultimate responsibility lies with the physician to ensure that the patient's tetanus prophylaxis is up to date.

Far more controversial and problematic is the issue of antibiotic prophylaxis. Despite the fact that 90% to 95% of all patients with uncomplicated lacerations do not acquire an infection, there remains an excessive use of prophylactic antibiotics.[1-5] As discussed subsequently, multiple large studies have failed to support the use of prophylactic antibiotics, and they may increase the risk for infection.

TETANUS PROPHYLAXIS

For all patients with an emergency wound or laceration, a decision has to be made about whether to administer tetanus prophylaxis. Although contaminated wounds with extensive devitalized tissue are considered more tetanus-prone than are clean minor wounds, one third of documented cases of tetanus have originated from seemingly trivial injuries.[6,7] A common portal of entry for tetanus is a puncture wound to the foot.[7] The importance of tetanus prophylaxis was underscored during a shortage of immunization doses in 2001.[8] During this period, the number of cases of tetanus increased.[9]

Despite widespread immunization programs, 40 to 50 cases of tetanus are reported each year. Tetanus occurs almost exclusively in patients who have never been immunized or who have never completed a proper immunization program.[10] Probably for this reason, most cases are reported in patients who are older than age 50.[10] A high proportion of older adults, when tested for serum tetanus antibody, have been shown to have inadequate levels of protection.[11,12] Young adults and children are more likely to have appropriate levels of protection because of widespread immunization programs that have been put into place in recent years. Regardless of the circumstances, a careful immunization history is taken for every patient with a minor wound. This history should establish whether initial immunization has been properly completed and should establish the date of the last tetanus toxoid dose.

Immunization Schedules

When patients present for wound care, the opportunity is taken to boost immunity to diphtheria and pertussis as well as tetanus. Diphtheria, although rare, still occurs, and a diphtheria toxoid booster will help maintain immunity.[13] Pertussis is more common, with 25,000 cases reported in 2005.[14] In 2005, a tetanus toxoid, reduced diphtheria toxoid, and acellular pertussis vaccine (Tdap) was approved for use in adults from ages 11 to 64 years.[13] DTaP, which contains a higher concentration of diphtheria and pertussis than Tdap, continues to be the primary vaccination agent for children. In 2010 the Advisory Committee in Immunization Practices (ACIP) of the Centers for Disease Control and Prevention recommended that Tdap could be safely given to children from ages 7 to 10 and for adults >64 years old.[15] Tdap is particularly important for patients <64 if they will have contact with children aged 12 months or less. These updated recommendations are reflected in Figure 21-1. The standard interval between doses of tetanus booster is 10 years. In regions with increased risk for pertussis, this interval can be as little as 5 years (2 years in Canada), if the patient has never received a Tdap as an adult. Thereafter, Td is given at 10-year intervals.[13] The ACIP recommends Td for pregnant women because of the lack of safety data for Tdap in pregnancy.[16] However, if protection from pertussis is considered important, Tdap can be administered as long as the patient is made aware of the lack of that safety data.[16]

Complications of Tetanus Toxoid and Tdap

Occasionally a patient reports an allergic reaction to a previously administered tetanus shot. In a study of 740 patients who claimed to be allergic to tetanus shots, the true incidence of allergy on skin challenge testing was low.[17] Of the 740 patients, 7 developed local reactions that were self-limited. One patient became syncopal, and one developed a fever that lasted for 4 days. Only 1 of 740 patients had a true urticarial response but still tolerated a full immunizing dose. Despite these reassuring figures, the possibility of a serious reaction still must be considered.[17] For patients considered at high risk for a reaction, tetanus immune globulin (250 to 500 U) is provided in the ED. Tetanus immune globulin confers immunity for that injury but not for future exposures. This preparation consists only of antitetanus antibody and does not cross-react with the toxoid. Referral to an allergist for skin testing and subsequent immunization with toxoid is recommended as prudent follow-up.

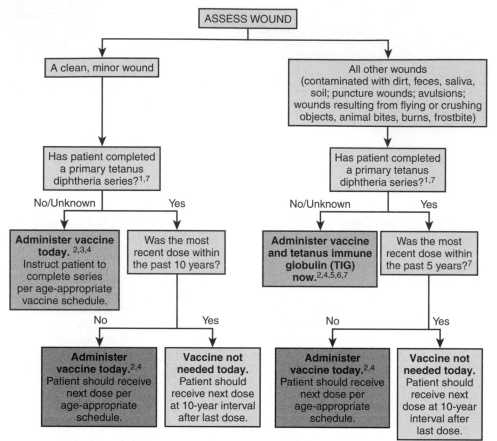

Figure 21-1. Summary guide to tetanus prophylaxis in routine wound management. *1,* A primary series consists of a minimum of three doses of tetanus- and diphtheria-containing vaccine (DTaP/DTP/Tdap/DT/Td). *2,* Age-appropriate vaccine: DTaP for infants and children from 6 weeks through 6 years of age (or DT pediatric if pertussis vaccine is contraindicated); Tdap for persons 7 through 10 years of age if they have not completed vaccination with DTaP; Tdap for persons >64 years of age if they have not previously received Tdap—otherwise, Td can be administered; and Tdap for persons 11 through 64 years of age, unless they have received Tdap previously. *3,* No vaccine or TIG is recommended for infants <6 weeks of age with clean minor wounds (and no vaccine is licensed for infants <6 weeks of age). *4,* Tdap is preferred for persons 10 through 64 years of age who have never received Tdap. Td is preferred over tetanus toxoid (TT) for persons 7 through 10 years of age or >64 years of age or for those who have previously received Tdap. If TT is administered, an adsorbed TT product is preferred to fluid TT. (All DTaP/DTP/Tdap/DT/Td products contain adsorbed tetanus toxoid.) *5,* Provide TIG 250 U for all ages. It can and should be administered simultaneously with tetanus-containing vaccine. *6,* For infants <6 weeks of age, TIG (without vaccine) is recommended for "dirty" wounds (wounds other than clean, minor). *7,* Persons who are HIV positive should receive TIG regardless of tetanus immunization history. (Modified with recommendations from Centers for Disease Control and Prevention: Updated recommendations for use of tetanus toxoid, reduced diphtheria toxoid and acelleular pertussis (Tdap) vaccine from the Advisory Committee on Immunization Practices, 2010, *MMWR Morb Mortal Wkly Rep* 60:13–15, 2011.)

Local and systemic reactions to Td are uncommon but occur in 7% to 9% of pediatric patients.[18] Pain, swelling, and erythema can occur at the injection site, but these reactions usually are self-limited. When Tdap and Td are compared, the safety and adverse event profiles are similar to one another.[13] Common local symptoms include pain at the injection site, erythema, and swelling. Systemic symptoms observed in both Tdap and Td are headache, body aches, fatigue, and nausea. No cases of Guillain-Barré were observed in the safety studies.[13]

PROPHYLACTIC ANTIBIOTICS FOR EMERGENCY WOUNDS

For small, uncomplicated, minor, nonbite wounds and lacerations, there is no convincing clinical evidence that systemic antibiotics provide protection against the development of wound infection.[5,19-21] A randomized, controlled study using oral cephalexin for prophylaxis showed no efficacy of the antibiotic for minor lacerations.[5] In two randomized, controlled studies using oral or parenteral cephalosporins for minor hand lacerations, there was no increase in the infection rate of non–antibiotic-treated patients compared with patients treated with antibiotics.[1,19,20]

In a study of 2834 pediatric patients, not only was there no protective effect, but there also was a significant increase in the infection rate in the antibiotic-treated patients.[22] Other studies also support this contradiction.[3,5,20,23] It is thought that selection for resistant organisms, rebound bacterial proliferation after the initial effect, or impairment of host defenses by the drugs might account for this paradox.

Although not all authorities agree, and there is no strong scientific evidence underlying any specific set of recommendations for wound antibiotic prophylaxis, clinical and empirical experiences suggest that there are wound characteristics and circumstances that warrant antibiotic intervention.[24-26] If antibiotics are indicated, there is some evidence that the initial dose has to be administered as soon as possible to obtain an effect.[23,25,26] Delays in treatment beyond 3 to 5 hours from injury have been shown in some studies to lead to an increase in the infection rate.[24] Other investigators have found little correlation between the interval between injury and antibiotic delivery and the ultimate risk of wound infection.

The following are guidelines for when antibiotics should be considered:

- *Wound age:* Relative indications include hand and foot wounds more than 8 hours old, facial wounds more than 24 hours old, and wounds at other sites more than 12 hours old.
- *Wound condition:* Crushing mechanism wounds for which extensive débridement and tissue revision are needed.
- *Contamination:* Wounds initially contaminated with soil, vegetative matter, and other particulates that require extensive cleaning and irrigation.
- *Suspected CA-MRSA contamination:* Risk factors for CA-MRSA include HIV, previous or current incarceration, previous MRSA infection, athletes, veterinarians, indigents, and children.
- *Mammalian bites:* See Chapter 15 for indications regarding wound prophylaxis in dog, cat, and human bites.
- *Vulnerable anatomic sites:* Wounds of cartilage (ear, nose), tendon, bone, and joint.
- *Circulatory impairment:* Wounds in impaired areas of drainage, such as lymphedema secondary to venous disease or surgical procedure (radical mastectomy).
- *Impaired host defenses:* Diabetes, immunosuppressive agents (corticosteroids, anticancer agents), and diseases with altered immune status.

- *Cardiac valvular disease:* Guidelines published by the American Heart Association should be followed relative to wounds in patients with cardiac valvular disease. Prophylaxis is not indicated in patients who have clean, uncomplicated lacerations.
- *Orthopedic implants:* Prophylaxis should be considered in patients with orthopedic implants who have contaminated wounds. Prophylaxis is not indicated for clean, uncomplicated wounds.

ANTIBIOTIC CHOICES

The choice of antibiotics for nonbite wound prophylaxis is based on the likely infecting organisms. Multiple studies have shown that for common, uncomplicated wounds and lacerations, *S. aureus* and *Streptococcus* species have been the most common infecting agents in more than 90% of cases.[20,21,23,27] In recent years, there has been an explosion of CA-MRSA cases.[28] More extensive wounds, involving contamination with soil, increase the spectrum to include gram-negative organisms and *Clostridium* species.[29] Wounds involving fresh water, including lakes, streams, and swimming pools, may be contaminated with *Aeromonas hydrophila*.[30,31] Injuries occurring in salt water can be infected with *Vibrio vulnificus*.[32]

- For prophylaxis to be effective, the initial dose should be delivered as soon after the injury as possible, preferably in parenteral form, to ensure an adequate level of antibiotic activity.[25,26,33,34] For a common, uncomplicated, nonbite wound requiring prophylaxis, the first-generation cephalosporin cefazolin (Ancef) can be administered parenterally, followed by a 3- to 5-day course of cephalexin (Keflex), cephradine (Velosef), cefadroxil (Duricef), or dicloxacillin. Cefadroxil has the advantage of once-a-day or twice-a-day dosing, which may encourage greater compliance.
- For patients allergic to penicillin and cephalosporins, an intravenous dose of clindamycin (Cleocin) followed with oral clindamycin provides coverage of common infecting organisms. Because of the short course, the risk of diarrheal complications from clindamycin is negligible. The macrolides, including erythromycin and azithromycin, are another alternative.
- If CA-MRSA is suspected, trimethoprim/sulfamethoxazole (TMP-SMX), clindamycin, or doxycycline can be used prophylactically.
- When the offending organism cannot be determined clinically, the combination of TMP-SMX with cefalexin will provide coverage for CA-MRSA, methicillin-sensitive *S. aureus,* and group A *Streptococcus.* Clindamycin is an alternative.
- If *A. hydrophila* is suspected, ciprofloxacin (Cipro), TMP/SMX (Bactrim, Septra), or an aminoglycoside provides adequate coverage. *V. vulnificus* is more difficult to treat but is sensitive to doxycycline (Vibramycin), chloramphenicol, and ceftazidime (Fortaz).

References

1. Cummings P, Del Beccarro MA: Antibiotics to prevent infection of simple wounds: a meta-analysis of randomized studies, *Am J Emerg Med* 13:396–400, 1995.
2. Gosnold JK: Infection rate of sutured wounds, *Practitioner* 218:584–585, 1977.
3. Hutton PA, Jones BM, Law DJ: Depot penicillin as prophylaxis in accidental wounds, *Br J Surg* 65: 549–550, 1978.
4. Rutherford WH, Spence R: Infection in wounds sutured in the accident and emergency department, *Ann Emerg Med* 9:350–352, 1980.
5. Thirlby RC, Blair AJ, Thal ER: The value of prophylactic antibiotics for simple lacerations, *Surg Gynecol Obstet* 156:212–216, 1983.
6. Brand DA, Acampora D, Gottleib LD, et al: Adequacy of anti-tetanus prophylaxis in six hospital emergency departments, *N Engl J Med* 309:636–640, 1983.
7. Furste W: Fifth international conference on tetanus, Ronneby, Sweden, 1978, *J Trauma* 20:101–105, 1980.
8. Zun LS, Downey L: Tetanus immunization shortage in the US, *Am J Emerg Med* 21:298–301, 2003.

9. Pascual FB, McGinley EL, Zanardi LR, et al: Tetanus surveillance—United States, 1998-2000, *MMWR Morb Mortal Wkly Rep Surveill Summ* 52(SS03):1-8, 2003.
10. Richardson JP, Knight AL: The management and prevention of tetanus, *J Emerg Med* 11:737-742, 1993.
11. Alagappan K, Rennie WP, McPherson P, et al: Seroprevalence of antibody levels to tetanus in adults over 65 years of age (abstract), *Acad Emerg Med* 2:373, 1995.
12. Crossley K, Irvine P, Warren JB, et al: Tetanus and diphtheria immunity in urban Minnesota adults, *JAMA* 242:2298-2300, 1983.
13. Kretsinger K, Boder RK, Cortese MM: Preventing tetanus, diphtheria, and pertussis among adults: use of tetanus toxoid, reduced diphtheria toxoid and acellular pertussis vaccine, *MMWR Recomm Rep* 55(RR17):1-33, 2006.
14. CDC: Final 2005 reports of notifiable diseases, *MMWR* 55:880-881, 2005.
15. CDC: Updated recommendations for use of tetanus toxoid, reduced diphtheria toxoid and acellular pertussis (Tdap) vaccine from the Advisory Committee on Immunization Practices, 2010, *MMWR Morb Mortal Wkly Rep* 60(01):13-15, 2011.
16. Appendix A: summary of ACIP recommendations for prevention of pertussis, tetanus, and diphtheria among pregnant and postpartum women and their infants, *MMWR Recomm Rep* 57(04):49-49, 2008.
17. Jacobs RL, Lowe RS, Lanier BQ: Adverse reactions to tetanus toxoid, *JAMA* 247:40-42, 1982.
18. Cody CL, Baraff LJ, Cherry JD, et al: Nature of adverse reactions associated with DTP and DT immunizations in infants and children, *Pediatrics* 68:650-660, 1981.
19. Grossman JA, Adams JP, Kunec J: Prophylactic antibiotics in simple hand lacerations, *JAMA* 245:1055-1056, 1981.
20. Haughey RE, Lammers RL, Wagner DK: Use of antibiotics in the initial management of soft tissue wounds, *Ann Emerg Med* 10:187-190, 1981.
21. Samson RH, Altman SF: Antibiotic prophylaxis for minor lacerations, *N Y State J Med* 77:1728-1730, 1977.
22. Baker MD, Lanuti M: The management and outcome of lacerations in urban children, *Ann Emerg Med* 19:1001-1005, 1990.
23. Worlock P, Boland P, Darrell J, et al: The role of prophylactic antibiotics following hand surgery, *Br J Clin Pract* 34:290-292, 1980.
24. Burke JF: The effective period of preventive antibiotic action in experimental incisions and dermal lesions, *Surgery* 50:161-168, 1961.
25. Cardany CR, Rodeheaver G, Thacker J, et al: The crush injury: the high risk wound, *J Am Coll Emerg Physicians* 5:965-970, 1976.
26. Edlich RF, Kenny JG, Morgan RF, et al: Antimicrobial treatment of minor soft tissue lacerations: a critical review, *Emerg Clin North Am* 4:561-580, 1986.
27. Day TK: Controlled trial of antibiotics in minor wounds requiring suture, *Lancet* 2:1174-1176, 1975.
28. David MZ, Daum RS: Community-associated methicillin-resistant *Staphylococcus aureus*: epidemiology and clinical consequences of an emerging epidemic, *Clin Microbiol Rev* 23:616-687, 2010.
29. Fitzgerald RH, Cooney WP, Washington JA, et al: Bacterial colonization of mutilating hand injuries and its treatment, *J Hand Surg* 2:85-89, 1977.
30. Gold WL, Salit IE: *Aeromonas hydrophila* infections of the skin and soft tissue: report of 11 cases, *Clin Infect Dis* 16:69-74, 1993.
31. Skiendzielewski WH, O'Keefe KP: Wound infection due to fresh water contamination of, *Aeromonas hydrophila*, *J Emerg Med* 8:701-703, 1990.
32. Chuang YC, Young C, Chen CW: *Vibrio vulnificus* infection, *Scand J Infect Dis* 21:721-726, 1989.
33. Morgan WJ, Hutchinson D, Johnson HM: The delayed treatment of wounds of the hand and forearm under antibiotic cover, *Br J Surg* 67:140-141, 1976.
34. Edlich RF, Rodeheaver GT, Thacker JG, et al: Revolutionary advances in the management of traumatic wounds in the emergency department during the last 40 years: part 1, *J Emerg Med* 20:1-11, 2009.

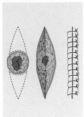

CHAPTER 22

Suture Removal and Wound Aftercare

Key Practice Points

- Suture removal times vary from 4 to 14 days depending on the location of the laceration.
- Sutures are removed from the face within 4 to 5 days to prevent the formation of epithelial plugs or "stitch" marks).
- Most repaired lacerations are minimally painful. Discomfort can be managed with acetaminophen or nonsteroidal antiinflammatories.
- Elevation of the wounded part can significantly reduce pain and swelling.
- Sutured or stapled wounds can be bathed (without immersion) in a shower within 12 to 24 hours after repair.
- Signs of wound infection include pain, swelling, redness, purulent discharge, and red streaks.
- A laceration can take up to 1 year to reach its final appearance. In the first few weeks, it can be red and swollen but eventually lose its red color and flatten out. Informing the patient of these phases can be very helpful.

Wound aftercare includes return scheduling for suture removal, aftercare instructions to the patient, and information on what to expect as the wound heals. When carefully and fully informed, most patients take good care of their wounds and dressings. Written instructions are followed best when reinforced with unhurried verbal explanations. Because each wound and patient differs, information about dressing care, limitations of activity, bathing, and suture removal has to be individualized. Patients often expect that healing is complete when the sutures are removed. If educated about the changes that a wound undergoes over months, patients are more likely to understand and accept the wound's appearance.

SUTURE AND STAPLE REMOVAL

Timing of Removal

The recommended intervals between wound repair and suture or staple removal are listed in Table 22-1. In the face, where cosmetic appearance is paramount, sutures are removed as early as possible; this is done with the knowledge that a facial wound has barely begun to gain tensile strength at the time of suture removal. Minimal accidental force can cause disruption and can dehisce the laceration. The application of wound tapes for continued support over healing lacerations is recommended. A return visit for tape removal and wound adhesive closure is not necessary.

If wound tapes are the primary method of wound closure, they can be left in place for 10 days without causing complications. Adhesives flake off in 5 to 10 days.

TABLE 22-1	Recommended Intervals for Removal of Percutaneous (Skin) Sutures

Location	Days to Removal
Scalp	6-8
Face	3-5
Ear	4-5
Chest/abdomen	8-10
Back	12-14
Arm/leg*	8-12
Hand*	8-10
Fingertip	10-12
Foot	12-14

*Add 2 to 3 days for joint extensor surfaces.

At minimum, these alternative closures should support the wound for the time recommended for sutures.

Suture punctures are small wounds. Epithelial cells invade these small wounds, leaving keratinized epithelial "plugs" caught in the healing suture wound. This phenomenon produces unsightly "railroad tracks" that can be avoided if sutures are removed in fewer than 7 to 8 days.[1,2] Skin tapes and wound adhesives as wound closure methods are alternative techniques to avoid suture tracking. The subcuticular and pull-out dermal closures described in Chapter 11 are other closure options.

In other areas of the body, where cosmetic appearance is not as important and wound healing is not as rapid as in the highly vascular face, sutures are left in place for longer periods. Extensor surfaces of joints require longer times before removal because of the mechanical forces brought to bear on the healing wound. Because of the dependency of the lower extremities and their relatively slower rate of healing, sutures in those lower extremity sites are left in place longer as well.

Technique for Removal

The technique for suture removal is illustrated in Figure 22-1. Staple removal is discussed in Chapter 14. The suture is cut under the knot, close to the skin surface, so that when it is pulled from the wound, the previously exposed and contaminated portion of the suture does not travel back through the wound. Although standard scissors can be used for most suture removal tasks, iris scissors or a no. 11 scalpel blade is recommended to cut the fine sutures used on the face. Bandage or commercial suture removal scissors have tips that often are too blunt to cut small, closely spaced sutures easily. Before removal, all dried coagulum is removed gently from the suture line with cotton swabs and hydrogen peroxide. Cleaning away the coagulum makes locating small sutures and knots much easier. In addition, it prevents the unnecessary tugging and pulling that often accompany suture removal when sutures are excessively crusted.

ANALGESIA

Pain after wounding can range from trivial to severe. Simple lacerations are well tolerated by the patient after repair and dressing. The pain of abrasions and partial-thickness (second-degree) burns can be unbearable. For most patients with uncomplicated lacerations, aspirin, acetaminophen, or other nonsteroidal antiinflammatory drugs relieve

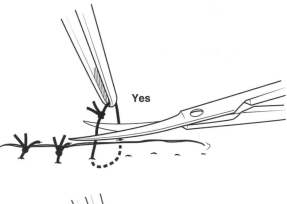

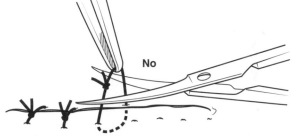

Figure 22-1. *Top,* Technique for correct removal of a suture. The scissors cut between the knot and the skin. The lower figure shows the incorrect technique to remove sutures. (Modified from Zukin D, Simon R: *Emergency wound care: principles and practice,* Rockville, Md, 1987, Aspen Publishers.)

residual discomfort after repair. Occasionally, codeine or hydrocodone is necessary. Burn victims require more powerful analgesics, such as oxycodone. In addition to drugs, elevation of the injured part, proper immobilization, and cool compresses applied to the affected area can greatly enhance pain relief.

The pain of lacerations and burns tends to subside significantly within 24 to 48 hours. A key follow-up instruction to the patient is to be concerned when pain increases or recurs. The most likely cause of this change in the pain pattern is wound infection. If pain increases, the physician must be notified immediately.

INSTRUCTIONS TO THE PATIENT

Wound Protection

Patients need to be instructed carefully in nonmedical terms about how to care for their wound at home. The key principles of home care are protection, elevation, and cleanliness. Most patients instinctively protect wounds from further trauma, but the caregiver should remind the patient that although sutures are in place, undue pressure or other mechanical forces on the wound can cause disruption and possible infection. Counseling and admonition against premature use of a repaired hand or foot are especially necessary for patients who are anxious to return to work or sporting activities.

Elevation is particularly important in extremity wounds. The tendency of lower extremities and hands to develop edema from lymphatic stasis is well recognized. Elevation helps prevent these complications, lessens pain, and improves wound healing. Lower extremity wounds have a higher rate of wound infection, a complication that can be abetted by edema and stasis. Crutches and slings for extremity wounds are useful adjuncts for home wound care.

Fresh healing wounds and repaired lacerations are vulnerable to direct sunlight. Excessive exposure can result in irreversible darkening or hyperpigmentation of the healing epidermis.[3] The wound is at risk for 1 year or until the scar fully matures.

Sunblock agents are recommended when prolonged exposure to the sun or ultraviolet light, such as in a tanning facility, is anticipated.

Dressing and Bandage Change Intervals

For uncomplicated, bandaged lacerations, the first change should occur 1 to 2 days after repair. The wound can be cleansed of dried blood and wound exudate. It can also be inspected for signs of infection. Complicated and contaminated wounds are undressed in 24 hours because of the higher likelihood of infection. Early recognition of infection is important for successful treatment. Subsequent bandage changes can be carried out at 2- to 3-day intervals.

Wound Cleansing and Bathing

Cleanliness is an important issue in wound aftercare. Sutured wounds of the scalp and face can be left open, provided that they are kept clean. In a controlled study of 200 head and neck incisions and traumatic lacerations, the investigators concluded that early washing (8 to 24 hours) after wound repair did not significantly alter wound healing or increase the potential for infection.[4] Wounds on other body sites can be cleansed gently after suture repair without ill effect.[5]

Patients can begin to bathe 12 to 24 hours after wound repair. They can be allowed to bathe once a day, or with each bandage change, provided that the wound is not immersed and soaked in water. Showers are preferable to tub baths. Gentle soaping and rinsing are followed immediately by patting the wound dry with a soft towel. Application of an antibiotic ointment or reapplication of a dressing is recommended after each washing.

Signs of Wound Infection

Most wounds heal without problems or complications. A few wounds become infected, however, despite compliance with accepted wound care procedures. In an analysis of more than 5000 patients, characteristics of wounds that became infected were identified.[6] The overall infection rate was 3.5%. Patients with wound infection were likely to be older or to have diabetes. Large wounds and wounds with visible contamination or foreign bodies also were at risk. Recommendations for prophylactic antibiotics are discussed in Chapter 21.

Every patient must be instructed in the signs of wound infection. If any of these signs develop, the patient needs to return immediately for examination. Signs of infection include the following:

- *Excessive discomfort:* Most minor wounds are only mildly uncomfortable.
- *Excessive swelling:* Swelling can accompany wound infection.
- *Discharge:* Continued drainage, particularly if it is purulent appearing, is a sign of infection.
- *Redness:* Erythema from neovascularization and capillary dilation accompanies most wounds. Redness that extends well beyond the wound margins (>5 mm) with accompanying swelling, induration, or tenderness does not occur in normal healing wounds.
- Lymphangitic streaks, local nodal enlargement, and fever all are signs of advanced infection.

If a wound becomes infected, sutures or staples act as foreign bodies and have to be removed. Attempts to remove alternate sutures and to start the patient on antibiotics are likely to fail. Chapter 21 discusses the care of infected wounds in greater detail.

Written Instructions

Patients should receive specific written instructions reinforcing and detailing general principles and any other specifics for the given wound problem. Follow-up visits, dates, and times have to be written clearly and understood by the patient and, whenever

WOUND CARE INSTRUCTIONS

You have been treated for a laceration. Please follow the instructions below to care for your wound.

TREATMENT

▫ **Sutures/staples**: Keep the wound and bandage clean. Bandages can be changed every 1 to 3 days. After removing the bandage, gently clean the wound with soap and water. A shower can be taken starting 24 hours after repair. After cleansing the wound, apply a coating of antibiotic ointment and a new bandage. Face wounds can be left uncovered.

Return or see your doctor for suture/staple removal in _____ days or on _____date.

▫ **Wound adhesives**: Adhesives do not need to be removed. The adhesive flakes off in 5 to 10 days. Do not pick at or rub the adhesive. Do not place adhesive tape, antibiotic ointment, or skin cream on wound. You may take a shower but do not soak wound in hot water. Return if the wound opens up.

▫ **Wound tapes**: Keep tapes dry and clean. Do not pick at or rub tapes. Do apply ointments or creams on tapes.

Keep tapes on for _____ days.

NOTIFY YOUR DOCTOR OR RETURN TO THE EMERGENCY DEPARTMENT IF YOU EXPERIENCE

Any signs of infection such as redness, swelling, drainage, increased pain, red streaks, or fever.

Figure 22-2. Sample discharge instructions for patients with lacerations.

possible, by accompanying family members. Figure 22-2 is an example of simple, yet effective, written wound care instructions.

UNDERSTANDING WOUND HEALING

Patients are most concerned about the size and appearance of the scar that will result from their laceration or wound. Because traumatic injuries occur randomly on the body surface, the final outcome, to a certain extent, is predetermined. It is the duty of the caregiver to advise the patient about the kind of scar he or she can expect. Candidly discussing various aspects of wound healing, such as the effects of wound mechanism, associated diseases, body region, and skin tension, allows the patient to accept and cope with the healing process better:
• Early (Inflammatory) Phase: Days 1 to 4
  • Wound is red, swollen, warm, and painful
  • Blood vessels dilate
  • Wound fluid (exudate) can be normal
• Early Scar Formation (Proliferative) Phase: Days 4 to 42
  • New vessels form
  • Early scar material (collagen) laid down by fibroblast cells

- Wound is swollen and red appearing
- Sutures or staples removed 4 to 14 days
- Wound strength low but increasing
- Remodeling Phase: 6 weeks to 1 year
  - Scar tissue gradually finds its final shape
  - Scar contracts 40% to 80% and flattens
  - Red color disappears. Scar slightly lighter than skin
  - Final tissue strength 80% of normal skin
  - Most patients satisfied with final scar appearance

References

1. Crikelair CT: Skin suture marks, *Am J Surg* 96:631–632, 1958.
2. Edlich RF, Rodeheaver GT, Thacker JG: Revolutionary advances in the management of traumatic wounds in the emergency department during the last 40 years: part 1, *J Emerg Med* 201–211, 2009.
3. Ship AG, Weiss PR: Pigmentation after dermabrasion: an avoidable complication, *Plast Reconstr Surg* 75:528–532, 1985.
4. Goldberg HM, Rosenthal SAE, Nemetz JC: Effect of washing closed head and neck wounds on wound healing and infection, *Am J Surg* 141:358–359, 1981.
5. Noe JM, Keller M: Can stitches get wet? *Plast Reconstr Surg* 81:82–84, 1988.
6. Hollander JE, Singer AJ, Valentine SM, et al: Risk factors for infection in patients with traumatic lacerations, *Acad Emerg Med* 8:716–720, 2001.

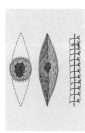

Index

Page numbers followed by *f* indicate figures; *b*, boxes; *t*, tables.